Seniors Guide to

Pain-Free Living

All-Natural **Drug-Free** Relief for Everything That Hurts!

by **Doug Dollemore** and the editors of **PREVENTION** *HEALTH BOOKS for SENIORS*

RODALE

Printed in the United States of America
Rodale Inc. makes every effort to use acid-free ∞, recycled paper ♲

The pain-scale information in "What to Tell Your Doctor" on page 20 is adapted from "Things to Tell Your Doctor" from *Relieving Cancer Pain*, published by Fred Hutchinson Cancer Research Center, 1993.

Library of Congress Cataloging-in-Publication Data

Dollemore, Doug.
    Seniors guide to pain-free living / by Doug Dollemore and the editors of Prevention Health Books for Seniors.
        p.   cm.
    Includes index.
    ISBN 1–57954–127–5 hardcover
    ISBN 1–57954–295–6 paperback
    1. Pain in old age—Popular works.   I. Prevention Health Books for Seniors.   II. Title.
RB127 .D65 2000
616'.0472'0846—dc21   00–024809

Distributed to the book trade by St. Martin's Press

2 4 6 8 10 9 7 5 3   hardcover

2 4 6 8 10 9 7 5 3   paperback

Visit us on the Web at www.preventionbookshelf.com, or call us toll-free at (800) 848-4735.

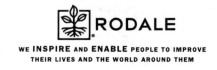

RODALE
WE INSPIRE AND ENABLE PEOPLE TO IMPROVE THEIR LIVES AND THE WORLD AROUND THEM

About *Prevention* Health Books

The editors of *Prevention* Health Books are dedicated to providing you with authoritative, trustworthy, and innovative advice for a healthy, active lifestyle. In all of our books, our goal is to keep you thoroughly informed about the latest breakthroughs in natural healing, medical research, alternative health, herbs, nutrition, fitness, and weight loss. We cut through the confusion of today's conflicting health reports to deliver clear, concise, and definitive health information that you can trust. And we explain in practical terms what each new breakthrough means to you, so you can take immediate, practical steps to improve your health and well-being.

Every recommendation in *Prevention* Health Books is based upon interviews with highly qualified health authorities, including medical doctors and practitioners of alternative medicine. In addition, we consult with the *Prevention* Health Books Board of Advisors to ensure that all of the health information is safe, practical, and up-to-date. *Prevention* Health Books are thoroughly factchecked for accuracy, and we make every effort to verify recommendations, dosages, and cautions.

The advice in this book will help keep you well-informed about your personal choices in health care—to help you lead a happier, healthier, and longer life.

Notice

This book is intended as a reference volume only, not as a medical manual. The information given here is designed to help you make informed decisions about your health. It is not intended as a substitute for any treatment that may have been prescribed by your doctor. If you suspect that you have a medical problem, we urge you to seek competent medical help.

Seniors Guide to Pain-Free Living Staff

EDITOR: Stephen C. George

WRITERS: Doug Dollemore, with Gale Maleskey, James McCommons, Eric Metcalf

CONTRIBUTING WRITERS: Alisa Bauman, Bill Doherty, Jennifer Bright Kaas, Bebe Raupe, Christine Seliga

ART DIRECTOR: Darlene Schneck

INTERIOR DESIGNER: Lynn N. Gano

COVER DESIGNER: Andrew Newman

ILLUSTRATORS: Molly Babich, Karen Kuchar

ASSISTANT RESEARCH MANAGERS: Sandra Salera Lloyd, Shea Zukowski

PRIMARY RESEARCH COORDINATOR: Anita C. Small

LEAD RESEARCHER: Jennifer Bright Kaas

EDITORIAL RESEARCHERS: Elizabeth A. Brown, Adrien Drozdowski, Lori Nudo George, Staci Hadeed-Sander, Grete Haentjens, Lois Guarino Hazel, Jennifer S. Kushnier, Paris Mihely-Muchanic, Paula Rasich, Terry Sutton-Kravitz, Holly Ann Swanson, Barbara Thomas-Fexa, Nancy Zelko

SENIOR COPY EDITOR: Karen Neely

COPY EDITOR: Kathryn C. LeSage

EDITORIAL PRODUCTION MANAGER: Marilyn Hauptly

LAYOUT DESIGNER: Donna G. Rossi

ASSOCIATE STUDIO MANAGER: Thomas P. Aczel

MANUFACTURING COORDINATORS: Brenda Miller, Jodi Schaffer, Patrick T. Smith

Rodale Healthy Living Books

VICE PRESIDENT AND PUBLISHER: Brian Carnahan

EDITORIAL DIRECTOR: Michael Ward

VICE PRESIDENT AND MARKETING DIRECTOR: Karen Arbegast

PRODUCT MARKETING MANAGER: Denyse Corelli

BOOK MANUFACTURING DIRECTOR: Helen Clogston

MANUFACTURING MANAGERS: Eileen Bauder, Mark Krahforst

RESEARCH MANAGER: Ann Gossy Yermish

COPY MANAGER: Lisa D. Andruscavage

PRODUCTION MANAGER: Robert V. Anderson Jr.

OFFICE MANAGER: Jacqueline Dornblaser

OFFICE STAFF: Julie Kehs, Mary Lou Stephen, Catherine E. Strouse

Contents

▶ PART THREE:
PAIN MAKERS—THE TOP 20

▶ PART FOUR:
PAIN MAKERS—EVERYDAY ACHES

PART FIVE:
PAIN MAKERS—CHRONIC ILLNESSES

RESOURCES

Introduction

A few years ago, an older gentleman who had excruciating pain in his right knee hobbled into his doctor's office in Baltimore, hoping to get some relief. Instead, the doctor disdainfully dismissed his complaint: "What do you expect? You're 78 years old."

The callousness of that statement says a lot of about aging, pain, and medical care in this country. The sad truth is that most doctors simply don't know that much about pain, particularly among older Americans.

"When I went to medical school, I had hours of lectures on obscure tropical diseases, but almost no lectures on pain," says Randall Prust, M.D., medical director of both the Center for Pain Management at El Dorado Hospital and the Pain Medicine Center at Tucson General Hospital, both in Tucson, and author of *Conquering Pain*.

Fortunately, there is a growing legion of doctors and other health-care professionals dedicated to eradicating unnecessary pain. These professionals know that pain is *not* an inevitable part of aging. They realize that in many instances herbs, prayer, exercise, and other natural remedies can be just as effective pain relievers as drugs or surgery.

To make this book the most comprehensive pain-relief book possible, we interviewed dozens of the nation's top pain-management specialists. We spent time in pain clinics throughout the United States and spoke with a myriad of patients who have learned to use a variety of natural techniques to relieve their discomfort.

We soon discovered that pain-free

living after age 60 is hardly a pipe dream. Instead, it is a goal well within the reach of the vast majority of older Americans. Even if you've been in pain for a number of years, the healing tips and techniques in this book can help dampen your discomfort.

In part one, Feeling Your Pain, we explore what causes pain and how attitude and lifestyle changes can help you cope with your aches. In addition, we take a critical look at painkilling drugs ranging from aspirin to morphine.

In Pain Takers, the second part of this book, you'll learn all about 30 natural ways to relieve pain, including prayer, meditation, acupressure, biofeedback, and yoga.

In part three, we take an in-depth look at treating the 20 most common aches and pains that afflict older Americans, including headache, backache, knee pain, cancer pain, muscle pain, and shingles. In part four, you'll discover dozens of new ways to cope with bruises, cuts, sore throats, and other nagging everyday aches and pains. Finally, in part five, you'll find an extensive guide to coping with a dozen chronic painful illnesses that afflict older Americans, including fibromyalgia, gallstones, and ulcers.

For your convenience, each chapter in these last three parts of the book includes a special feature called "For Fast Relief" that highlights the remedy that doctors deem the simplest and swiftest way to relieve the pain of a particular disorder. Additional remedies that require more sustained treatment are listed under "For Lasting Relief." Many chapters also include tips for preventing painful disorders from developing or recurring. Sprinkled throughout the book are inspirational stories of people just like you who have discovered how to overcome their pain.

We sincerely hope this book helps you conquer your aches and pains and, in turn, allows you to retain the self-confidence and independence you need to live a full and active life.

PART | ONE

▶

Feeling Your Pain

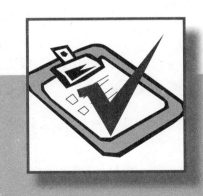

Pain and Aging

In his heyday, Edward H. Gibson was a star attraction for just one reason. He never—except for an occasional headache—felt an ache or pain in his life. Not that he didn't try. In a fit of rage, he once broke his nose by banging it on a piano. In another instance, he was accidentally struck in the head with a hatchet. Nothing hurt him.

In the 1920s, Gibson made much of this distinction, touring on the vaudeville circuit as "The Human Pincushion." Twice a day, dressed only in shorts, he would go out on stage and ask a volunteer from the audience to stick as many as 60 pins into him in a single performance. Then, in front of the audience, Gibson would calmly pull the pins out one by one.

You may think that it would be wonderful to be like Edward Gibson and never feel pain. But it wouldn't be. Without the ability to sense pain, you'd be more prone to burns, infections, and injuries. But more to the point, you probably wouldn't be around long enough to get a senior discount.

"Generally, the few people who are born without the ability to perceive pain don't live very long," says Stephen W. Harkins, Ph.D., professor of gerontology, psychiatry, psychology, and biomedical engineering at the Virginia Commonwealth University in Richmond. "Pain plays an important part in self-protection and self-preservation. Without it, a person tends to take great risks that others wouldn't."

TOO MUCH OF A GOOD THING?

A certain amount of pain is vital for survival. But as we get older, pain often seems to spin out of control. Instead of being a useful sensor that keeps us out of harm's way, it can become the equivalent of an annoying car alarm that howls incessantly for no apparent reason. Over time, unrelenting pain in your back, hips, and other parts of your body takes its toll, causing depression, sleep disturbances, mobility problems, and other difficulties that can diminish the quality of your life, says Randall Prust, M.D., medical director of both the Center for Pain Management at El Dorado Hospital and the Pain Medicine Center at Tucson General Hospital, both in Tucson, and author of *Conquering Pain*.

In fact, persistent, unrelieved pain is the most common complaint among older Americans, according to the American Geriatrics Society. Up to 50 percent of seniors report significant pain that interferes with their daily lives. But before you indict Father Time, you should know this: Aging probably has little to do with your pain.

"Many people—patients, families, and even some health-care providers—believe that pain is just an expected consequence of aging, and if it is happening to you, you have to learn to live with it because nothing can be done to stop it. That's not true at all," says Keela Herr, R.N., Ph.D., a pain researcher and associate professor of nursing at the University of Iowa College of Nursing in Iowa City. "Chronic pain is not an inescapable part of growing old."

Lifestyle, not the aging process, is the real underlying culprit that triggers many of the painful diseases such as arthritis, osteoporosis, and sciatica that become more common in later life, doctors say.

"We tend to pretend that we don't have to do anything to maintain our health, and that eventually catches up with us," says Margaret A. Caudill, M.D., Ph.D., co-director of the department of pain medicine at the Dartmouth-Hitchcock Medical Center in Manchester, New Hampshire, and author of *Managing Pain Before It Manages You*.

POTENT PAIN PREVENTERS

Inactivity, poor nutrition, smoking, drinking too much alcohol, and being overweight are just a few of the things that can aggravate any ache in your body, Dr. Prust says. But, as doctors point out, all those are lifestyle factors that you can change, too.

"It is not too late for older Americans to prevent existing aches and pains from getting worse, nor is it too late to prevent the onset of new aches and pains," says Risa Lavizzo-Mourey, M.D., director of the University of Pennsylvania Institute on Aging and chief of the division of geriatric medicine at the University of Pennsylvania Medical Center, both in Philadelphia.

Here are a few potent, natural lifestyle changes you can start making right now to help prevent or even relieve aches and pains throughout your body.

"These are lifestyle changes that will help in the long run," Dr. Prust says. "It's not like taking a pill and the pain will go away tomorrow. But if you stick with these changes in lifestyle, gradually over the next few months, you will start feeling better and better, and stronger and stronger."

Keep churning. Regular physical activity is one of the best things you can do to prevent or relieve incessant pain, Dr. Prust says. In fact, the less you do, the more intensely you'll feel pain.

"When you're sedentary, your muscles turn into butter. And when that happens, your bones lose all of their structural support, and that's going to make your pain feel worse," he says. "It's like a building: The bones are the columns, and the muscles are the brick and mortar. Without the brick and mortar, the building will collapse."

In addition, regular activity bolsters bloodflow to areas that do hurt, helping the body heal itself faster, Dr. Prust says. Try to do an activity you enjoy—no matter if it's golf, tennis, swimming, walking, or gardening—for at least 20 minutes, 3 or 4 days a week.

"You have to pick something you like; that's the key," he says. "Personally, I love water exercises. The water is very soothing, and I think people like it because it takes the weight off their joints. I tell people to just start walking in the pool every day. That is the simplest exercise you can do." Check with your local pool to find out if it offers water stretching, yoga, or aerobics classes.

Eat the right fuels. Without good nutrition, you'll be more prone to chronic aches and pains, Dr. Prust says.

"You need every cell in your body to be in tip-top shape in order to fend off pain," he says. "If you don't eat a well-balanced diet, your body won't have all of the building blocks it needs to do that."

He suggests eating a daily diet that includes 6 to 11 servings of breads, cereals, rice, and pastas; 3 to 5 servings of corn, carrots, and other vegetables; 2 to 4 servings of oranges, bananas, strawberries, and other fruits; 2 to 3 servings of milk, yogurt, and other low-fat dairy products; and 2 to 3 servings of meat, poultry or fish, eggs, nuts, or dry beans. Remember, don't go overboard. A portion doesn't have to be huge—one banana or one slice of bread counts as a serving.

Call in reinforcements. Glucosamine, a sugar that is one of the body's natural building blocks, and chondroitin, another natural chemical, are an important dynamic duo that can keep your joints pain-free, Dr. Prust says. These two chemicals, which naturally diminish in your body as you age, help maintain cartilage and other vital connective tissues surrounding your joints.

Specifically, glucosamine helps repair damaged cartilage tissue, and chondroitin moisturizes cartilage so that it doesn't become brittle, he says. To picture how these chemicals work, imagine that your cartilage is a well-manicured lawn. As you age, you may be more prone to get crabgrass or dry, brown spots on that lawn. Glucosamine helps your body get rid of the crabgrass, and chondroitin eliminates dry, brown spots. As a result, your cartilage stays healthy and your joints remain pain-free.

You'd have to eat far too much to get enough glucosamine and chondroitin in your diet, so supplements are your best bet. Look for 500-milligram tablets of glucosamine sulfate and 400-milligram tablets of chondroitin sulfate. The dosage depends on your weight. If you weigh up to 110 pounds, Dr. Prust recommends taking two tablets of glucosamine and two tablets of chondroitin daily; 110 pounds to 200 pounds, take three tablets each of glucosamine and chondroitin each day; more than 200 pounds, take four tablets of glucosamine and four tablets of chondroitin daily. These supplements can be taken with or without food, but it's a good idea to take the entire dosage at a single meal like breakfast or dinner simply because it helps you remember to do it. It will take 2 to 6 months before you notice a difference, he says.

"People who use these supplements tolerate them very well," Dr. Prust says. "I even have my parents, who are in their seventies, taking glucosamine and chondroitin."

Clear the air (and your lungs). Smoking is one of the worst things that you can do if you are in chronic pain, Dr. Prust says. Nicotine, the active ingredient in tobacco, causes blood vessels to clamp down, cutting off the flow of oxygen and nutrients to your nervous system. Nicotine also may block the release of endorphins, your body's natural painkilling hormones. People who smoke use more narcotics to relieve pain than nonsmokers.

"I have patients who smoke who can literally feel the pain intensify every time they take a puff," he says. "If there was ever a reason to quit, there it is."

Although smoking is a difficult addiction to break, there are plenty of ways to do it successfully. For starters, Dr. Prust suggests that you try nicotine patches and gums—two of the most effective methods—which are available over the counter.

Decaffeinate your life. Like smoking, drinking too much caffeine cuts bloodflow to your joints and can heighten your sense of pain throughout your body. Limit yourself to no more than two cups of regular coffee or three cups of regular tea, Dr. Prust says. You can drink as many decaffeinated beverages as you like, since most of the caffeine has been removed. Be aware that certain foods like chocolate and sodas also contain caffeine, so read food labels carefully.

Close down the tavern. Some older people believe that they can drink their pain away, Dr. Prust says. But in reality, alcohol damages your nerves, diminishes the effectiveness of pain medication, and disrupts your body's repair mechanisms.

"Even in small quantities, alcohol can cause problems if you have chronic pain," he says. "Any nerves that are damaged by alcohol are probably going to be raw, inflamed, and hurt like heck. I tell most of my patients, 'I don't know if one drink a day is going to be bad, but there is no question that drinking more than two drinks a day is going to harm nerves and increase your susceptibility to chronic pain syndromes. So if I had my druthers, I'd wish that you didn't drink.'"

Shed the overload. Excessive weight puts unnecessary strain on every single joint in your body and can trigger pain, Dr. Prust says.

"If you have to use a lot of energy just to maintain all the fat in your body, then you're not going to have a lot of energy to fight pain," he says. "If you're overweight, that's like carrying around a 30-, 40-, or 50-pound bag of dog food with you everywhere you go. Who really wants to do that? Of course, that makes it much more likely that you're going have a lot of aches and pains."

Small changes in your eating habits and activities can make a big difference in your weight, Dr. Prust says. So to kick-start your weight-loss effort, begin your meals with a fibrous food like an apricot, a slice of whole-grain bread, or a raw carrot. Fibrous food like fruits, vegetables, beans, and grains are packed with nutrients and usually have few calories. Fiber also adds bulk to your diet, so your stomach will fill up faster and you'll eat less. As for activity, when you go to your shopping mall, for instance, park as far as you can from the entrance, he says. The walk to the door will help burn extra calories.

Reach out to others. An idle mind is a painful mind, Dr. Prust says. If you have too much time on your hands, you'll probably dwell on your aches and feel worse. So stay as socially active as you can.

Find something to do every day that will occupy your mind. Volunteer at your local library, for instance, or another agency in need. Take a class at a community college. If you enjoy music, join a community band.

"Maintaining social activity decreases pain because the activity helps take your mind off the pain," Dr. Prust says. "The most common time for patients to have pain is first thing in the morning or at night, when other people aren't around. So companionship or social activity of some kind is necessary to divert the brain from the pain."

Imagine there's no pain. Imagery, a powerful mind/body technique you'll learn more about in this book, can help you pre-

vent aches and pains from creeping up on you, says Dennis Gersten, M.D., a psychiatrist and medical director of the Gersten Institute for Higher Medicine in Cardiff-by-the-Sea, California, and author of *Are You Getting Enlightened or Losing Your Mind?*

To try it, take a couple of deep breaths, then imagine that you are holding a ball of mercury (the silvery liquid found in thermometers) in your hands and that it can draw pain out of your body like a magnet. Then imagine that any pain developing in your body—even if you don't feel it right now—is sucked into this magnetic ball of mercury and disappears into the ball. Then let the ball, which is full of pain, dribble onto the floor and flow out of sight.

Do this for 1 minute twice a day to keep pain under wraps, Dr. Gersten suggests.

The Two Sides of Pain

His vivid imagination working in high gear, Robert Louis Stevenson thrashed about so wildly in bed one night that his frightened wife woke him up. Infuriated, Stevenson yelled, "I was dreaming a fine bogey tale!"

Writing feverishly for the next 3 days, the famed Scottish author transformed his nightmare into a classic novel: *The Strange Case of Dr. Jekyll and Mr. Hyde*, the story of a good man who unwittingly unleashes an evil personality that lurks within him.

Like Dr. Jekyll, pain has its good side. Bang your knee, smash your finger in a doorjamb, or cut yourself on the hand, and that instantaneous pain sends you a clear message: Ouch! Stop! Tend to this injury now!

It's called acute pain. To soothe it, you might apply ice to the swelling, use a soothing antibiotic ointment, or cover the wound with an adhesive bandage. In a few minutes or a few days, the wound heals and the pain disappears.

Even when the problem is more serious, such as a kidney stone, pain is doing a good deed. This acute, excruciating pain is telling you to do something about it—in this case, seek immediate medical care. Once the crisis passes, the pain withers away.

But, like Dr. Jekyll, acute pain also has a demonic twin. Chronic pain—the Mr. Hyde of this story—lingers on long after the body has healed. In some cases, the pain persists for years or even decades. Often, doctors can find no underlying cause for it. Chronic pain affects more than 50 million people in the United States. People over 60 are twice as likely to suffer from chronic pain conditions as their younger counterparts. Nearly one in five older Americans take pain medication to combat it. And the reasons for its prevalence and tenacity are as compelling and mysterious as any "fine bogey tale" that Robert Louis Stevenson ever dreamed up.

ACUTE PAIN JANGLES YOUR ALARM BELLS

For most of us, especially when we're enduring it, all pain seems the same. No matter if it stings, burns, throbs, or grates, we only know two things: It hurts, and we want it to go away. But before you can begin to soothe any discomfort, it's important to know more about the differences between acute pain and chronic pain, and about how they are treated.

"Acute and chronic pain have absolutely nothing in common except for the word *pain*. They are quite distinct," says Robert N. Jamison, Ph.D., director of the pain-management program at Brigham and Women's Hospital in Boston and author of *Learning to Master Your Chronic Pain*. Acute pain is a message that some-

thing is wrong and you need to tend to it. Chronic pain really isn't very helpful. It's a signal that's hard to turn off.

Normally, acute pain is as predictable as a gothic novel. It has a beginning, a middle, and, most important, an end. Rest, a bit of heat or cold on the injury, an over-the-counter analgesic like ibuprofen, and the passage of time are usually enough to get you through the worst of it.

"People usually recover from acute pain in a finite and reasonably limited time span," says Margaret A. Caudill, M.D., Ph.D., codirector of the department of pain medicine at the Dartmouth-Hitchcock Medical Center in Manchester, New Hampshire, and author of *Managing Pain Before It Manages You*.

Consider, for instance, what happens when you have blood drawn. As soon as pain receptors in your skin sense the prick of the needle, they begin transmitting information to a network of nearby nerve cells. Like runners in a relay handing off a baton, these nerve cells pass the pain signals along pathways into your spinal cord. Although this happens almost instantaneously, some of these nerve pathways are faster than others, and that can make a difference in the type of pain you feel.

As the needle pierces your skin to draw

blood, for example, the sensation travels through your nervous system at about 40 miles per hour and produces a sharp pain that is focused right where the needle puncture is located, Dr. Caudill says. Meanwhile, the pain signals produced by a mildly upset stomach may slog along at about 3 miles per hour, causing a dull, aching feeling in your gut that is hard to pinpoint.

In any case, once a pain signal reaches your spinal cord, researchers theorize, it passes through a complex series of specialized nerves cells that act like gates. If the pain isn't particularly bothersome, these gate cells can diminish or even cancel the signal before it gets to your brain. But if the pain is intense enough, as in the case of being jabbed by a needle, these "gates" open up and allow the signal to pass along your central nervous system from your spinal cord to your brain, says Randall Prust, M.D., medical director of both the Center for Pain Management at El Dorado Hospital and the Pain Medicine Center at Tucson General Hospital, both in Tucson, and author of *Conquering Pain*.

In your brain, the thalamus, a sorting and switching station, sends out two messages. One travels to your cerebral cortex,

the thinking part of your brain, which assesses the damage that is causing the pain and spurs your body's repair mechanisms into action. You may, for instance, instinctively begin rubbing the area where the needle was inserted. This is soothing because rubbing stimulates another set of nerves in the skin, ones that carry touch and pressure messages to your brain that can override or block the acute pain messages.

The second message that your thalamus sends goes to the injury or wound, ordering the pain receptors to stop sending out messages. After all, once your brain knows you are hurting, it doesn't need to be told over and over again. To ensure that this order is carried out, your body releases morphinelike hormones called endorphins and enkephalins that help dampen pain. In fact, during a blood test, you might notice that the pain is virtually gone even before the needle is withdrawn from your skin, Dr. Prust says. Of course, if the injury is severe—like a broken leg—the pain receptors will likely disregard this order and continue sending out intense distress signals that will encourage you to seek medical care.

Pain, as you probably know, also is linked to your emotions. In fact, in your brain, the lines between the physical and

When to Go to a Pain Clinic

No matter how skilled and experienced they are, sometimes even the finest family physicians can't unravel what's hurting you. In fact, sometimes no single specialist may be able to relieve your pain. That's when it's time to call in reinforcements.

When all else fails, a comprehensive pain-treatment center often can do wonders to eliminate or dampen persistent pain, says Harris McIlwain, M.D., a pain-management expert in Tampa, Florida, and coauthor of *Winning with Chronic Pain*.

At a comprehensive pain center, you'll be cared for by a team of physicians and other health professionals who together can develop a pain-management program that is right for you. A typical team at one of these centers might include doctors who specialize in treating the brain, muscles, bones, and joints. In addition, you might be treated by an occupational therapist, physical therapist, or even a dentist. This multidisciplinary approach allows doctors to fully evaluate the causes of your pain and offers you the best chance of finding

the emotional blur. The cerebral cortex, for instance, controls body functions like breathing, muscle tension, and heart rate. But the cortex also sends and receives messages from your brain's limbic center, which produces emotions such as sorrow, anxiety, and anger in response to the pain. These emotions can stimulate the cerebral cortex

relief, Dr. McIlwain says. Treatments range from simple stretching exercises to highly complex surgery, depending on the extent and severity of your problem.

When is it time to go?

Like any journey, you'll have to take a few steps before you get there. Start with your family physician, Dr. McIlwain suggests. If that doesn't solve the problem, ask for a referral to a specialist. If that doesn't help, then ask for a referral to a comprehensive pain center.

"If you are not getting the pain relief you need from your family doctor, chiropractor, or other health-care provider, then be upfront about it. Just say, 'Listen doc, things aren't working out here. I need to go someplace else,'" says Randall Prust, M.D., medical director of both the Center for Pain Management at El Dorado Hospital and the Pain Medicine Center at Tucson General Hospital, both in Tucson, and author of *Conquering Pain*.

But because Medicare may only pay for some of the costs of treatment at a pain clinic, be sure to double-check which services will be covered *before* you agree to any care, says Dr. Prust.

and, in turn, quicken your pulse rate and cause other physiological changes that can heighten your susceptibility to acute pain.

If acute pain seems complex, you're right. But in most instances, pain does its job and then fades away. When it doesn't, that's when the real troublemaker, chronic pain, can set in.

Chronic Pain: The Ache That Runs Amok

Sisyphus, according to Greek mythology, was a cunning king who outwitted Death. As a result, he was condemned to repeatedly roll a huge stone up a hill only to have it roll down again as soon as he had managed to get it to the summit. Why Sisyphus was punished in this particular way—can you imagine the aches and pains he must have felt after an eternity of stone rolling?—has been lost to antiquity. But in many ways, chronic pain is just as senseless and baffling.

"Chronic pain is garbage in the brain. It is not useful information that the body can use in any meaningful way," says Norman J. Marcus, M.D., medical director of the Norman Marcus Pain Institute in New York City and the Princess Margaret Hospital Pain Treatment Center in Windsor, England, and author of *Freedom from Chronic Pain.*

Unlike acute pain, which lasts from a few seconds to a few weeks, chronic pain can last for months, years, or even decades. Although it may have begun as acute, useful pain—a symptom warning you to rest an inflamed back muscle, for instance—over time, chronic pain transforms itself into a disease, much like gentle Dr. Jekyll turned into venomous Mr. Hyde.

Like many relentless diseases, chronic pain plunders your vitality, shatters your self-esteem, and consumes your life. Yet strangely enough, a medical examination of a person who complains about chronic pain often reveals that the body has healed and that the physiological changes such as increased heart rate that accompany acute pain have returned to normal, Dr. Marcus says. But that doesn't mean the pain is a figment of your imagination. It is quite real.

"If you feel pain, you've got pain," says Nelson Hendler, M.D., director of the Mensana Clinic in Stevenson, Maryland, one of the nation's first pain clinics. "The reason you have chronic pain is you still have something wrong with you."

But what that "something" could be remains elusive. Doctors simply aren't sure how or why the body's nervous system runs amok and causes chronic pain.

"According to conventional wisdom, when pain lasts more than 3 months, it shifts from the acute phase into the chronic phase. What happens during that transition? That's what we don't know," says Jeffrey Ngeow, M.D., associate attending anesthesiologist and former director of the pain-management program at the Hospital for Special Surgery in New York City.

Nerve damage or diseases such as arthritis and diabetes all can contribute to the development of chronic pain. But it also can occur without a known injury or disease. Whatever the cause or causes, it is clear that the gateways that regulate pain sensation are blocked open, allowing nerves to continue sending their torturous messages on a fast track to the brain. Plus, all of the emotional and psychological responses to acute pain are magnified when it becomes chronic, leading to a cycle of insomnia, fatigue, irritability, anger, and sadness that can aggravate your condition.

Doctors also know that many of the standard treatments for acute pain—rest, heat, cold, and medication—aren't always the best choices for relieving chronic pain.

While rest is beneficial for acute pain, it actually can make chronic pain worse, Dr. Marcus says. Excessive rest can lead to flabby muscles, frail bones, and substantial weight gain. All of these things can strain your joints and cause even more aches and pains. In turn, these new aches and pains can convince you that you need more rest. But in reality, the more you rest, the more chronic pain you feel. So cancel the lounge act, and stay as active as you can.

In the long run, painkillers are often ineffective against chronic pain, Dr. Marcus says. Instead of relieving your torment, these drugs can actually lower your pain threshold. So even if you get higher doses, ultimately, you may get less relief.

"Pain medication is only useful for chronic pain if you're using it to improve and facilitate activities of daily living," he says. "If you're taking a medication that doesn't help you function any better, what good is it?"

While heat and ice packs often can reduce the swelling that accompanies acute pain, when you have chronic pain, the swelling is usually long gone, so heat and ice simply aren't going to be as effective, says Michelle Bricker, M.D., director of the University Center for Pain Medicine and Rehabilitation at Hermann at the University of Texas Medical Center in Houston.

So what does combat chronic pain? Plenty, including exercise, relaxation techniques, and other therapies and remedies we will discuss in this book.

"Even if you are older and have developed chronic aches and pains, it is not too late to do something about it," Dr. Prust says.

Where Does It Hurt?

Max Lerner thought that he and his doctors were on the same wavelength. So imagine how Lerner, a longtime columnist for the *New York Post*, felt when he checked into a hospital and discovered that the simple biopsy he had agreed to was actually a major procedure that involved sawing through a rib to gain access to one of his lungs. Dismayed, to say the least, he lashed out at his physicians.

"I had been—with the best of intentions—sandbagged," Lerner wrote in his memoir, *Wrestling with the Angel*. "I felt trapped. I could say with the narrator in T. S. Eliot's poem, 'This is not what I meant at all. This is not what I meant at all!'"

Even under the best of circumstances, communication is a fragile thing. And under the stress and strain of medical care, communication often crumples as easily as a dry leaf. Yet when you are in pain, nothing—absolutely nothing—is more critical than finding the right words to help your doctor understand your agony.

"Communicating with your health-care provider about your pain is the most important thing you can do to take an active role in your own care. It's vital for an older person to make their doctor or nurse aware of exactly what is going on," says Keela Herr, R.N., Ph.D., a pain researcher and associate professor of nursing at the University of Iowa College of Nursing in Iowa City.

BRIDGE THE COMMUNICATION GAP

Your doctor can't feel your pain. Neither, for that matter, can your friends or relatives.

It isn't like a rash that everyone can see and touch. Nor does pain feel the same to all people. A sprained ankle may hardly bother one person but can be unbearable to another. And although grimaces, twinges, and other nonverbal expressions of pain can give doctors a pretty good idea of how much you hurt, they really won't know unless you speak up. In fact, if you are stoic enough, your pain can be virtually invisible to others.

"Far too many older Americans needlessly endure pain because they don't talk to their doctors about it. They either mistakenly believe that their doctors can't do anything about it or they simply don't know how to describe their pain," Dr. Herr says. "Many times, they feel that nurses and doctors, because of their experience, know when they hurt. And if something could be done, they would be doing it without being asked. Unfortunately, that's not true. In many instances, nothing will be done unless you bring your pain to their attention."

But many Americans, particularly those of us who are older, are reluctant to do that. In fact, more than one in four people surveyed say there have been times when they wanted to talk to a doctor about a health problem but were reluctant to do so. Yet in that same survey, 9 out of 10 doctors agreed that serious medical problems such as pain could be averted if patients were willing to talk more freely. And 2 out of every 3 doctors said that it is difficult to treat patients who are hesitant or too embarrassed to talk about their health problems.

"Doctors aren't mind readers. We have to be told when you are in pain, what your pain is like, and what affects it. And the only person who can accurately do that is you," says Paul Blake, M.D., a pain-management expert and outpatient-services director at Meridian Point Rehabilitation Hospital in Scottsdale, Arizona. Here are some ways you can bridge the communication gap and help your doctor understand your pain.

BEFORE YOU GO

Chart a course. Take a few minutes *before* you visit the doctor to sketch out an agenda of what you'd like to discuss during the appointment, suggests Judson J. Somerville, M.D., an interventional pain-management specialist in Laredo, Texas. It could simply be a written list of your five major symptoms and concerns. At the appointment, hand your list to the doctor as he walks into the examination room.

"Frequently, what happens is that the doctor will speak very fast, throw a lot of questions at you, and then move on to the next patient. A list of symptoms is something that might slow the doctor down a

SPOTTING EMERGENCY PAIN

If you whack your head on the door of a kitchen cabinet, it hurts. Most pains are like that. They're easily explainable and quickly go away without treatment. But certain pains should never be ignored, says Stuart Farber, M.D., a geriatrician, pain-management expert, and clinical assistant professor of family medicine at the University of Washington in Seattle. Seek immediate medical attention if:

▶ You have pain in your chest that spreads into your neck, jaw, or left arm. This symptom also may be accompanied by shortness of breath, dizziness, nausea, vomiting, sweating, or generalized weakness.

▶ You develop a sudden, severe headache accompanied by numbness, dizziness, tingling.

▶ You have difficulty walking, seeing, speaking, or swallowing.

▶ You develop sudden back pain or lower-abdominal pain and feel light-headed or dizzy.

▶ You have constant abdominal pain that is in the lower-right area of your belly or that lasts for more than an hour and is accompanied by fever.

▶ You have painful urination accompanied by back pain, blood in your urine, or the urge to urinate more frequently.

▶ You have any other new, unexplainable pain that lasts more than a week.

little bit so that he will spend some extra time with you," he says.

The list will help you organize your thoughts so that you won't forget to mention a bothersome symptom or side effect of your treatment. From the doctor's standpoint, a written list—typewritten, if possible—will help him quickly address your concerns and spot telltale symptoms that may refine your diagnosis and treatment.

Make your first shot count. A typical person gets only about 18 seconds to explain a medical problem before the doctor interrupts with questions.

To make the most of that time, you need to clearly and concisely state what you expect out of the visit, says Margaret A. Caudill, M.D., Ph.D., codirector of the department of pain medicine at the Dartmouth-Hitchcock Medical Center in Manchester, New Hampshire, and author of *Managing Pain Before It Manages You.*

So before your appointment, take some time to imagine that your doctor has just walked into the examination room. What would you like to say in two or three sentences? Write that down. Now imagine how you'd like your doctor to reply to you. Do you want advice, reassurance, compassion, information, or a combination of these things? Try rewriting your opening statement so that it includes a clear request for what you expect your doctor to do for you.

You might, for example, say, "I'm scared, so I would appreciate it if you would reassure me" or "I don't expect miracles, but I would like some advice about coping better with flare-ups without using drugs."

"Many times, people come in and say, 'My pain is worse. It's terrible. I can't take it anymore.' End of story. They don't come right out and ask for what they really want," Dr. Caudill says. "It is very helpful to know exactly what a patient is looking for right up front."

Take five. Anticipate the five questions your doctor is most likely to ask you about your pain, suggests Michelle Bricker, M.D., director of the University Center for Pain Medicine and Rehabilitation at Hermann at the University of Texas Medical Center in Houston. If you can, jot down your responses to the following questions and take them with you when you visit your doctor.

◗ Where do you feel the pain, and what does it feel like?

◗ When did you first notice the pain you are experiencing now?

◗ Is there anything—such as changing your body position—that seems to make the pain feel better or worse? If so, what?

◗ Does the pain come and go, or is it persistent?

◗ Does it hurt more in the morning than in the evening?

WHAT TO TELL YOUR DOCTOR

Photocopy this page and have it with you when you talk with your doctor or nurse.

1. How strong is your pain? Mark a "W" on the pain scale below to show how your pain is at its worst. Mark a "U" on the pain scale below to show how your pain is at its usual level.

0	1	2	3	4	5	6	7	8	9	10
No pain			**Mild**			**Moderate**			**Severe pain, as bad as can be**	

2. Where is the pain? On the picture below, mark the places where you feel pain.

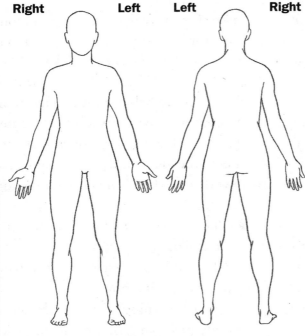

Right   **Left**   **Left**   **Right**

3. What does the pain feel like?
[ ] Pressure   [ ] Burning
[ ] Aching   [ ] Sharp
[ ] Throbbing   [ ] Shooting
[ ] Cramping   [ ] Tingling

4. Does the pain make it harder for you to:
[ ] Walk   [ ] Enjoy life
[ ] Sleep   [ ] Eat
[ ] Sit   [ ] Be active
[ ] Work   [ ] Be with family or
                  friends

5. When is the pain worse?
[ ] In the morning
[ ] During the night
[ ] I can't predict when it will get worse
[ ] Before my next dose of medication
[ ] With activity

6. What other problems are you having?
[ ] Constipation
[ ] Dry mouth
[ ] Sleepiness
[ ] Nausea or vomiting
[ ] Other symptoms
_____

If you're prepared for these questions beforehand, it can save time and help you to clearly communicate your needs, Dr. Bricker says.

Keep track of your aches. Often, it is difficult to convey to your doctor in a short office visit how much the pain really hurts in your everyday life. So keep a pain diary and take it with you each time you see your physician, Dr. Caudill suggests. Record your pain level on a 0-to-10 scale (10 being the worst pain you can imagine) three times a day at regular intervals, such as morning, noon, and bedtime. Do this for at least 3 months, Dr. Caudill says, and you may start noticing patterns of pain that you can point out to your doctor.

Keep time on your side. If you suspect that you'll need more than a 15-minute appointment to discuss your aches and pains, let the doctor's receptionist know that when you make your appointment, Dr. Caudill suggests. That way, you and your doctor will feel less hurried.

IN THE EXAM ROOM

Be succinct. Whenever you are describing your pain, stick to the pertinent facts, suggests Stuart Farber, M.D., a geriatrician, pain-management expert, and clinical assistant professor of family medicine at the University of Washington in Seattle. "You can't tell your life story and expect the doctor to pay attention," he says.

So avoid straying off the subject. If you're describing how you injured your back while gardening, for instance, avoid going into the details about the type of flowers you were planting or asking the doctor about his gardening habits. Instead, focus on how the injury occurred and how you feel now. So you might say, "I was gardening when I felt this awful twinge in my lower back that felt like a firecracker exploding. It's been 3 days since that happened, and it still hasn't gone away." That approach will grab your doctor's attention, Dr. Farber says.

Let your doc feel it, too. Just saying "It hurts" isn't going to help your doctor understand your pain. Be specific—let the doctor know precisely how the pain is disrupting your life, Dr. Farber suggests. So if you have a sore ankle and it is preventing you from doing daily activities such as walking, playing tennis, puttering in the garden, or even doing household chores, speak up.

"When you break down pain into a personal experience so that the physician can understand how it is really affecting you, it's a much more persuasive motivator for the doctor to help you do something about it," Dr. Farber says.

Know the lingo. The more accurately you can describe your pain, the better the chances are that your doctor can help you find relief, Dr. Farber says. Use simple words like stinging, burning, throbbing, aching, cramping, or jabbing to help the doctor pinpoint the problem.

A sharp, stabbing pain in your legs and back that goes all the way down to your toes, for example, will probably need to be treated differently than a burning, scalding pain that begins in your hip and travels down the front of your thigh. "Details like that can help your doctor understand the mechanism of your pain and what can be done about it," Dr. Farber says.

Pick a target. If you have more than one ache or pain, zero in on the most bothersome one first, suggests Norman J. Marcus, M.D., medical director of the Norman Marcus Pain Institute in New York City and the Princess Margaret Hospital Pain Treatment Center in Windsor, England, and author of *Freedom from Chronic Pain.*

"If you tell the doctor that you hurt everywhere, you can forget about getting good care. Everything doesn't hurt everywhere in exactly the same way," he says. "You're better off saying something like, 'Yes, I do have a lot of aches and pains, but this one is unique, and here's why it's unique. It's not like most of my other pains

that just feel achy. This pain feels like somebody is jabbing in my lower back. It comes on when I do this or when I don't do that. It doesn't respond to medication the way my other pains do.' Information like that will give your doctor something to work with."

Question authority. If an explanation or procedure puzzles you during the exam, ask your doctor for clarification. Otherwise, he will assume that you understand what is going on, Dr. Blake says.

You might say something like, "I still don't quite get what you're trying to tell me. Can you explain it again?"

"Some older people are reluctant to ask their physicians to repeat instructions they don't fully understand," Dr. Blake says. "But you have to keep in mind that your physician is there to educate you as well as treat you. So it's okay to keep asking questions until you fully grasp it."

Push the rewind button. Similarly, if your doctor doesn't seem to understand you, ask him to repeat what you just told him about your aches and pains, Dr. Somerville says. If it doesn't match what you said, try restating your problem until the doctor gets it.

"Just take one step back and say, 'Somehow, doctor, I'm not conveying to you what is wrong with me. Is there some way I can explain it to you better or differently?'" he says. "That way, the doctor won't feel as if you're attacking him and then react defensively to your comments."

Say, "Show me." Ask your doctor to use pictures and other visual aids that will make your pain and its treatment easier to comprehend, Dr. Somerville suggests.

Get it in writing. Ask your doctor for pamphlets, step-by-step instructions, or other written materials. These handouts can help you understand your condition and help you recall exercises and other techniques he suggests for relieving your aches and pains, Dr. Blake says.

BEFORE YOU LEAVE

Let it all simmer. After your appointment ends, take a few minutes to sit down in the doctor's waiting room to jot down notes or go over any written materials you were given during the visit. If you don't understand something, particularly the diagnosis, testing procedures, treatment, or even when you are supposed to return for a follow-up visit, ask a nurse for clarification, Dr. Somerville suggests. If you're still confused after that conversation, ask to speak briefly with the doctor.

Know how to connect. Physicians, like most of us, tend to be busier at certain times of the day than at others. So be sure to ask a nurse when the best time would be to telephone your doctor if you have a question or need advice between appointments, Dr. Somerville suggests. If you phone and leave a message, let the doctor know when you'll be available so he can contact you. If you have access to a computer, you also might ask if the doctor has e-mail.

Ask for seconds. If, after talking to the doctor, you are still uncomfortable about some aspect of your diagnosis or treatment, ask for a second opinion, Dr. Blake says. "There is nothing wrong with getting a second opinion for a complicated problem like pain. You're not necessarily going to hear the same thing from a second doctor. Most doctors won't get upset with you if you ask for another opinion."

If you do ask for a second opinion, before you leave the office, be sure to sign a release form and request that your doctor forward a copy of your medical records to the consulting physician.

Adopting
a Pain-Free Attitude

His hands deformed by an aggressive form of rheumatoid arthritis, Pierre-Auguste Renoir still managed to produce more than 400 paintings in the last 25 years of his life. Even when this famed nineteenth-century French artist awoke at night crying out in pain, he would ask for his brushes and palette and begin to create small paintings on wood as he sang or hummed tunes from the great operas.

Renoir lived much of his life in pain, but he never allowed pain to become his life.

"He had a good attitude. Renoir knew he had things that he could do while he waited out the pain. It wasn't an ideal situation, but he wasn't going to be beaten down by it," says Margaret A. Caudill, M.D., Ph.D., codirector of the department of pain medicine at the Dartmouth-Hitchcock Medical Center in Hanover, New Hampshire, and author of *Managing Pain Before It Manages You*.

"Attitude can make all the difference in the world. If one has a hopeful, self-assured attitude, it helps one feel less overwhelmed or managed by the pain," she points out. "Attitude really sets the tone of how one perceives the ability to manage the symptoms."

You may not have a choice about when or where you hurt, but you certainly can choose how you react to your pain. And that reaction—that attitude—has as much to do with your pain as any mangled nerve or spasmodic muscle in your body.

ENDING PAIN POSITIVELY

Virtually every negative emotion—fear, depression, anxiety—sparks an incredible biological assault on your nervous system, says Dharma Singh Khalsa, M.D., a pain-management expert in Tucson, Arizona, and author of *The Pain Cure*. Your heart beats faster, your body secretes stress hormones, your muscles tense, your blood vessels constrict, and neurotransmitters in your brain are overly stimulated. As a result, your pain threshold plunges, and your body's ability to counteract your discomfort is diminished.

This pain often is a self-perpetuating cycle that is hard to break. But you can do it.

"I have a quote scribbled on my desk that reads, 'I know it's going to be a good day because I know how to make it a good day.' A patient told me that once, and I thought it was brilliant," Dr. Caudill says. "I'm not saying positive thinking will make all of your pain go away. But you have more control than you think when you're in the midst of a pain problem."

Among other things, a positive attitude triggers the release of endorphins, powerful morphinelike substances in your brain that relieve pain, says Stanley Chapman, Ph.D., a psychologist at the Emory Clinic Center for Pain Management in Atlanta.

In addition, a brighter attitude helps move the pain and suffering from the forefront of your thinking into the background, says Emmett Miller, M.D., who practices in Los Altos and Nevada City, California, and is the author of *Deep Healing: The Essence of Mind/Body Medicine*. And when that happens, a pain that once seemed unbearable might become a mere nuisance and seldom disruptive.

"Miracles happen when your outlook changes," says Robert N. Jamison, Ph.D., director of the pain-management program at Brigham and Women's Hospital in Boston and author of *Learning to Master Your Chronic Pain*. "If your perception of the pain changes, then the pain itself may actually go down."

Here are a few ways you can foster a pain-free attitude.

Ax the four-letter words. The words *pain* and *hurt* are associated with fear, helplessness, and isolation. So use more neutral terms such as *discomfort* or *sensation*, which imply that you can help yourself and stay active, Dr. Miller suggests. Sure, it's a subtle change, but it can make a huge difference in your attitude.

Take a look at the big picture. On a blank piece of paper, jot down all of the things that you deeply desire from life. If you want to go on a long-delayed cruise along the Mexican Riviera, for instance, write that down. If you want to spend more time with your grandchildren, jot that down, too. Record whatever pops into your head. Keep in mind that there are no right or wrong answers. As you do this, you'll probably begin to see that there is much more to your life than just overcoming the pain. Once you realize this, it may have a profound effect on your attitude toward your discomfort, Dr. Khalsa says.

This goal-setting exercise, called psychic clustering, will help you regain control of your destiny and cast off attitudes that have allowed pain to dominate your life, he says.

Seeing is believing. Visualization, a powerful mind-control technique, can help you dampen pain and reshape your attitude toward it, Dr. Khalsa says. In a study done at a major pain clinic, 20 percent of people with severe chronic pain attained total relief after just 4 weeks of visualization training.

"Visualization literally reprograms the brain and alters perception of pain," he says.

To try it, sit down in a quiet place that is free of distractions. Close your eyes, breathe deeply, and relax as much as possible, Dr. Miller says. As you relax, imagine that in front of you, several feet away, is a movie screen. Imagine that you can see any part or area of your body that you wish. If there is an area of your body that has been having unpleasant sensations, picture this part of your body on the screen. If you wish, you may even picture the word *pain* on that screen.

As you look at that shape you are projecting on that screen, notice what color it is or give it a color that matches the sensation. See the color clearly. See the size and shape of this area. Is it a bright color or dull? Are its borders smooth or irregular? Does it look flat or bumpy? Is it the same color throughout or does it vary in color? As you continue to relax, let the color and the image fade. As this happens, the unwanted sensation will continue to fade along with it, becoming less and less as you slip into a deep, comfortable state of peace.

Next, imagine that you are entering the very deepest part of your mind, Dr. Miller says. Imagine that you can picture it as a control room with switches and knobs that control the amount of awareness of any sensation. By adjusting these controls, you turn down the sensations in your body so they fade far, far away. Notice that there is a knob that controls your awareness of that sensation that was projected out on that screen in front of you. Grasp this knob now and begin to turn it down so that the sensation disappears more and more, as though it is dissolving into a cloud of peace and relaxation.

Do this for 10 to 15 minutes twice a day, Dr. Miller suggests.

Go with the flow. Meditation is one of the best ways to rise above pain and forge a positive attitude, Dr. Khalsa says. It increases your mental energy, so your brain can launch an effective counterattack against the pain. In addition, meditation allows you to slip into a state of absolute calm, called the sacred space, that triggers regeneration and healing of your mind, body, and spirit.

Find a quiet, comfortable spot where you won't be disturbed. Close your eyes and take several deep, relaxing breaths. If any thoughts intrude, let them drift away, and refocus your attention on your breathing.

To help focus the physical energy of your brain, press the tip of your left thumb on your forehead, between your eyebrows, Dr. Khalsa suggests. This is the area of the brain where your highest thought processes occur. Then with your thumb still pressing on your forehead, make a fist, but leave your little finger extended. Grasp your extended little finger in the palm of your right hand, and extend the little finger of your right hand. Hold this position for 3 minutes as you continue to breathe deeply. Then lower your hands; you should feel more focused and aware of your body.

Keep breathing deeply through your nose—about 8 to 10 breaths per minute.

As you do, focus your attention on an area in your body that hurts. Notice how the discomfort waxes and wanes, Dr. Khalsa says. Then focus on areas of your body that do not hurt. Pay attention to the comfort you feel there and realize that this sensation is just as real as the pain. Don't become attached to the comfort or repulsed by the pain. Just accept these sensations as they are. Allow peace of mind and spirit to grow with each breath. And as it does, feel tension, worry, and discomfort wash away.

Do this meditation for 10 to 15 minutes twice a day, Dr. Khalsa suggests.

Accentuate the positive. Affirmations can change how you think about your pain and actually help keep it in check, Dr. Khalsa says. So at least three times a day—at breakfast, lunch, and supper—take a few minutes to state how you would *like* to feel. You might, for example, try telling yourself, "I'm in power, not my pain." Or "My healing has already begun."

The more you repeat these affirmations, the more powerful they will become, and the greater the likelihood they'll become a natural way of thinking.

Use your body wisely. Treat pain like money. You have so much to spend, and you have to decide what is worth spending it on, says Eric Willmarth, Ph.D., a pain-management expert and president of Michigan Behavioral Consultants, based in

Grand Rapids. Suppose, for instance, you were invited to your grandson's wedding. You may be standing a lot and may be in pain afterward. Is that worth it? Probably. On the other hand, if you're invited to a neighborhood block party, you might not want to spend your pain that way. Thinking about activities this way will help you regain a sense of control over your pain, he says, and, in turn, it makes it easier for you to maintain a positive attitude.

Keep a checklist. Keep a written list of strategies that make you feel better during flare-ups, Dr. Caudill says.

"It's so funny how people may have a back problem and cope with it fine. But if they develop a neck problem, they get unhinged because they don't appreciate that the same things apply," she says. "Having these strategies written down acknowledges that you're going to have flare-ups and acknowledges that you have successfully coped with them in the past."

Flip a switch. Whenever you have a negative thought about your pain, jot it down on a notepad. Take a hard look at that thought. Now think of a rational, positive response to that statement, then write that down next to the first one, Dr. Caudill suggests. You might think, for instance, "I can't do anything because of this pain." Your response might be, "If I take frequent breaks, I can still do many things I enjoy."

After a couple of weeks of doing this on a regular basis, you might be surprised to find that your negative thoughts have been replaced by positive ones.

"When you're in chronic pain, you tend to think the same negative thoughts over and over again," she says. "Many people who go through this exercise tell me they discover that everything needn't be black or white or horrific in their lives. You can really see the lights go on."

Carry a trump card. After you've listed your negative thoughts, you'll probably start seeing the same phrases over and over again. If this happens, jot down five of your most common negative thoughts about your pain on one side of an index card. Then on the other side, write down five replacement thoughts for each of these negative attitudes. Carry this card with you. When one of these thought pops into your head, pull out the card and use one of the replacement phrases to drown out the negative one, Dr. Jamison suggests.

So if you typically think, "This is unbearable," write that phrase on one side of the card. On the flip side, jot down phrases like "I've gotten through this in the past, and I'm going to get through this again."

Follow the crowd. Socialize. Go to the bowling alley or a nearby coffee shop. Get out to where people are on a daily basis, Dr. Jamison says.

"If you have nothing going on except the four walls around you and an ever-present silence, your pain is apt to overwhelm you," he says. "But if you get out and do things that occupy your mind, it will help diminish your discomfort and help you feel more connected with the world." If it's not possible to get out and about, pick up the phone and talk to a friend or get together for a game of cards or lunch. Take up a hobby to help keep your mind active and involved. The Internet can also be a great way to bring the world to you by looking up subjects that interest you. You can even chat with your friends and family online.

Spot a smile maker. Find a heartwarming experience in each day, Dr. Willmarth suggests. Watch a toddler picking a dandelion. Take time to contemplate a rainbow.

"The more ammunition you can give yourself for developing a positive attitude, the better off you'll be," he says. "Train yourself to observe beauty, humor, compassion, and other good things around you."

Exercise your funny bone. Laughter is a powerful weapon against pain, Dr. Jamison says. It relaxes tense muscles, decreases the production of stress-related hormones, and distracts your mind from the pain. So if you're having a particularly rough day, imagine how your favorite comedian would describe it. It will help you laugh it off. Reserve a portion of your refrigerator or bulletin board for cartoons and funny pictures or sayings. Stockpile a library of humorous writings and videos you can turn to when your pain flares up.

"Humor helps a lot. Pain is so deadly serious and it makes you so miserable that it is hard to distance yourself from it," he says. "But laughter can renew your sense of why life is worth living. So any way that you find humor in your existence is important."

The Good and Bad of Drugs

War is hell. You should know; you're waging a battle against pain. And just like soldiers on a real battlefield, you need to use the best weapons in your arsenal to win. In this war, that often means painkilling drugs. But like any weapon, a drug can be self-destructive as well as useful. Even the ancient Greeks recognized that drugs were a double-edged sword. Their word for drugs, *pharmakos*, meant both "remedy" and "poison."

But you have an important ally on your side: knowledge. Doctors and pharmacists now know far more about limitations and dangers of drugs than at any other time in history. They know, for instance, that the risk of addiction to painkilling medications is extremely low when they are used appropriately. They know that older Americans react differently to painkillers. They

know that taking pain medication is not a sign of weakness.

And by the time you finish reading this chapter, you'll know these things, too. This knowledge will help you overcome fears and misconceptions you may have about using these medications as part of an overall battle plan to conquer your pain.

DRUGS, PAIN, AND YOU

As you get older, one of the most important things you need to know is that your body reacts differently to drugs than it would have when you were younger. This fact raises some issues of which you need to be aware.

Your metabolism may be slower. Part of the reason drugs have a different ef-

30

TAKE PAINS TO ASK THESE QUESTIONS

Here are the three most important questions to ask your doctor about a medication, according to Isaiah Florence, M.D., director for the Center for Pain Management at Englewood Hospital and Medical Center in New Jersey.

▶ Does this interact with my other medications?
▶ What are the side effects?
▶ What can I expect this medicine to accomplish for me?

fect on older people is that most drugs tend to hang around longer in the system of a senior than in a younger person, says Max A. Schneider, M.D., director of education at the Positive Action Center at Chapman Medical Center in Orange, California; chairperson of the board of directors of the National Council on Alcoholism and Drug Dependence; and former consultant to the Drug and Alcohol Advisory Committee of the FDA. As you age, your body's filtration system—your kidneys and liver—can be affected by disease or age and can take longer to filter drugs out of your system. Also, most seniors weigh less than the average person, so the same amount of drug will have a greater effect in them than in younger people, who weigh more.

You may be mixing a lot of different drugs. This is one of the greatest issues of concern for experts on pain and aging, says Dr. Schneider. Consider this: Americans over age 65 take more drugs than any other age group, according to the FDA. In fact, two-thirds of older Americans take two or more medications each day. And any time you mix more than one drug, it elevates your risk of adverse reactions because medications frequently compete with

THE KEYS TO THE MEDICINE CHEST

As many brands compete for your medication dollars, the number of special features they tout has begun to rival those of Mercedes and BMWs. Do you want tablets? Caplets? Capsules? Will that be enteric-coated? Buffered? Time-released?

What does it all mean? How do you choose?

The choice between tablets, caplets, and capsules is purely one of personal preference. "There are some people who have difficulty swallowing certain shapes, which is why the drug companies offer so many choices, explains Mark Baugh, Pharm.D., a pharmacist at San Diego Hospice and author of *Sports Nutrition: The Awful Truth.* "Some people have trouble swallowing something round, whereas something long and narrow they don't have as much trouble with.

your liver's ability to detoxify them, thus slowing their excretion. It's much like taking a chemistry set and randomly mixing compounds together. Unless you know what you're doing, you could trigger a reaction in any number of organs in your body.

"It's critical to bring a list of your medications to the doctor every time so that the doctor can look at it and find out what you're taking, especially if you're seeing more than one doctor. You need to make sure that doctor A is not accidentally poisoning you because of what doctor B is giving you," Dr. Schneider says.

You're a prime candidate for drug side effects. It's a logical, if scary, progression: Because older men and women

That's the secret. Just pick the one you can swallow the best." Here's a primer for the choices.

Buffered. This means an antacid has been added to the medicine to protect your stomach. Experts say that it really doesn't do much to save your stomach, but it does help the pill dissolve faster than normal.

Enteric-coated. These pills are less likely to cause stomach upset because they will dissolve in your intestines instead of in your stomach. But that also means they will take about 15 minutes longer to start working.

Time-released. This may also be called delayed-release or extended-release. They all mean the same thing. The effect is scientifically designed so that some of the medicine dissolves fast, then the inner core is designed to release over an extended period of time. They won't provide the quick pain punch of other analgesics.

are more sensitive to the actions of drugs, they're more likely to experience side effects, some of which can be serious enough to warrant a trip to the emergency room. "If you take something and it makes your heart race, or if you start to perspire, have trouble breathing, or your throat constricts, go to the emergency room right away," says Mark Baugh, Pharm.D., a pharmacist at San Diego Hospice and author of *Sports Nutrition: The Awful Truth*.

Be sure to call your doctor immediately if you develop rashes, indigestion, vomiting, sour stomach, diarrhea, balance problems, black or bloody stools, ringing in the ears, double vision, or loss of appetite or sense of taste, says Dr. Schneider. These, too, are signs of adverse reactions.

DRUG/HERB COMBINATION CONCERNS

In general, herbs cause fewer side effects than drugs. But don't forget: They're still powerful medicines and are capable of interacting with other medications and supplements. Jennifer Brett, N.D., a naturopathic physician and chairperson of botanical medicine at the University of Bridgeport College of Naturopathic Medicine in Connecticut, offers these rules for safe herbal healing.

▶ Don't use herbs with drugs that have similar ingredients or that act on the body in similar ways. For instance, don't combine willow bark or aspirin with an anticoagulant such as warfarin (Coumadin).

▶ Try not to take herbs and other medications or supplements at the same time, just in case they might interact with one another.

▶ Avoid herbs that increase or decrease the amount of time it takes other medications or supplements to be absorbed in your body. Licorice, for example, lengthens the time it takes to clear prednisone (Orasone) from the body.

Here are 11 of the most well-known and widely used herbs, along with their known drug or supplement interactions.

1. Black cohosh   May interfere with effects of low-dose oral contraceptives or hormone-replacement therapy

2. Garlic   Can intensify the effect of blood thinners like warfarin (Coumadin)

3. Ginger   May inhibit the effectiveness of heart medications, anticoagulants, and diabetic medications

4. Ginkgo   Do not use with antidepressant MAO-inhibitor drugs such as phenelzine sulfate (Nardil) or tranylcypromine (Parnate), aspirin or other nonsteroidal anti-inflammatory medications, or blood-thinning medications such as warfarin (Coumadin)

5. Ginseng (Panax)   Can interact with phenelzine and MAO inhibitors; don't take with coffee or caffeinated beverages, antipsychotic drugs, or hormone treatments

6. Kava kava   Intensifies the effects of alcohol, antidepressants, and antihistamines

7. Licorice   Can interfere with hormone therapy; avoid if you take drugs that already leave you prone to potassium loss (thiazide diuretics)

8. St. John's wort   Do not use with antidepressants; may increase photosensitivity effect of sulfa drugs or antibiotics like tetracycline

9. Uva-ursi   May irritate bladder when taken with acidic agents like fruit juice or supplemental vitamin C

10. Valerian   Can intensify the effect of sleep-enhancing or mood-regulating medications such as diazepam (Valium) or amitriptyline (Elavil)

11. Willow bark   Can interact with blood thinners such as warfarin (Coumadin) or with barbiturates or sedatives; can cause stomach irritation when taken with alcohol

BANISHING THE BIG THREE

Of all the side effects that can strike, nausea, constipation, and heartburn are the three that most often plague seniors. Certainly, these side effects should be discussed with your physician, but here are a few things you can do to dampen them on your own.

Treat nausea gingerly. "Nausea is very common with nonsteroidal anti-inflammatory drugs. It also happens frequently with narcotics," explains Mark Beers, M.D., senior director of geriatrics and editor of the *Merck Manuals* in West Point, Pennsylvania. The best trick to combat it is to take the medicine with food. A tall glass of flat, cold, caffeine-free soda like ginger ale also may help. As your body adjusts to the medication, the nausea should dissipate, usually within a day or two after you begin taking the drug. Nonetheless, many older people are not able to tolerate these drugs, admits Dr. Beers.

Go over the counter for constipation. Constipation is another common side effect, especially with narcotics. "When you're taking narcotics, constipation needs to be treated with a stimulant laxative," Dr. Beers says. "No other kind of laxative will work well because of the way narcotics directly cause the muscles of the bowel to slow down." Look for products containing bisacodyl, such as Correctol, or sennosides like Ex-Lax at your drugstore, and follow the package instructions.

Douse the fire. A third common side effect for seniors is heartburn. Try antacids, suggests Dr. Beers. "If you have heartburn, you need to buffer the gastric irritation. Try Mylanta, Maalox, or Tums." Be sure to follow the package instructions.

TO PRESCRIBE OR NOT TO PRESCRIBE

Drugstores boast a dizzying array of over-the-counter pain medications, but maybe what you need is a prescription. Which is better? Which is cheaper? Which is safer?

The general rule of thumb is: Treat a minor pain such as a simple headache, bruises, or aches from straining first with acetaminophen as directed on the label, says Dr. Baugh. If that doesn't work after 24 hours, stop taking it and try a nonsteroidal anti-inflammatory drug, the most common of which is ibuprofen. The over-the-counter strength is 200 milligrams. If you take two tablets, you get 400 milligrams, which is equivalent to the lowest dosage available by prescription. If that doesn't work within 24 hours, the next logical step is to see a doctor for a prescription.

Today's arsenal of prescription pain relievers includes Cox-2 inhibitors (a new generation of nonsteroidal anti-inflammatory drug) and narcotics. Medications developed for other uses, such as anticonvulsants, antidepressants, and corticosteroids, also can relieve some types of pain. But for many older Americans who fear addiction, prescription narcotic painkillers present a disquieting option.

THE TRUTH ABOUT ADDICTION

One of the greatest fears most people have about taking painkilling drugs is that they'll become addicted. And while it's certainly a reasonable concern, it is often an exaggerated one, explains Isaiah Florence, M.D., director for the Center for Pain Management at Englewood Hospital and Medical Center in New Jersey. Before you ever reach a state of being addicted, you have to pass through several levels first. To begin with, there's tolerance, which means that after taking a drug for an extended period of time, you'll need more of it to get the same pain relief. Then there's physical dependence, which means that if you take a drug for a while

and then stop, you'll develop withdrawal symptoms such as irritability, sweating, and chills.

The difference between physical dependence and the next step, addiction, is huge, says Richard Patt, M.D., president of the Patt Center for Cancer Pain and Wellness in Houston and coauthor of *You Don't Have to Suffer*. For someone to be addicted, they have to experience three conditions. First, they have an overwhelming desire for the drug for reasons other than pain control. Second, they want the drug despite the threat of physical or psychological harm. And third, they lack control over their medication use. If taking your pain medication makes you work better and think clearer, then you're using it appropriately, he explains. Drug addicts become less functional and more isolated. If that sounds like you, it's time to talk to your doctor.

KNOW YOUR WEAPONS

As it is, you may be taking numerous drugs for pain, or you may be wondering what other drug options exist for pain as well as what side effects or risks they might pose. The following drug profiles will help address those concerns.

DRUG PROFILES

▼ Acetaminophen

What Is It?

Available over the counter, acetaminophen alleviates pain by inhibiting the production of prostaglandins, hormonelike substances that lead to swelling and help transmit pain signals to the brain. It's best for minor aches and pains, pain with bruising, and muscle pain.

Active Ingredient (Common Brand)

Acetaminophen (Tylenol)

Common Side Effects

None

Safe Use

Don't exceed the dosage recommended in package directions—too much can cause liver and kidney damage. If you suspect that you've taken too much, contact the nearest poison information center. Do not drink alcohol if you'll be taking more than two doses of acetaminophen.

Hidden Benefits

Research suggests that when a woman takes a single dose on a daily basis, acetaminophen may reduce her risk of ovarian cancer by half.

Not Recommended For

Heavy drinkers or people with liver damage. If you consume alcoholic beverages, consult your physician before using acetaminophen, since it is hard on the liver.

Special Hints

Keep your acetaminophen out of damp places, including your bathroom medicine cabinet. Heat and moisture cause it to break down. Many heavily advertised names can be more expensive; check into store brands. Don't waste your money using this medicine for the swelling of arthritis—it isn't as effective against inflammation as other medications. Save it for headaches and other minor aches and pains.

DRUG PROFILES

▼ Anticonvulsants

What Are They?

Anticonvulsants are medications prescribed to control seizures. They can be helpful for nerve pain, especially burning, stabbing pains due to diabetic neuropathy and postherpetic neuralgia.

Active Ingredients (Common Brands)

Carbamazepine (Tegretol) and gabapentin (Neurontin)

Common Side Effects

Clumsiness, dizziness, light-headedness, drowsiness, nausea, vomiting, or irregular, pounding, or unusually slow heartbeat and chest pain

Safe Use

Take this medicine as prescribed for a specified pain only. Do not use it to treat minor discomforts. These agents are not simple analgesics and should not be taken casually.

Hidden Benefits

Carbamazepine has been used to treat the acute phase of schizophrenia when other agents have failed.

Not Recommended For

People who are allergic to tricyclic antidepressants and those with liver or bone marrow disease should avoid taking carbamazepine.

Special Hints

Keep this medicine out of damp places, including your bathroom medicine cabinet. Heat and moisture cause it to break down.

DRUG PROFILES

▼ Combination Drugs

What Are They?

These nonprescription pain relievers have more than one ingredient. Caffeine is added to enhance the absorption of the aspirin or acetaminophen, so it gets to your brain—and stops pain—faster. They work best for arthritis when using aspirin or for tension headaches when using acetaminophen.

Active Ingredients (Common Brands)

Acetaminophen, aspirin, and caffeine (Excedrin Extra-Strength); aspirin and caffeine (Anacin); and acetaminophen and caffeine (Aspirin-Free Excedrin)

Common Side Effects

Abdominal cramps or stomach pain, heartburn or indigestion, nausea and vomiting, slowed blood-clotting time (for medicines containing aspirin), and jitters and trouble sleeping (for medicines containing caffeine)

Safe Use

Before medical testing, tell your doctor that you're taking these drugs.

Hidden Benefits

Research suggests that a single daily dose of acetaminophen may slash the risk of ovarian cancer in half.

Aspirin is approved by the FDA to reduce the risk of subsequent strokes and adverse cardiovascular events. It reduces the risk of death from heart attacks, prevents second heart attacks, and diminishes the risk of heart attack in people with angina.

Not Recommended For

If you consume alcoholic beverages, consult your physician before using these drugs, especially because both acetaminophen and alcohol are hard on the liver. Medications containing aspirin are not recommended for people with asthma, nasal polyps, high blood pressure, bleeding disorders, severe liver or kidney disease, stomach ulcers, or history of hemorrhagic stroke.

Special Hints

To prevent gastrointestinal side effects, take with meals.

DRUG PROFILES

▼ Corticosteroids

What Are They?

Corticosteroids are prescription medicines that provide relief of inflammation. They provide pain relief by reducing swelling, itching, redness, and allergic reactions. They work best for arthritis, cancer pain, and surgical pain, especially when there is inflammation.

Active Ingredients (Common Brands)

Betamethasone (Celestone), cortisone (Cortone Acetate), dexamethasone (Decadron), prednisolone (Predalone 50), and prednisone (Orasone)

Common Side Effects

Increased appetite, indigestion, restlessness, nervousness, and trouble sleeping

Safe Use

Since steroids may lower your immune function, infections may be harder to treat. Be sure to talk to your doctor if you develop symptoms of another infection such as fever, difficulty breathing, or pain in your kidneys or bladder. To prevent stomach problems, take with food. Don't drink alcoholic beverages while taking steroids.

Hidden Benefits

None

Not Recommended For

People with active tuberculosis, fungal infections, herpes infection of the eyes, or peptic ulcer disease

Special Hints

Since side effects occur with prolonged use of corticosteroids, avoid using these medications for long periods of time. Sometimes steroids can be taken every other day or at varying doses to lessen side effects. Check with your doctor to see if this is right for you. Avoid people with influenza, chickenpox, measles, or who have recently taken an oral polio vaccine. While your immunity is compromised by the steroids, these people could easily pass these illnesses on to you, even if you already had them once.

DRUG PROFILES

▼ Cox-2 Inhibitors

What Are They?

Hailed as the new generation of nonsteroidal anti-inflammatory drugs (NSAIDs), Cox-2 inhibitors promise to relieve the pain of arthritis without causing the gastrointestinal problems of older NSAIDs. Cox—short for cyclooxygenase—is an enzyme that controls the production of hormone-like substances called prostaglandins that lead to swelling and transmit pain to the brain. There are two types of the enzyme: Cox-1 and Cox-2. Cox-1 controls prostaglandins that help to create the protective mucus of the stomach, so if it's suppressed, damage to the stomach can result. Cox-2 regulates prostaglandins that cause inflammation and pain, so if it's suppressed, you have less pain. While older NSAIDs block both Cox-1 and Cox-2, Cox-2 inhibitors only block the prostaglandins that you want to block, the ones that cause pain.

Active Ingredients (Common Brands)

Celecoxib (Celebrex) and rofecoxib (Vioxx)

Common Side Effects

Gastrointestinal bleeding, skin rash, weight gain, and fluid retention

Safe Use

If you are prone to stomach ulcers, don't use Cox-2 inhibitors until the ulcers are completely healed and your doctor says it's okay.

Hidden Benefits

They're more gentle on the gastrointestinal system than other pain medicines, and they may slow the progression of cancer and Alzheimer's disease. Unlike other NSAIDs, Cox-2 inhibitors don't appear to increase the risk of uncontrolled bleeding.

Not Recommended For

People who have had reactions to aspirin or other NSAIDs such as wheezing hives or allergies, or those who are allergic to sulfonamides

Special Hints

These drugs are expensive. Only use them if you have drug-induced ulcers and can't take NSAIDs.

▼ Local Anesthetics

What Are They?

These drugs are given by injection to cause loss of sensation. They are used by a medical professional, usually before and during surgery.

Active Ingredients (Common Brands)

Lidocaine (Dilocaine) and prilocaine (Citanest)

Common Side Effects

Skin rash, hives, itching, and allergic reactions

Safe Use

These drugs are typically used during dental surgery. If the numbness and tingling in your mouth doesn't go away within a few hours or you can't open your mouth, call your dentist.

Hidden Benefits

None

Not Recommended For

Those who have had adverse reactions to local anesthetics or epinephrine in the past or who are allergic to sulfites or PABA (para-aminobenzoic acid). Typical adverse reactions include very high fever, fast and irregular heartbeat, acute asthma attacks, muscle spasms, and breathing problems.

Special Hints

Take care with any part of your body that has been numbed by an injection. Since you won't feel pain in that area, it's very easy to hurt yourself.

DRUG PROFILES

▼ Narcotics/Opioids

What Are They?

Potent drugs that suppress activity in the central nervous system and relieve pain. These drugs are available by prescription only. They are usually reserved for moderate and severe pain, especially bone and muscle pain, cancer pain, pain during surgery, or times when other medications haven't been able to relieve unrelenting pain.

Active Ingredients (Common Brands)

Codeine, hydrocodone, fentanyl (Sublimaze), morphine (Duramorph), methadone (Dolophine), propoxyphene (Darvon), hydromorphone (Dilaudid), and meperidine (Demerol)

Common Side Effects

Dizziness, light-headedness, drowsiness, nausea, vomiting, and constipation

Safe Use

Don't combine narcotics with alcohol or other medicines, such as antihistamines, that slow down the nervous system.

Hidden Benefits

These medications can also reduce anxiety.

Not Recommended For

People with severe asthma or those with fluid in their lungs from congestive heart failure

Special Hints

Dry mouth is a common side effect. To combat it, try chewing candy or gum, melt ice in your mouth, or use a saliva substitute.

DRUG PROFILES

▼ Nonsteroidal Anti-Inflammatory Drugs (NSAIDs)

What Are They?

These drugs halt the production and release of prostaglandins, hormonelike substances that lead to swelling and help transmit pain to the brain. They work best for mild to moderate pain accompanied by swelling.

Active Ingredients (Common Brands)—Prescription

Indomethacin (Indocin), nabumetone (Relafen), sulindac (Clinoril), flurbiprofen (Ansaid), and others

Active Ingredients (Common Brands)—Nonprescription

Ibuprofen (Advil), ketoprofen (Orudis KT), and naproxen (Aleve)

Common Side Effects

Abdominal or stomach cramps, diarrhea, drowsiness, dizziness, lightheadedness, headache, heartburn, indigestion, nausea, vomiting, and high blood pressure. Since gastrointestinal damage from NSAIDs can occur at any point, short-term use isn't necessarily safer. In fact, long-term use may actually allow gastric mucous membranes to adapt, reducing the chance of stomach problems.

Safe Use

Never mix NSAIDs with the cancer medication methotrexate (Mexate), which is sometimes prescribed to treat psoriasis and rheumatoid arthritis. This combination can be fatal.

Hidden Benefits

May offer protection against Alzheimer's disease and colorectal cancer.

Not Recommended For

People with gastrointestinal, liver, or kidney problems or those taking medication for high blood pressure. NSAIDs should not be combined with alcohol, because they can increase stomach bleeding, or with diuretics, because they can cause an increased risk of kidney failure, especially in seniors.

Special Hints

Take with a full 8-ounce glass of water. To avoid irritation after swallowing, remain upright for 15 to 30 minutes after taking it.

DRUG PROFILES

▼ Salicylates

What Are They?

These prescription and nonprescription drugs relieve swelling, stiffness, and joint pain by halting the production and release of prostaglandins, hormonelike substances that lead to swelling and help transmit pain to the brain. They work best to ease symptoms of both types of arthritis, headaches, muscle aches, and dental pain.

Active Ingredients (Common Brands)— Prescription

Salsalate (Disalcid) and choline and magnesium salicylates (Trilisate)

Active Ingredient (Common Brands)— Nonprescription

Aspirin (Bayer, Bufferin)

Common Side Effects

Abdominal cramps, pain, or discomfort; indigestion; heartburn; nausea; vomiting; and high blood pressure

Safe Use

Call your doctor if you have headaches or a ringing or buzzing in your ears. These may be signs that you're taking too much of this medicine. Do not use it for more than 10 days without consulting your doctor.

Hidden Benefits

Aspirin is approved by the FDA to treat strokes and may prevent future cardiovascular events. It reduces the risk of death from heart attacks, helps prevent second heart attacks, and reduces the risk of heart attack in people with angina. It prevents ischemic strokes, the kind that happen when blood clots clog the arteries that supply blood to the brain. Preliminary evidence suggests aspirin users have fewer lung and breast cancers.

Not Recommended For

People with asthma, high blood pressure, bleeding disorders, severe liver or kidney disease, ulcers, or history of hemorrhagic stroke

Special Hints

Beware of aspirin products that smell like vinegar—they could be breaking down.

DRUG PROFILES

▼ Tramadol

What Is It?

This medication is prescribed to relieve severe pain, particularly after surgery. It works on the brain to decrease pain, and it's best used for moderate to severe pain.

Active Ingredient (Common Brand)

Tramadol (Ultram)

Common Side Effects

Abdominal or stomach pain, anxiety, confusion, nervousness, dizziness, sleep trouble, diarrhea, constipation, nausea, vomiting, excessive gas, dry mouth, skin flushing, headache, heartburn, hot flashes, itching, skin rash, loss of appetite, loss of energy, sleepiness, and sweating

Safe Use

Take this medication precisely as instructed by your physician.

Hidden Benefits

Side effects are less likely than with other drugs.

Not Recommended For

People who are allergic to narcotic medications

Special Hints

Seniors should not take more than 300 milligrams daily.

▼ Tricyclic Antidepressants

What Are They?

Prescribed to relieve depression, these drugs can also alleviate pain, probably by affecting the part of the brain that controls messages between nerve cells. They're most often used for postherpetic pain, diabetic neuralgia, and other conditions resulting in nerve damage.

Active Ingredients (Common Brands)

Amitriptyline (Elavil), imipramine (Tofranil), and doxepin (Sinequan)

Common Side Effects

Dizziness, drowsiness, dry mouth, headache, increased appetite, nausea, tiredness, weakness, unpleasant taste, weight gain, and accentuated memory loss

Safe Use

These medicines may cause sun sensitivity. Stay out of direct sunlight or at least wear protective clothing, sunblock, and sunblock lip balm. Take with food and take only as directed by your doctor.

Hidden Benefit

Improved sleep

Not Recommended For

People who drink excessive amounts of alcohol or those who have glaucoma. If you consume alcoholic beverages, consult your physician before using this drug.

Special Hints

To lessen stomach upset, take this medication with food, even for your bedtime dose.

The Pain-Free Lifestyle

Dust accumulates. Dirty dishes mount. Laundry piles up. Garbage collects. Spills happen.

Life goes on, no matter how much pain you feel. And it's important—make that *vital*—that you make every effort to continue living as full a life as possible.

"Cooking, cleaning, shopping—such everyday activities can help maintain your body and dampen your pain," says Randall Prust, M.D., medical director of both the Center for Pain Management at El Dorado Hospital and the Pain Medicine Center at Tucson General Hospital, both in Tucson, and author of *Conquering Pain*. "We've known that for a long time. Years ago, doctors used to keep patients bed bound after surgery. As a result, they didn't heal as fast, they developed more complications, and experienced more pain. The same thing can happen if you don't stay active in your everyday life."

In fact, the mundane tasks of everyday living can have an extraordinary impact on pain, says Neal Barnard, M.D., president of the Physician's Committee for Responsible Medicine in Washington, D.C., and author of *Foods That Fight Pain*. Just staying active around the house helps your body produce natural painkillers called endorphins that are as potent as morphine without causing any of that drug's nasty side effects. In addition, household chores and other everyday tasks strengthen muscles, ligaments, and tendons surrounding your joints and help make your whole body less susceptible to pain.

People in pain who continue to do everyday tasks also increase blood supply to the areas of their bodies that hurt, Dr.

49

(continued on page 54)

STRETCH YOUR LIMITS

Regular exercise, such as stretching, walking, and strength training, is an important component of the pain-free lifestyle, says Paul Blake, M.D., a pain-management expert and outpatient-services director at Meridian Point Rehabilitation Hospital in Scottsdale, Arizona. Staying in shape helps keep your muscles and joints strong and limber, enhances your ability to do daily tasks, and bolsters your pain tolerance.

"Regular exercise makes you healthier, stronger, and fitter. And an older person who meets that description is going to be able to tolerate pain and its underlying condition much better," Dr. Blake says.

Always stretch before and after doing any strenuous activity including housework, he says. In addition, walk, bike, or swim 20 to 30 minutes a day four or five times a week. Remember, it doesn't have to be done all at once. So you could take a 15-minute walk in the morning and then a 15-minute bike ride or swim in the afternoon.

Don't neglect strength training either. If you don't have any equipment, simply lifting common household objects like food cans or milk jugs is a terrific way to strengthen your body and increase your mobility, Dr. Blake says. For example, start with an object, such as a 12-ounce soup can or an 18-ounce jar of peanut butter, that you can comfortably lift 10 times. Add one lift each time you exercise if you can, until you reach 25. Then, try a slightly higher weight at 10 repetitions and repeat the cycle.

Here are a few specific strengthening exercises for your arms, shoulders, and lower legs. These exercises can be done safely by most people but may have to be modified if you have problems such as some types of arthritis or other medical conditions that affect your muscles, bones, or coordination. You should always consult with your doctor before beginning an exercise program, but Dr. Blake suggests that it is especially important to check with a physician first if you have any of these problems.

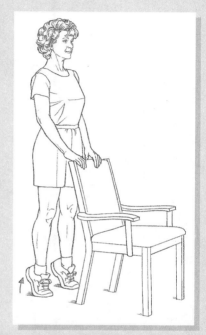

Plantar flexion. Stand straight, with your feet flat on the floor and spaced shoulder-width apart, behind a chair or table, holding on to the edge for balance. Stand as high up on your tiptoes as you can; hold for 1 second, then take 3 seconds to slowly lower yourself back down. Do this exercise 8 to 15 times; rest; then do another set of 8 to 15 repetitions.

As you become stronger, do this exercise first on your right leg only, then on your left leg only, for a total of 8 to 15 repetitions on each leg. Rest, then do another set.

Arm raise. Sit in a chair with your back straight, your feet flat on the floor and spaced shoulder-width apart. In each hand, hold a 12-ounce soup can or a 1- to 2-pound hand weight down at your sides, with your palms facing in. Lift both arms out sideways until they are parallel to the ground. Your hands should be slightly in front of your body, not straight out to the sides. Hold for 1 second. Take 3 seconds to lower your arms. Pause. Repeat 8 to 15 times. Rest; do another set of 8 to 15 repetitions. This exercise can also be done while standing.

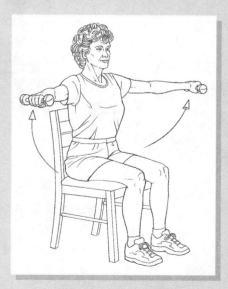

(continued)

STRETCH YOUR LIMITS—CONTINUED

Dip exercise. Sit in a sturdy chair with armrests. Lean slightly forward, keeping your back and shoulders straight. Hold on to the arms of the chair. Your hands should be level with the trunk of your body, or slightly farther forward. Place your feet slightly under the chair, with your heels off the ground and the weight of your feet and legs resting on your toes and the balls of your feet.

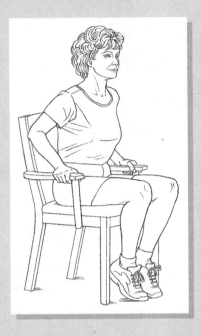

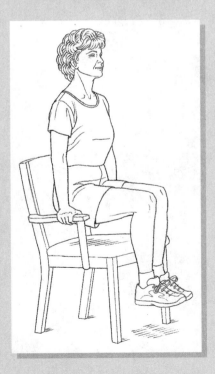

Using your arms, slowly lift yourself up as high as you can, keeping your back straight. Many people won't be able to push themselves up off the chair when they first try it. This pushing motion will work your arm muscles even if you aren't able to lift yourself up off the chair. Don't use your legs or feet for assistance. Slowly lower yourself back down. Repeat 8 to 15 times. Rest; repeat another 8 to 15 times.

Dumbbell row. Stand next to a sturdy chair or weight bench. With your left leg, kneel on one end of the chair, while keeping your right foot flat on the floor. Keep your right knee slightly bent. Support yourself with your left arm. Your back should be slightly arched. Hold a 1- to 2-pound hand weight in your right hand with your arm down at your side, palm facing your body. Take 3 seconds to lift your right hand toward your chest by bending

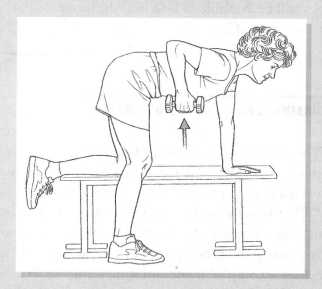

your elbow. Lift it until your elbow is a few inches higher than your back. Hold this position for 1 second. Take 3 seconds to lower your hand to the starting position. Pause, then repeat until you have done the exercise 8 to 15 times. Rest, then do the same on your other side.

Prust says. And more blood means that more oxygen, vitamins, and other vital nutrients will be available to help heal the underlying cause of the pain.

DRAINING PAIN OUT OF YOUR BRAIN

The pain-stopping power of everyday life reverberates in your brain, the organ that actually perceives and reacts to pain.

"What seems mundane and what most of us take for granted—keeping a clean house, doing the grocery shopping—becomes an accomplishment and something to strive for when you are in constant pain. It's part of what keeps you going," Dr. Prust says.

Older people in chronic pain who, with their doctor's approval, find ways to accomplish these routine tasks usually have a better quality of life than those who don't, says Stanley Chapman, Ph.D., a psychologist at the Emory Clinic Center for Pain Management in Atlanta. They develop a hardy I-can-do-it attitude that motivates them to do more. The more you accomplish despite discomfort, the more tasks you'll be willing to tackle. The more tasks you tackle successfully, the better your self-esteem. Better self-esteem means less de-

pression and a better quality of life, despite the presence of pain.

BREAKING DOWN THE BARRIERS

Certainly, there are limits. Even light dusting can be a challenge when you are in pain, and there are going to be days when you hurt so much that you won't feel up to doing these everyday tasks. That's fine. The important thing is to do as much as you can as often as you can.

"Nothing is perfect," Dr. Barnard says. "But we all can try to do our best. You can do things despite the pain."

But because you are in pain, you may have to make a few changes in your household routine—like using lightweight cookware instead of heavy cast-iron skillets in the kitchen—in order to get these tasks done. And that's okay, too, says Jan I. Maby, D.O., medical director of the Cobble Hill Health Center in Brooklyn, New York.

"It's all well and good to talk about how you used to do five loads of wash on laundry day. It's quite another thing to expect yourself to continue doing it when you are in pain," Dr. Maby says. "You need to have realistic expectations for yourself. If you enjoy cleaning, do a light dusting, but

PACE YOURSELF

As you do daily activities such as washing dishes, vacuuming, or cleaning up the bedroom, take note of how long it takes for your pain to flare up. When it does, stop and do something else, like phoning a friend, reading the newspaper, or paying a few bills, says Margaret A. Caudill, M.D., Ph.D., codirector of the department of pain medicine at the Dartmouth-Hitchcock Medical Center in Manchester, New Hampshire, and author of *Managing Pain Before It Manages You.*

Notice how long it takes for your pain to subside to a point that you feel like going back to your previous chore. If you can fold laundry, for instance, for 10 minutes before your pain stops you, write that down. If you need 15 minutes to recover, jot that down, too.

Once you've established the working and rest periods you need for the majority of your activities, try this: Set a timer and do an activity for only that amount of time. Then reset the timer and do a restful activity until the alarm goes off. Over time, you'll probably find that the amount of time you can do an activity without pain will increase, and the amount of time you need to rest will decrease, Dr. Caudill says.

Researchers suspect that pacing yourself like this helps relieve pain because you're not pushing your mind and body to the point of exhaustion. Pacing yourself also can prevent pain from spreading to other parts of your body.

don't try to move the furniture. Be satisfied that you dusted your home and it looks better. Scrubbing the kitchen floor on your hands and knees isn't necessary. You can mop it and still have a very clean floor. Same thing with washing your hair. You don't necessarily have to do it every day anymore. You might try washing it every other day if the pain outweighs the benefit."

Yet many older Americans resist these changes because they are seen as concessions to age and discomfort. If you're among them, give yourself a break, Dr. Maby says. Stubbornly clinging to habits and routines that aggravate your pain isn't beneficial. If anything, you'll probably stop doing these everyday tasks because it hurts too much. Once that happens, you may tumble into a downward spiral of inactivity that can lead to the loss of your independence.

Think of it this way: Nobody begrudges you because you wear eyeglasses in order to see better. So why should you feel guilty about changing how you do things around your home so that you can live pain-free?

In fact, even subtle adaptations in the bedroom, bathroom, or kitchen, which most family and friends probably won't notice, can make a huge dent in your pain and greatly enhance the quality of your life, Dr. Prust says.

One of Dr. Prust's patients has severe pain in her arms. "But every day she gets up, she washes her hair, and she puts on her makeup," he says. "It's almost second nature for her to do it the way she is doing it now. She has learned to adapt so that she can continue doing *all* of her normal everyday activities."

Your doctor or an occupational therapist can suggest adaptations that are best suited to your individual needs. But here is a room-by-room compendium of ideas to help you get started.

IN THE BEDROOM

Smooth out the wrinkles. To make it easier to make your bed, before you get out of bed, use your feet to smooth the sheets at the bottom of the mattress, suggests Shelia Goodwin, P.T., a physical therapist and clinical director of the Workplace, a rehabilitation center in Birmingham, Alabama. For better accessibility, keep your bed away from walls. Nylon tricot sheets are lightweight, stretch without tugging, and can be put on with one hand. Use a wooden pizza paddle or a large spatula to tuck bedding under the mattress.

If making a bed is too painful, you can forgo sheets and blankets altogether, Goodwin says. Simply curl up in a sleeping

Brainstorm Pain Stoppers

On a sheet of paper, jot down a list of household chores you normally perform in a week. Check off the three activities that cause the most pain, says Jan I. Maby, D.O., medical director of the Cobble Hill Health Center in Brooklyn, New York. Then take a few minutes to concentrate on the most painful of these three tasks. List any ideas—no matter how offbeat—that you might have for minimizing the pain when doing this chore.

If doing the laundry is a problem, for instance, you might do smaller loads or break the job up so you do it several times a week instead of all at once. If you feel stumped, ask friends and family for advice.

Pick one of these ideas that you think will work, and give it a try. If it doesn't help, try another approach. Keep trying new ideas until you hit upon one that works, Dr. Maby suggests. Do this for all three tasks. Then pick another three painful chores to conquer.

bag on top of the mattress. In the morning, just fold the bag over and stuff it into a closet.

Easy on, easy off. Elastic waistbands eliminate the need for belts and can make pants easier to slip on and off, says Denyse Hernaez, O.T., an occupational therapist at the Hospital for Special Surgery in New York City. Instead of slipping a T-shirt over your head, cut open one side, including the sleeve, and attach Velcro so you can slide the shirt sideways and then fasten it shut. Velcro can be found at most sewing stores. When purchasing clothing, particularly pullover sweaters, consider getting them a size or two too large. It will help make dressing easier.

Reach for a stick. If bending is painful, a dressing stick or a reacher can help you pull up pants, put on pullover shirts, or retrieve hard-to-reach clothes, says Debbie Nakayama, a certified occupational therapist assistant at Christ Hospital and Medical Center in Oak Lawn, Illinois. Dressing sticks and reachers are available in most medical supply stores and rehabilitation/adaptive-equipment catalogs.

Beat the buttons. If you have difficulty using buttons, have someone sew Velcro on clothing. For appearance's sake, you can permanently attach buttons to the top side of the hole while still using Velcro as the actual fastener underneath, Hernaez says. You also can hook large paper clips over buttons to ease their insertion through button holes.

Sock it to 'em. If you have difficulty putting on your socks, consider buying a sock aid, Nakayama suggests. To use it, slide your sock onto the sock aid form. Then, firmly grasp the ends of the cord and allow the toes of the sock to drop to the floor. Slide your foot onto the shell and pull the sock gently on with the cord. Then remove the aid. Sock aids are also available in many medical supply stores and rehabilitation/adaptive-equipment catalogs.

Horn in. A long-handled shoehorn can help maneuver your feet into your shoes, Hernaez says. Soft cushion inserts or gel soles can prevent aching feet and lessen the strain on your legs and back.

When buying shoes, look for a pair that has Velcro closures, a toe area wide enough to prevent rubbing or crunching of your toes, and heels no more than 1 inch high.

Simplify the essentials. For women, if a girdle is necessary, look for one that has a zipper or other features that allow you to put it on with one hand, recommends Goodwin. If your fingers hurt, wear knee-high stockings. Panty hose require more finger strength and dexterity to put on.

For men, clip-on ties can eradicate painful struggles with the Windsor knot, she says.

IN THE BATHROOM

Take a seat. Sitting is preferable to standing in the bathroom, Hernaez says, because it is less tiring and usually less painful. So sit in a chair when brushing your teeth, shaving, or putting on makeup. In the tub, use a bath board or a waterproof lawn chair. When you clean the toilet or bathtub, sit on a stool and use a long-handled scrub brush.

SPREAD OUT THE LOAD

Use larger joints to prevent strain and pain in your smaller ones, urges Denyse Hernaez, O.T., an occupational therapist at the Hospital for Special Surgery in New York City. Use the palm of your hand, for instance, instead of a fingertip to push down on spray cans. Close lids with your palm as well. To wring out a wet towel or washcloth, drape the item over a faucet and squeeze out the excess water between the palms of your hands.

Work up a lather. A shower caddy within easy reach will cut down on the need to bend, twist, or stoop in the shower, Nakayama says. Store liquid soap, shampoo, and conditioner in pump dispensers rather than squeeze bottles. If you insist on using bar soap, consider soap on a rope.

Wring yourself out. After bathing, wrap yourself in a terry cloth robe and allow it to soak up the water as you pat yourself dry, Nakayama suggests. This one-step technique is less painful for many older people than the awkward contortions of towel drying.

Crank up the commode. The toilet often is the lowest seat in the house. Sitting down and getting up from such a low point can be tricky as you age, especially if you are in pain. A raised toilet seat with armrests, available at most medical supply stores, can make getting up and down off the commode a much easier task, Nakayama says.

Get a grip. Apply cylindrical foam tubing, available at most medical supply stores and rehabilitation/adaptive-equipment catalogs, to combs, toothbrushes, and other bathroom essentials. The foam tubing will increase the size of the handles and make them easier to grasp. Foam tubing also can be used on kitchen utensils, Nakayama says. As for makeup, put tubing onto eye-liner and mascara handles for a better grip.

IN THE KITCHEN

Conquer chaos. An efficient kitchen is a pain-free kitchen, Goodwin says. So store equipment and supplies that you regularly use between eye and hip level. It will minimize bending, stooping, reaching, and other painful movements. Stash bread, cereal boxes, and other dry breakfast foods on a counter near the toaster and refrigerator. Hang a pegboard near your stove for cooking utensils like skillets and spatulas. Cluster dry goods, mixing bowls, and measuring tools in one spot. Plan storage so that one item can be removed without lifting or sifting through others. Store canned goods, for instance, so that the same items are lined up behind one another.

Get a go-cart. A rolling utility cart is a vital kitchen tool if you have chronic pain, Goodwin says. All the essentials for a meal can be loaded onto the cart and wheeled to the dining table, eliminating several trips to the kitchen. After a meal, dishes can be collected from the table in one trip.

Crack it open. Install a jar opener that will grip lids so that you can use both hands to turn jars, Nakayama suggests. Like many items, jar openers are available at most specialty housewares stores.

To open frozen foods and other bagged items, place the bag on its side and use a sharp serrated knife to open the end, Goodwin suggests. Instead of using your thumbs to open milk cartons, use the heels of your hands to push back the flanges of the spout, then use a knife to pull the spout out. Open flip-top cans with a butter knife.

Seal it shut. Many foods such as cheese are sold in resealable packages these days. But these packages can be torturous to close if your hands ache. If you have this problem, remove the food from its original container and store it in a way that is more convenient for you, Nakayama says. You could, for instance, simply store the cheese in a plastic sandwich bag, fold the top of the bag over, and seal it with a clothespin.

Slice chopping pain. A food processor or onion chopper can streamline slicing and dicing foods, Hernaez says. Instead of a knife, try using a pizza wheel to cut various foods. If you must use a knife, consider getting one with an angled handle. It will put less strain on your wrist and fingers. These specialized knives are available at most housewares stores.

Spray and slide. If you use cooking pots, place the pot on the counter next to the sink, then use a spray attachment to fill the pot. Then, slide the pot along the counter to the stove or slip it into a cart and wheel it over. This way, you'll avoid lifting heavy pots, Goodwin says. Once the water is heated, place the food you want to cook into a frying basket and lower it into the pot. When the food is done, simply lift the frying basket out and let it drip-drain over the pot. After the pot has cooled, you can slide it back to the sink and drain it.

Maximize frugality. One-pot meals require less cleanup and can be served in the same containers in which they were cooked, Nakayama says. Serve foods on paper plates and line pans with aluminum foil to cut down on dishwashing.

Mop, but don't drop. Long-handled brooms, mops, and dustpans take the strain off your back and knees, Nakayama says.

IN THE REST OF THE HOUSE

Shrink your laundry loads. Line your hamper with a small plastic grocery bag, Goodwin suggests. When it is full, simply remove the bag by the handles and carry it to the washing machine. The bag will remind you to do smaller, lighter loads of laundry. Avoid overloading the bag.

Douse the dust. Keep your fingers flat and extended while dusting, Goodwin says. Use both arms to distribute the workload. A dusting mitt is worth the investment.

Can the canister. Upright vacuum cleaners require less physical energy than canister or tank models, Goodwin says. If you must use a canister vacuum, try nudging it around the room with your feet rather than pulling it with your arms. It's less stressful on your joints and muscles.

Bottle the nozzle. Aerosol spray nozzles can be difficult to use if you're in pain. Look for cleaners in easy-to-use containers or invest in an adaptor, Goodwin says. Adaptors replace the spray buttons with easier-to-use pump handles that can be switched from one can to another. Spray-can adaptors are available at many housewares stores.

Take up a collection. As you clean, place items that belong elsewhere in a basket. Then when you're done cleaning each room, carry the basket with you and drop the items in their appropriate places as you go about your chores, Hernaez suggests. It will help clean more efficiently and conserve energy.

To order self-help aids through the mail, write to the Rehabilitation Division of Smith and Nephew at 1 Quality Drive, Germantown, WI 53022-4422 and ask for their free consumer-products catalog. Or write to the Customer Service Department of Sammons Preston at P.O. Box 5071, Bolingbrook, IL 60440-5071 and ask for their enrichments catalog.

PART TWO

▶ Pain Takers

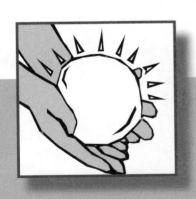

Finding Natural Relief

Most people coping with pain eventually learn the limitations of traditional medicine. If you're taking medications, you may discover that some have unpleasant side effects or simply don't work as well after a time. Arthritis medications, for example, can eat away at the lining of your stomach. Some headache medications actually cause rebound headaches. Other pain-relieving drugs make you so "out of it" that you need to take some additional drug simply to stay awake. That's not exactly the kind of life most of us want.

If you've had surgery for a pain problem, you may find that it, too, offers only limited help or, sometimes, no help at all. Surgical nerve blocks, for instance, once popular for a variety of painful, hard-to-treat conditions usually caused by damaged nerves, are now seldom used. They rarely work, or they cause other health problems just as bad as the ones they're meant to solve—numbness, sweating, even incontinence or impotence.

If you're feeling depressed or anxious because of pain, you may get help from drugs and psychological counseling. But you may still be grappling with how to regain the fullness of your life, to gain and grow from your experience.

So there are lots of reasons people become disillusioned with traditional medicine and what it has to offer someone in chronic pain. They want more, and many of them find it in complementary medicine—the kind of "alternative" medicine that adds multiple dimensions to traditional care.

"Surveys show that many people who seek out alternative medicine do so because they are in pain and are not getting relief from their problems," says Brian Berman, M.D., director of the Center for Complementary Medicine at the University of Maryland School of Medicine in Baltimore. "Traditional medicine tends to focus on pain only as a physical problem, and we know that pain, especially chronic pain, is a multidimensional problem, with physical, emotional, mental, and, some would say, spiritual aspects." People who receive only a drug or a nerve block, he says, "aren't getting all the answers they are seeking, and that's why a lot of them turn to complementary medicine. It does take a whole-person approach—physical, emotional, spiritual."

Even among doctors, there's a growing sense that drugs and surgery often aren't the answer. "Many of us believe that lingering or chronic pain actually is better treated with nondrug approaches: exercise, physical therapy, cognitive and behavioral therapies, lifestyle changes that improve emotional well-being and overall health," Dr. Berman says.

No one therapy is likely to be the sole solution to your pain, but any can be an important part of the whole, he says. Look to see what combination of therapies works best for you. Your program might include elements from a long list, including but not limited to chiropractic care, yoga, massage, prayer, aromatherapy, music therapy, hypnosis, and acupuncture.

If you're lucky enough to have a doctor who knows both traditional and complementary medicine, ask your doctor for advice as you delve into the world of alternatives available to you, Dr. Berman suggests. You can also do some of your own research to see what alternative treatments appeal most to you and have been proven helpful for your condition.

Reading all of the chapters in this section will also give you a feel for which complementary therapies are most helpful for certain conditions, which have scientific studies to back up their claims, and which may be helpful but have yet to be fully evaluated.

Consider your pain both a crisis and an opportunity, Dr. Berman suggests. By necessity, your pain may become an opportunity for you to really start taking care of yourself. And alternative medicine can offer you the tools to do that. "Realistically, you can hope that it will improve the quality of your life, your ability to cope with your problem, as well as give you confidence that you can make certain changes in your life, change certain behaviors so that you can be more active with less pain," Dr. Berman says. "There is research to back that up. It is possible."

Acupressure

This relaxing, pain-relieving technique is sometimes called acupuncture without needles. It involves applying pressure to about 360 points throughout the body. According to oriental medicine, the points are located along meridians, or channels of energy, called *qi* (pronounced "chee"). An acupressurist will select certain points, based on your symptoms, and press the points with his fingertips.

"The acupressurist's job is to assess the points and decide which ones to work on, both by judging tenderness and tension at the point and by what's going on in a person's body," says Joseph Carter, L.Ac., a licensed acupuncturist and acupressurist, and an instructor at the Acupressure Institute in Berkeley, California.

Acupressure might be used instead of acupuncture for conditions that don't require as direct and invasive an approach, such as muscle aches, tension headaches, or stiff arthritic joints. But acupressure's real utility and advantage over acupuncture is that it's something most people can do on themselves anytime they need pain relief. "It literally is pain control at your fingertips," Carter says. And if you have trouble using your hands, there are even knobby wooden tools, often sold as massagers, that you can use to apply pressure.

How Does It Ease Pain?

Eastern medical philosophy takes the position that pain is a result of blocked energy flow, and that acupressure, like

67

ORIENTAL "GATEWAYS" TO PAIN RELIEF

You can stimulate body-wide pain relief using potent acupressure points on your hands and feet, says Kathy Moring, a certified oriental bodywork instructor and an instructor at the Acupressure Institute in Berkeley, California.

In the webbing between your thumb and index finger on each hand is a spot called Large Intestine 4 (LI4). Squeeze the webbing, angling the pressure toward the bone that connects your thumb with your index finger. Take long, slow, deep breaths as you continue to press this spot for 30 seconds. Then do your other hand.

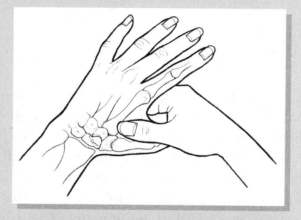

An equivalent spot on each of your feet, Liver 3 (LIV3), is found between the bones that connect your big toe and second toe. Press this point with your finger or thumb, or use the heel of your other foot to press and rub the spot for 30 seconds.

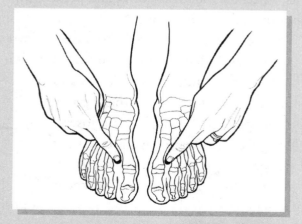

acupuncture, helps to unblock the energy, restoring energy flow. In doing so, the pain associated with the blockage is relieved.

From a Western scientific and medical point of view, several theories have been proposed to explain how acupressure relieves pain and induces relaxation. One theory holds that when pressure is applied to specific points, a countersensation diverts the brain's attention away from the pain or discomfort. Another theory is that acupressure triggers the brain to release endorphins, natural chemicals that reduce perception of pain. Indeed, researchers in China found elevated levels of endorphins in people who had received acupressure.

Acupressure doesn't just help kill pain, it may also speed healing. Researchers at the University of Virginia in Charlottesville found that women who received a combination of massage and acupressure after surgery had lowered levels of the stress hormone cortisol 5 days after the surgery, compared with women who did not receive the treatment.

"Although elevated stress hormone levels are initially helpful in recovering from the trauma of surgery, long-term elevation is detrimental to healing because it depresses the immune system and slows the formation of collagen, a connective tissue used in wound healing," explains Martha Menard, Ph.D., the study's main author and a massage therapist in Charlottesville.

Like massage, acupressure also helps to improve circulation and the flow of lymph throughout the body, says Kathy Moring, a certified oriental bodywork therapist and an instructor at the Acupressure Institute. And it can often be used in situations where massage might not be appropriate, such as when you have an acute injury or severe swelling. While it's not used directly on the site, acupressure can be used to get blood flowing through the injured area again, reducing swelling and promoting healing, Moring adds.

In addition to physical benefits, acupressure has psychological benefits, Moring says. "People tense themselves up and breathe very shallowly when they are in pain, and acupressure relaxes them," she says.

HOW IS IT DONE?

An acupressure practitioner is often also a massage therapist (sometimes one who specializes in shiatsu, a form of Japanese massage) or even an acupuncturist. Acupressure is often done as part of a massage session. You undress, or at least partly undress, and are provided with a sheet, towel, or gown. You lie on a comfortable, padded massage table, and only the part of your body being worked on is uncovered.

During a session, the acupressurist may assess your body with his fingers, feeling for points that need stimulation, and then "working," or applying pressure to, those points. "The trick is to be able to figure out what that point needs," Carter says. "If it is tender, it may not need all that much pressure. As you press, you can feel the muscle underneath relax and the area get warm as circulation improves." Those are signs of improved energy flow. "Sometimes, the action is as simple as pressing and gently holding the point; sometimes, it involves pressing and rubbing with more vigor," he says.

The acupressurist may press with his fingers or the edge or the heel of his hand, but he might also rock an elbow back and forth over a pressure point, push with a knee, or gently drum on a point. There's even a style called barefoot shiatsu, where you lie on a mat on the floor while massage therapist works on you with his feet or knees. "Full weight is seldom used, but this might be used for very tight muscles on the backs of the thighs," Carter says. "Standing on one foot and using the heel of the other foot to loosen up those muscles can be more effective than using your hands alone to work the area."

As for how long the pressure is applied, "often, the practitioner coordinates the movement with the person's breathing, stimulating each point in the time it takes the person to complete one full breath," Carter says.

WHAT DOES IT FEEL LIKE?

Since it often stimulates tender points or knotty muscles, acupressure may hurt somewhat at first, but then pain gently eases off as the muscles relax. "But it should 'hurt good'—kind of like the discomfort you might feel with massage or stretching," Carter says. "It should not be painful." Your practitioner should ask you, "How is that pressure?" And after about 30 seconds to a minute at any point, any amount of pressure should feel good as the muscle relaxes and the *qi* flows.

WHAT RESULTS CAN YOU EXPECT?

Acupressure can completely relieve pain in some cases. People in severe pain can use it in addition to other methods of pain control, Moring says. "I've worked with people who have bone cancer and are taking morphine, and it's helpful because it's something people can do for themselves to get some instant additional relief when they need it. It gives them some sense of control."

How often you need acupressure depends on your symptoms, Moring says. "For headaches, it can be used every day. For chronic pain conditions, pain relief may not last long at first, but it lasts longer and longer as treatment is continued."

Who's Qualified to Do It?

The Acupressure Institute trains and certifies practitioners and can refer you to a practitioner in your area. Contact the institute at 1533 Shattuck Avenue, Berkeley, CA 94709-1516. Look for credentials such as licensed acupuncturist (L.Ac.), licensed massage therapist (L.M.T.), and membership in the American Oriental Bodywork Therapy Association (AOBTA).

What Does It Cost?

Treatments generally range between $35 and $80 and last for 30 to 90 minutes. Some medical insurance does not pay for acupressure treatments, but larger insurance carriers cover it or are considering covering it in the near future.

Acupuncture

The word *acupuncture* comes from two Latin words: *acus*, which means needle, and *punctura*, which means pricking. The treatment itself, however, originated as an ancient Chinese method of healing and pain relief that involves the insertion of very thin needles into specific parts of the body called acupuncture points.

HOW DOES IT EASE PAIN?

In traditional Chinese medicine, it's believed that pain or illness comes from a blockage or imbalance of the body's vital energy flow, called *qi* (pronounced "chee"). Acupuncture works to unblock the energy flow or correct an imbalance, thus relieving pain and illness. *Qi* is thought to flow along pathways called meridians, and acupuncture points are found along these meridians.

There is no Western or known scientific basis for *qi* or meridians, but there's evidence to show that using acupuncture along those meridians really works, says Gary Kaplan, D.O., medical director of the Kaplan Clinic, a comprehensive chronic pain center in Arlington, Virginia, and director of the Medical Acupuncture Research Foundation in Los Angeles.

"Research shows that acupuncture stimulates the release of endorphins, your body's natural pain relievers," he says. "And other research indicates that acupuncture primes your nervous system to keep releasing these pain-blocking endorphins, even when you aren't receiving acupuncture treatments." Research has also documented changes in other hormones and brain chemicals, such as serotonin, which may affect your perception of pain.

Acupuncture apparently even changes the pattern of bloodflow in your body. "It can increase the amount of blood flowing to an area where there is muscle spasm and pain. This will help reduce the spasm of the muscles in that area and, in turn, reduce the pain," Dr. Kaplan explains.

Additionally, researchers at the Hospital of the University of Pennsylvania in Philadelphia found that acupuncture affects areas of the brain that are associated with controlling and relieving pain.

Acupuncture tends to work best on the kinds of aches and pains that are also eased by standard Western treatments such as anti-inflammatory medicines, ice, rest, and physical therapy, Dr. Kaplan says. These include dental pain, migraine and tension headaches, osteoarthritis, back pain, muscle overuse or injury, tendinitis, bursitis, and wrist, ankle, and foot problems. Problems normally treated with antispasmodic drugs, such as facial pain, neuralgia, muscle spasms, and irritable bowel syndrome, also respond well to acupuncture, as does phantom limb pain (which can occur after amputation) or pain that sticks around long after an injury has healed. Studies also demonstrate that acupuncture is effective for nausea associated with chemotherapy or anesthesia.

HOW IS IT DONE?

You lie on a padded examination table, faceup or -down, depending on the sites selected for needles. Or you may sit in a recliner. You may need only to loosen your clothes, or you may need to undress and get into a gown or robe.

Your body has about 360 traditional or classically defined acupuncture points and more than 2,000 nontraditional acupuncture points that clinicians have worked with successfully over the years. The points your doctor or licensed acupuncturist selects are based on the type of acupuncture he uses and the symptoms you have. He may use as few as 2 needles, but seldom more than 30. To reduce the risk of transmitting infection from one patient to another, only disposable needles should be used. If he doesn't use them, look for someone who does.

The needles are very thin, ranging from 0.03 to 0.1 millimeter, barely more than the diameter of a hair. Most of the needles used are ½ to 1½ inches long and may be inserted from ⅛ inch or less up to 1 inch or more.

"How far in depends on where you are placing the needles and the effect you want," says Stephen M. Taylor, D.O., director of the Forest Park Institute in Fort Worth, Texas. "If you are inserting the needle in a finger, you'll put it in only a millimeter or two. If it's going into a spot where there's plenty of padding, such as the buttocks, you'll put it in up to an inch or so." Dr. Taylor sometimes even uses a 4-inch needle that is inserted at a very shallow angle just under the skin in the hip near the sciatic nerve. Because the needles are so thin, most people feel little, if any, pain. "They are not uncomfortable at all," he says.

After the needle is in place, it may be twisted or infused with electrical current. Some doctors use a process called moxibustion, holding a smoldering cylinder of a pungent herb, mugwort, near a needle to heat it up. The needles are left in place 15 to 30 minutes while you relax in a quiet, warm room.

What Does It Feel Like?

While there might be some initial sting or zing to the process, once the needle is in, it should not hurt. "If it does hurt, the needle is misplaced and needs to be removed and replaced," Dr. Kaplan says. Some people describe an initial discomfort and then a heaviness or pressure from the needles; others feel al-most nothing. If electrical stimulation is used, you'll feel a tingling or tapping sensation. With moxibustion, the area will feel warm. During the treatment, you should feel a reduction in your pain and feel mostly relaxed, with a sense of well-being.

Afterward, you should continue to feel relaxed and in less pain, although how long you'll feel that way varies from person to person. "The effect may last only a couple of hours or days initially, but as treatments continue, the effect lasts longer and longer," Dr. Kaplan says. People seeking relief from chronic pain may come in once or twice a week to begin, but ultimately, the goal is a pain-free life with no need for continued treatment.

"We tell people we can't cure them, but we can reduce the pain cycle so it doesn't continue to escalate," Dr. Taylor says. "We can reduce its intensity, get it under control so that it recedes into the background of your life again."

What Results Can You Expect?

Of course, not everyone is helped by acupuncture, and it's not clear why some people respond and others don't, Dr. Kaplan says. If a person hasn't gotten relief after 10 sessions, the therapy isn't working and should be stopped, according to a National Institutes of Health consensus panel.

WHO'S QUALIFIED TO DO IT?

The amount of training required to be licensed as an acupuncturist varies. Those with the most extensive training generally have graduated from one of the country's 37 colleges of acupuncture. Medical doctors (M.D.'s) and doctors of osteopathy (D.O.'s) in the United States can be licensed as acupuncturists in most states with 200 hours of training. (New York and New Jersey currently require 300 hours, and some states ask for additional licensure requirements.) Non-M.D. practitioners certified by the National Certification Commission for Acupuncture and Oriental Medicine have had at least 3 years of training and have passed a test. The American Academy of Medical Acupuncturists is a good source for locating one of the more than 1,500 medical acupuncturists throughout the United States and Canada. Write to them at 5820 Wilshire Boulevard, Suite 500, Los Angeles, CA 90036-4500 to request the name of a medical acupuncturist near you.

WHAT DOES IT COST?

Treatments generally range between $35 and $80 and last for about an hour. Medical insurance generally does not pay for acupuncture treatments.

Aromatheromy

Aromatherapy is the use of oils made from plants such as rose or lavender to help you feel relaxed, calm, or revived, and to help relieve pain, congestion, depression, stiff joints, and sore muscles. These oils, known as essential oils, are extremely concentrated and very fragrant—that's where the "aroma" part of the therapy comes in, and that's what makes aromatherapy so enjoyable.

"I think that of all the therapies in complementary medicine, this is without a doubt the most pleasurable, not just to receive but to give," says Jane Buckle, R.N., an instructor in the holistic nursing program at College of New Rochelle in New York; senior lecturer at Oxford Brookes University in Oxford, England; and author of *Clinical Aromatherapy in Nursing*.

Essential oils are distilled from blossoms, leaves, or roots. They can be diffused into the air and inhaled, mixed with water and used as compresses on the skin, added to bathwater, or diluted with another oil and massaged into the skin. Most essential oils are toxic and should never be taken internally.

HOW DOES IT EASE PAIN?

Aromatherapists believe that the fragrance of oils has a soothing effect on your brain's limbic system, the area involved in memory, emotions, and hormone control. "Pain is closely linked to feelings. Feelings such as anxiety and despair are known to heighten pain, and pleasure and relaxation appear to decrease pain," Buckle says.

"Aromatherapy enables people to get in touch with feelings of relaxation and pleasure through smell and touch. Feeling more relaxed and peaceful helps people to let go of their pain as much as possible."

Some research supports aromatherapy's potential, at least when it comes to attitude adjustments. Doctors at the Memorial Sloan-Kettering Cancer Center in New York City, for instance, found that people who inhaled intermittent puffs of the vanilla-like aroma of heliotrope had significantly less anxiety while undergoing magnetic resonance imaging scans than people not exposed to the fragrance.

In another study, researchers at Duke University in Durham, North Carolina, found that women exposed to pleasant smells (in this case, mint, orange, almond, or chocolate) showed improvements in mood even if they didn't particularly like the scents.

Some essential oils may also help ease pain if they are applied to the skin. Lemongrass, for instance, is thought to have an analgesic effect similar to opium-derived drugs. "The active ingredient causing the analgesic effect, myrcene, is also found in rosemary, frankincense, juniper, rose, ginger, and verbena, all of which have been used traditionally for their analgesic qualities," Buckle says.

And some oils simply work by reducing whatever symptoms are causing your pain. If your head hurts because your sinuses are clogged up, sniffing vapors from eucalyptus oil will help relieve the congestion. Or if your belly aches because of nausea and vomiting, inhaling the scent of ginger or peppermint may help.

How Is It Done?

The simplest way to do aromatherapy is to put a few drops of undiluted essential oil on a cotton ball, tissue, or handkerchief and hold it under your nose for about 5 minutes. "I've done this with people who've had extreme nausea from chemotherapy or surgery, using peppermint or ginger, and it works nicely," Buckle says. Inhaling fumes from an essential oil may also be the best route for colds and sinus headaches.

If you're looking for a more subtle ambience—say, you're trying to make a sickroom less oppressive—you can use a diffuser, which uses heat to evaporate the oil so that it diffuses into the air. There are many types of diffusers. Some use candles as a heat source, some use electricity. Some have fans. Some are part of a humidifying system, which can provide added comfort to someone who's sick. You can find diffusers at health food stores and wherever aromatherapy oils are sold. They range in price from $15 to $50.

"The candle diffusers are very nice and add another element of pleasure, but the safest ones are electric," Buckle says. Citrus oils—tangerine, orange, grapefruit—are useful for lifting depression, while sweet marjoram, lavender, or neroli (orange blossom) are calming.

You can also mix essential oils with a base oil such as almond, apricot kernel, or grapeseed oil and rub it into your skin as part of a gentle, soothing massage. This way, you get the benefits of both the fragrance and absorption. Simply mix 1 to 5 drops of essential oil to 1 teaspoon of the base oil, and you have an aromatic massage oil.

Caution: Essential oils *must* be mixed with a base oil; applying them full-strength to the skin without first diluting them will cause burning and irritation.

Base oils are available at health food stores and wherever essential oils are sold.

"The analgesic aspects of essential oils come to the front when they are applied topically," Buckle says. You may want to try this approach for arthritis or back, neck, or knee pain. Try using rosemary, ginger, or black pepper.

The oils can be mixed with water and used as compresses on your skin. To make a compress, add 5 drops of oil to 1 table-spoon of whole milk, which allows oil and water to mix, Buckle explains. Then add the oil-milk mixture to a bowl containing 1 cup of hot water. Put a washcloth in the bowl to absorb the water, wring it out, and place it where you hurt, she adds. Wrap or cover the cloth with plastic wrap, then a towel, and finally, place a heating pad set on low or a hot-water bottle on top. Settle back and relax for 10 to 15 minutes.

For full-body pain relief, draw a comfortably hot bath and add the oil-milk mixture to the water. For osteoarthritis, for example, add 2 drops each of rosemary, lavender, and eucalyptus to 1 tablespoon of whole milk and put that in the water, Buckle says. "This way, you are breathing in the volatile oil as it vaporizes with the steam of the bath, but also it is being absorbed topically." Relax in the bath for 20 minutes. If you can't manage a full bath, try soaking your feet or hands.

WHAT DOES IT FEEL LIKE?

Think of aromatherapy as a pleasurable addition to your pain-relieving regimen. It's not necessarily a replacement for pills, exercise, ice packs, or whatever it is you use to stay comfortable.

"It's not going to replace morphine, but it may lift your mood enough so that your pain drugs work better or you need less of a painkilling drug," Buckle says. This is because certain essential oils may enhance the effectiveness of barbiturates and opiates, she explains. You may start to feel better almost instantly and may continue to feel better for a few hours afterward.

What Results Can You Expect?

Don't underestimate the pain-relieving potential of a pleasurable, caring treatment, says Buckle. "I was carrying out some research in an intensive-care unit, looking at two different types of lavender, and I asked one man I had treated if he wanted to add any comments to the study. He said, 'You are the first person here who didn't hurt me.'"

"People in pain often undergo painful, invasive, and embarrassing procedures," she says. "Being able to actually offer something that is very pleasurable makes you both feel good."

Who's Qualified to Do It?

Anyone can do aromatherapy—practitioners are certified in Europe but not in the United States. But it's best to look for someone who has taken a course at a school such as Bastyr University in Seattle or through a professional organization. To find a qualified practitioner, you can contact the American Society of Aromatherapy, P.O. Box 95, Wallingford, PA 19086-0095; or the National Association for Holistic Aromatherapy, P.O. Box 17622, Boulder, CO 80308-0622. Massage therapists are most likely to incorporate aromatherapy into their practices, but more nurses and other health-care professionals are learning to do it as well.

If you want to try aromatherapy yourself, use a book as a guide and buy a few simple oils for starters, such as lavender, peppermint, ginger, and neroli, or buy scents you like, recommends Buckle.

What Does It Cost?

You can hire a professional aromatherapist for $50 to $100 per session. Medical insurance does not pay for aromatherapy. If you're doing it yourself, your main cost will be the essential oils. It's best to buy the oils directly from a supplier, not a health food store, and to buy them "straight" and dilute them yourself as needed, Buckle says. This way, you're more likely to get fresh, high-potency oils. These oils range in price from $3 or so per ¼ ounce for eucalyptus to $200 plus for rose and jasmine.

Biofeedback

Remember mood rings, with stones that change from black to blue depending on your skin temperature? Well, these bits of kitschy pop culture are a simple form of biofeedback.

"A temperature-sensitive liquid crystal in the ring changes color according to the temperature of your skin," says Steven M. Baskin, Ph.D., director of the New England Institute for Behavioral Medicine in Stamford, Connecticut. "If you're tense, the blood vessels in your hands constrict, making your fingers cool." And if you literally warm up to a person or situation, your hands show it.

The term *biofeedback* was coined in 1969 to describe a technique in which people learned to alter their brain-wave activity, blood pressures, muscle tension, and heart rates—bodily functions that, before that time, doctors didn't think could be consciously controlled.

Some of the first subjects tested in biofeedback experiments included master yogis from India, who claimed to be able to raise their body temperatures or reduce their heart rates. Scientific monitoring confirmed that, indeed, they were capable of these feats.

"But so were regular Midwestern folks in the neighborhood who were also enlisted for these experiments," says Peter Parks, Ph.D., a psychophysiologic therapist at the Menninger Clinic in Topeka, Kansas. "Biofeedback is a learned skill, and most people can learn to develop a substantial degree of control over their bodies."

Most biofeedback uses sensitive instruments that can measure muscle tension, brain-wave activity, exhaled carbon dioxide, skin temperature, or moisture, says

Stu Donaldson, Ph.D., director of Myosymmetries, a private clinic in Calgary, Alberta, Canada. The instruments translate changes in these measurements into understandable signals such as a line graph that moves up or down on a video screen, a beep that increases or decreases in pitch, or a change in color.

"The machines can detect a person's internal bodily functions with far greater sensitivity and precision than most people can do alone and can help them to monitor and control body functions they might not normally be aware of or have under control," Dr. Donaldson says.

HOW DOES IT EASE PAIN?

Biofeedback can help relieve pain by helping people recognize when they are tense and then helping them learn to relax those specific muscles in their bodies, says Dr. Baskin. It also may change brain pain mechanisms.

Some practitioners, such as Dr. Donaldson, use it to help people "rebalance" their muscles after injuries or strokes, to start using muscles they aren't using, which in turn allows overworked, strained muscles to relax. "Learning to use muscles or to relax certain muscles can relieve problems,

such as constipation and urinary incontinence, and can be used to help people relearn to walk after a spinal cord injury or to swallow after a stroke," he says.

Certain forms of biofeedback help people to relax their whole bodies, even to change the way blood flows through their bodies, Dr. Parks says. For instance, hand-warming, a technique in which you send more blood to your hands, literally warming them up, is used as a way to drop blood pressure and help prevent migraine headaches. For some people, hand-warming is a way to induce whole-body relaxation, a technique that helps people learn to reduce anxiety and regulate pain.

"It is a way to consciously calm the sympathetic nervous system, the system that activates when we are fearful," Dr. Parks says. Learning such a technique can help people stay cool, calm, and collected even when their environments seem to be conspiring to get them. "People often make things more uncomfortable for themselves than need be—a result of their mental, emotional, and physical response to a situation," he explains. "You can still be angry about a decision someone has made, for instance, but at the same time, you can notice your automatic response to the situation and learn how to control it. You can choose not to tense up

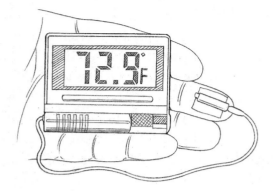

Using a tiny thermometer that measures and displays the temperature of a finger, people can learn to warm up their hands. For many people, hand-warming leads to total-body relaxation and a reduction in the sensation of pain.

your neck muscles so much that you get a headache."

How Is It Done?

The biofeedback practitioner should first explain to you what biofeedback is and the rationale behind it, Dr. Parks says. "I want people to understand that I am not doing something to them. I am teaching them a skill that they can use to modify their responses to stressful situations."

Next, you are attached to the biofeedback

machine, using sensor pads attached to lead wires (a painless process similar to that used if you were getting an electrocardiogram or electroencephalogram). If your muscles are being monitored, the pads are attached over specific muscles. If your hand temperature is being monitored, you will get a heat-sensitive sensor wrapped around your finger. A wire from the sensor goes to a machine that gives a digital temperature readout.

The biofeedback practitioner will first show you what is happening in your body, how your muscles tense and relax, or how your hand temperature may fluctuate with your thoughts and feelings. "You begin to get a sense of what it feels like in your body when it reacts this way," Dr. Parks says.

The next step, an ongoing process for many sessions, is to learn how to make your body react the way you want it to. Your biofeedback practitioner may instruct you in different relaxation and stress-management techniques to get you there, and the coaching aspect of biofeedback is important to the process, Dr. Parks says.

"I would begin to teach them some diaphragmatic breathing skills, and once people are comfortable with that, their hands often start to warm," he says. "Once they know they can have an impact on their hand temperatures by changing their breathing, we might start working on imagery skills, helping them begin to imagine things that are comforting or soothing. This leads to an increase in hand-warming skills." Some people like to experiment with imagining difficult or uncomfortable situations, which might cool their hands down, and then, imagining something that warms them up again. "They see what is involved in changing their physiology and changing their thoughts and feelings. And once that makes sense to them, then we just practice," he adds.

The goal, ultimately, is to be able to relax or contract your muscles, warm your hands, or perform some other feat, without needing the machine to tell you you're doing it right. "People eventually become much more sensitive to what's going on in their bodies and have much more control over their bodies," Dr. Parks says.

What Does It Feel Like?

Biofeedback itself doesn't feel like anything. The monitoring itself has no sensation. What you feel is what you do with your body during biofeedback. So you might feel your neck muscles relax or feel your hands become warmer or feel that you are able to isolate certain areas or functions in your body and control them.

What Results Can You Expect?

A standard treatment schedule is 6 to 10 weekly 1-hour sessions, with daily practice of 20 to 30 minutes. By the end of that time, the majority of people will have learned biofeedback well enough to be able to do it on their own to help control their symptoms, Dr. Parks says.

Results can vary widely, depending on what condition you are treating and your ability to learn the process, experts say. For a few health problems, the results of biofeedback are well-established. For migraine headaches, for instance, "there are numerous studies that establish that a typical person can experience a 40 to 50 percent drop in the frequency of their headaches," Dr. Baskin says. "In general, I'd say that about half the people with chronic pain who use biofeedback will experience significant relief. That is, they'll have at least a 50 percent reduction in their pain and an increase in quality of life, based on pain diaries that they keep."

Who's Qualified to Do It?

There is no licensing requirement for biofeedback practitioners. "Anyone who is trained to can do it," Dr. Baskin says. This includes psychologists, psychiatrists, dentists, nurses, physical and occupational therapists, social workers, educators, and counselors.

You may want to look for a practitioner who is certified by the Biofeedback Certification Institute of America. This organization offers certification based on a number of educational and training requirements. To receive a free list of certified practitioners in your state, send a self-addressed, stamped business-size envelope to the Biofeedback Certification Institute of America at 10200 West 44th Avenue, Suite 310, Wheat Ridge, CO 80033-2840.

It's also a good sign if someone belongs to the Association for Applied Psychophysiology and Biofeedback, a professional organization that provides ongoing education. Ask your doctor or dentist for a referral, or the psychology or psychiatry departments at local universities may be able to help you. To receive information on biofeedback and a free list of certified practitioners in your area, send a self-addressed, stamped envelope to the Association for Applied Psychophysiology and Biofeedback, 10200 West 44th Avenue, Suite 304, Wheat Ridge, CO 80033-2840.

WHAT DOES IT COST?

There is a wide price range, from $60 to $150 per 30- to 60-minute session. Some medical insurance companies will pay for biofeedback sessions if you have a doctor's referral and you have a condition, such as migraine headaches, that is well-established as treatable by biofeedback, Dr. Baskin says.

Breathing

We all know what breathing is, but most of us don't pay much attention to it. As a result, over the years, we tend to breathe more shallowly, using only our upper chests. "Especially when we are in pain, we tend to tense up and breathe quickly and shallowly," says Robert Fried, Ph.D., professor of biopsychology at Hunter College of the City University of New York and director of the Stress and Biofeedback Clinic at the Albert Ellis Institute, both in New York City; and author of *Breathe Well, Be Well.*

There are many different kinds of breathing techniques, often called breath work. But if you are dealing with pain and its accompanying muscle tension and anxiety, the best thing you can do is deep diaphragmatic breathing, Dr. Fried says. In this technique, you relax your abdomen and allow your diaphragm to move freely up and down. You learn how to exhale fully, then breathe in more deeply, lower in your abdomen, contracting your diaphragm downward into your belly and filling your lungs. The result is that you take in more air with each breath.

How Does It Ease Pain?

When you do deep breathing, "the message you are giving your body is that you are breathing like a very relaxed person. And when your body gets that message, it really does relax," says Dr. Fried. Muscle tension is reduced, blood vessels dilate so that blood pressure drops, your heart rate slows, and stress hormone levels drop.

"One of the most significant contributions to pain is muscle tension. So you can see that by relaxing your muscles, you will reduce your pain," he says. "The message gets around."

Deep breathing won't always get rid of pain, but it can make acute episodes more tolerable. It's something to try when your pain is bad and other things aren't helping enough, if your pain is making you anxious and tense, or when pain makes it difficult to sleep or move around, Dr. Fried says.

A particular form of deep breathing, what experts at the International Breath Institute in Boulder, Colorado, call Transformbreathing, may help relieve symptoms of fibromyalgia, premenstrual syndrome, asthma, depression, even nicotine and alcohol addictions.

"Chronic pain has an emotional component or may be the result of injury that someone still has a lot of negative feelings about," says Caron Goode, Ed.D., the institute's codirector. "We believe that you can use your breath to help release emotions associated with your pain, emotions that may be enhancing your perception of the pain."

ing, but the simpler and more natural the technique is, the better, Dr. Fried says.

Breathing is not intended to treat acute pain that may be a signal of a serious medical emergency. Breathing helps most in chronic pain and needs to be practiced regularly so that you can use it when needed.

It is possible to combine deep breathing with imagery or visualization that focuses on "breathing through" a painful area in your body, Dr. Goode says. In this case, you might imagine your breath blowing through your tight muscles, expanding, warming, and softening them. Or you might imagine your pain as clouds of fog, and as you breathe in and out, you let your breath roll the fog away.

Some techniques, such as Goode's Full-Wave Breath and yoga's three-part breath, use belly breathing as the first step in a flowing series of three steps that fill first your belly, then your chest, and then rises to your collarbones.

HOW IS IT DONE?

There are endless variations to get you to the same end point, deeper breath-

WHAT DOES IT FEEL LIKE?

For some people, deep diaphragmatic breathing is instantly pleasant and relaxing, just like a big sigh. "However, it may feel

INS AND OUTS OF PAIN-RELIEVING BREATHING

This exercise helps you learn to breathe more deeply, lower in your lungs. Start out doing one round for 3 to 4 minutes a day. Then add more rounds until you are doing two or three rounds a day.

Sit comfortably in a straight-back chair or lie down on a relatively flat surface. Place your right hand over your belly button and your left hand on your chest, over your sternum. Allow yourself to exhale just a bit longer than usual. Inhale fully. Imagine filling your belly up with air like a balloon, allowing your diaphragm to contract or move downward. Your right hand, on your belly, should move out. Your left hand, on your chest, should move as little as possible. After a brief natural pause, exhale again, extending your exhale a bit longer than usual.

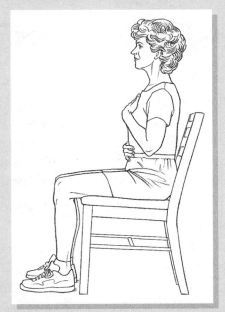

unnatural and difficult to do at first," Dr. Fried says. You may be one of those people who needs to work at it until it becomes relaxing.

Some people find themselves flooded with emotion if they are breathing deeply for the first time in many years, Dr. Goode says. "When you breathe deeply, you might feel like crying or laughing. This is a good thing, and you should just let it happen."

People with emphysema or with serious heart problems or diabetes should not do deep diaphragmatic breathing without expert supervision, Dr. Fried says. People with emphysema may damage their lungs after deep inhalations. People with diabetes or heart or kidney problems may have a metabolic need (acidosis) to breathe faster. Don't do breathing exercises right after surgery.

WHAT RESULTS CAN YOU EXPECT?

You should expect to feel less anxious and more in control of your pain. Deep breathing is appropriate to try before you reach for a pain pill, especially for relatively minor pain. And deep breathing is a tool that helps you feel more open to life and alive, even when you are in pain, Dr. Goode says.

WHO'S QUALIFIED TO DO IT?

Anyone can draw breath, of course, but you can learn more about deep dia-phragmatic breathing from some psychologists, respiratory therapists, and yoga instructors. The International Breath Institute offers training sessions as well and offers training certification to healthcare professionals, called certified breath facilitators. Contact the institute at 2525 Arapahoe Avenue, Suite E4-287, Boulder, CO 80302-6726 for a free list of facilitators and more information on breathing.

WHAT DOES IT COST?

Oxygen is free; so is breathing. But if you want to go beyond the few simple steps here, prices can vary widely, from less than $15 if you take a group yoga class to $80 to $200 if you work with a psychologist to $1,800 if you do a 4-weekend personal-development, professional-certification, and training program with the International Breath Institute.

Chiropractic

Chiropractors have been called the mechanical engineers of medicine. Their focus is the proper alignment of the spine, muscles, joints, and bones in your body. They believe that when these things are all in balance, functioning in proper relationship with each other, your body will be much healthier and more resistant to painful conditions. And if you are ill, with proper alignment, your body's own systems have a better ability to help you maintain optimum health.

Chiropractic care revolves around the spine, neck, head, and pelvis and is distinguished by physical procedures called spinal adjustments, or manipulations. These adjustments may be quick thrusts with the hands, traction, pressure, or gentle stretches that are intended to correct minor misalignments of the spine.

In addition to adjusting the spine, chiropractors may adjust other joints. Some, for instance, specialize in the bones of the skull and may use these techniques to relieve jaw pain, headaches, and sinus problems.

Chiropractors may also offer additional treatments for musculoskeletal disorders, including recommendations for stretching and strengthening exercises, suggestions to improve posture and movement, and lifestyle counseling.

"Every chiropractor tailors his approach to the individual patient because each person, after all, is different," says Jerome McAndrews, D.C., spokesperson for the American Chiropractic Association.

HOW DOES IT EASE PAIN?

The traditional theory is that spinal manipulations correct subluxations, subtle misalignments or locking of the vertebrae in the spine that interfere with proper movement and function of your spine, says Gerard Clum, D.C., president of Life Chiropractic College West in San Lorenzo, California.

"The key to chiropractic is the relationship between structure and function and the neurological consequences of improper spine mechanics," he says. Chiropractors believe—and there's some evidence to support this—that fixing physical misalignments in your body can help restore proper function of your brain, spinal, and nervous system, and that includes the elimination of pain signals that may travel through your nervous system.

The idea makes sense. The ability of nerves to transmit messages through your body can indeed be affected by injuries to your spine, causing nerve and muscle symptoms like shooting pains, numbness, weakness, or paralysis. A misalignment of your sacrum, the triangular-shaped bone at the base of your spine formed by five fused vertebrae, can result in muscle imbalance in your pelvis. This imbalance can cause spasms that alter an opening through which the sciatic nerve, a long nerve running down each of your legs, passes. That

can cause pain or weakness down your leg, Dr. McAndrews says.

No matter what theories lie behind chiropractic, it has been proven to work, at least for some kinds of pain. The largest and most impressive study found that people with chronic lower-back pain who were treated at chiropractic clinics ended up with less pain and more mobility than those treated in hospitals. Chiropractors also point to another big study, which concluded that people with certain types of acute lower-back pain could significantly boost their odds of recovering within 3 weeks by getting chiropractic treatment. Yet another study reported that people with lower-back pain who received chiropractic manipulation had a similar improvement in symptoms at 4 weeks.

Other studies offer support for the use of chiropractic to treat head, neck, and shoulder pain; migraine headaches; carpal tunnel syndrome; menstrual pain; and backache associated with pregnancy.

HOW IS IT DONE?

If it's your first visit to a chiropractor, the practitioner will begin with a case history and physical examination. Then he will likely examine how you stand and move, see whether you can bring your knees up to your chest, touch your toes, twist your torso easily from side to side, and turn your head from side to side. He'll check to see if your legs and arms are the same lengths, if your shoulders or pelvis are tilted, where your posture could stand some improvement. He'll check for muscle weaknesses or imbalances. He'll move your body with his hands, especially around your spine and sacrum.

Many chiropractors do a complete set of x-rays of your spine before doing any adjustments. Additional tests might also be useful to determine whether certain chiropractic techniques should be modified for a particular condition. For example, if you're at risk for osteoporosis, your chiropractor may ask you to have a bone-density test done. People who have lost just a little bone density can still get spinal adjustments, but the adjustments will be less forceful, Dr. Clum says. People with severe osteoporosis, however, should not get some forms of chiropractic adjustments.

For the actual spinal adjustments, you usually lie on a padded adjustable table, facedown, on your side, or face-up, as the doctor works on your back and neck. Some adjustments are done from the front. For one common procedure, you cross your arms in front, and the doctor presses on your arms to create pressure on your back.

The adjustment, often a brief, downward thrust, is very controlled and deliberate, and something chiropractors spend years learning, Dr. Clum says. "Each adjustment is done in a very specific direction with a controlled amount of force and is seeking to correct a specific problem in the spine."

People often hear popping or cracking during an adjustment, but it's not bones popping. It's the sound of tiny gas bubbles exploding as the fluid-filled joint space suddenly expands, much the way a champagne bottle pops when its cork is pulled out.

What Does It Feel Like?

Chiropractors say that a spinal adjustment feels like cracking a knuckle. So you feel some pressure, and then a release and sense of opening that feels good. And the adjustment should not hurt. People whose muscles are very tight may have some brief muscle spasms after an adjustment, but nothing that doesn't usually resolve quickly. A little massage or ice can help in those rare cases where relief is needed.

What Results Can You Expect?

In some cases, especially if you've just recently thrown your back out, you'll get instant relief from a chiropractic adjustment. If it's been a long time since you injured your back, though, it will probably take longer, depending on the age of the injury.

Most treatments do involve a series of visits. A typical range would be between 3 and 15 visits, depending on the severity and length of the problem. In the days following your first adjustment, you should see a reduction in pain, and improved mobility or range of motion. You should also sleep better and feel more comfortable moving around. "If you haven't had improvement in 2 weeks of three to five adjustments a week, your chiropractor will likely make a referral to a chiropractic who specializes in your condition or to a medical physician," Dr. McAndrews says.

WHO'S QUALIFIED TO DO IT?

Chiropractors are licensed in all 50 states and must have graduated from an accredited chiropractic college. Entrance to the 4-year program requires a minimum of 2 years of undergraduate work with emphasis on the sciences.

To find a good chiropractor, you can ask for a referral through your doctor, or you can call your state's chiropractic board of examiners (in the telephone book under state government listings). The board can tell you if the chiropractor you are considering seeing is licensed in your state and is up-to-date with continuing-education requirements, and whether he has a record of disciplinary actions.

WHAT DOES IT COST?

The cost of an initial visit may range from $50 to $100 (diagnostic tests are extra), and subsequent visits, $20 to $50 for a 10- to 25-minute visit. Most major medical insurers (including Medicare) will pay for some chiropractic care, and it is covered in all state workers' compensation acts. Since insurance plans vary, check with your provider to see if your plan offers chiropractic benefits. A doctor's referral may be necessary.

Cold

Cryotherapy is the fancy name for putting a bag of ice on a bee sting, plunging your leg into a whirlpool of cold water, or wrapping an ice pack around a sore joint. Cryotherapy simply means the application of cold to treat an injury or disease.

Numbing pain with ice or cold water undoubtedly goes back to the earliest human beings, who probably didn't understand why an icicle or glacial pool made their smashed toes feel better, only that it did. Medical science and sports medicine, of course, have provided us with a lot more science about cryotherapy. Today, it's commonly used to reduce inflammation, shorten recovery time in acute injuries, and reduce pain after reconstructive joint surgery.

HOW DOES IT EASE PAIN?

Ice is the first therapy for any acute injury: a sprain, bruise, or any type of swelling, such as from an allergic reaction, says Andrew Spitzer, M.D., associate surgeon at the Kerlan-Jobe Orthopaedic Clinic in Los Angeles.

Picture what happens to your ankle after a severe sprain. Blood vessels break, tissues tear, and blood and lymph fluids leak into spaces between cells. Your ankle blows up like a balloon, and the pressure exerts force on nerves and joints. The clinical name for this swelling is edema, and its damaging effects can go on for hours, even days, after the initial injury, says Dr. Spitzer.

By putting ice on your ankle, you reduce bloodflow, hold down swelling, and

93

temporarily numb the injured part. "Probably the most important effect ice has is to constrict those blood vessels and slow down circulation," he says. "By doing so, you immediately begin to limit the damage being done."

"Swelling around the joints can be especially painful," he adds. "Your joints are enclosed spaces, so when they start getting squeezed, it's going to hurt."

Bringing down swelling isn't the only way cold relieves pain. Cold also slows down pain messages running to the brain.

If your pain is more chronic, inflammation may be the culprit. Ice is the quickest way to douse that fire, too. "I tell my patients to use ice as a preventive," says Dr. Spitzer.

Cold also has the capacity to break muscle spasms. Spasms can be especially painful when muscles clamp down on a sensitive nerve, such as the sciatic nerve in your lower back. Cold quickly cools spasming muscles. That loss of mobility is the reason your body feels stiff and clumsy in very cold water.

HOW IS IT DONE?

Many physical therapists and chiropractors use prefabricated cold packs, rubber pouches of a soft gelatin kept in a freezer between applications. In your home, a bag of frozen peas works nearly as well, says Patrick Waters, D.C., a chiropractor at the Waters Chiropractic Clinic in Dallas.

Frozen veggies are cold and easily molded around a knee or elbow. An elastic bandage holds the bag in place. Ice cubes work well if you crush the cubes to decrease the air spaces between the chunks. That way, more cold contacts the hurt, suggests Dr. Waters.

Don't place the cold pack directly on your skin, however. Always create a thin barrier by wrapping a towel around the area to be treated. Typically, an ice pack should stay on for at least 20 minutes and no longer than 45 minutes. Any longer could freeze your skin and cause damage.

"The standard prescription is to give yourself a 60- to 90-minute break before icing again," says Dr. Spitzer.

Ice massage is one way to apply ice directly to your skin. You make an ice stick or ice block by freezing a foam or paper cup full of water and then tearing away the top of the cup to expose the ice. Hold the cup at the bottom and then rub it over your skin, keeping it moving at all times, suggests Dr. Waters. "When first applied, the ice feels cold. This is gradually replaced by a burning sensation, which lasts about 3 minutes. Then there will be an ache for just a short bit before the area goes numb. This whole process will occur within 5 minutes. When either the numbness occurs or the 5 minutes are up, the procedure is stopped," he says.

If it's possible to immerse your painful area, you could also try a mixture of ice and water. As you may imagine, an ice bath can be a little shocking, even painful. Ease yourself into it by immersing for 20 to 30 seconds and then withdrawing, sort of like dipping in a toe before going swimming. Sometimes, it's easier to soak towels in the ice bath and then wrap those around the painful spot. This method of cryotherapy should be used only for the extremities—fingers, toes, feet, hands, ankles, and elbows, says Dr. Waters. "The mixture of ice and water for the bath should be at a temperature between 50° and 60°F. As with ice massage, having direct contact with the ice will decrease treatment time to 5 to 10 minutes," he says.

The advantage of immersing your pain is that there is 100 percent contact between the injured area and the ice, causing a global cooling of the area. It is used for the first 24 to 72 hours (depending on severity) after the injury is incurred, and then heat is introduced," says Dr. Waters.

Heat complements cold therapy nicely, especially in the treatment of strains. It provides a sort of "pumping" effect, explains Dr. Waters. The cold slows everything down and anesthetizes the area as well as decreases circulation to the strain. The heat warms everything back up, loosens some of the stiffness brought on by the cold, and brings fresh blood and nutrients to the area by increasing circulation.

After you've applied ice for 10 minutes, apply a heating pad for 10 minutes. Alternate the ice and heat once more for 10 minutes each, and end with a cold application. You can do this anywhere from once a day to every hour. As long as you feel you are benefiting from it, continue to do it. Instead of using an ice pack and heating pad, you can alternate between a tub of ice and a tub of comfortably hot water. But don't ever use an ice tub with an electric heating pad, cautions Dr. Waters.

WHAT DOES IT FEEL LIKE?

Cold feels, well, cold. At least at first, anyway. But that frigid feeling is soon replaced by a burning sensation that many people find particularly uncomfortable, says Dr. Waters. The burning sensation lasts a short while before becoming a mild aching sensation. Then, the numbness begins.

"A lot of people remove the ice before it gets to the fourth stage, numbness. They put it on for just 5 minutes or so. Then it gets uncomfortable, so they take it off," he explains. "That's just not long enough to get the full beneficial effect."

Although it feels uncomfortable, that burning actually is a pain buster. It stimulates your brain to secrete endorphins, your body's natural narcotic. And it creates a counterirritant that so busies your brain with nerve impulses that it essentially blocks out other pain signals. Your brain feels the cold and burning and begins to ignore the other hurt.

"Ice is a powerful pain blocker, but it only works if you keep it on long enough," Dr. Waters says.

If you have any circulatory problems, you probably want to avoid the use of cryotherapy. People with diabetic conditions and loss of sensation in their limbs may be unable to tell the difference between cold that can help and cold that can cause further damage, says Dr. Waters. Anyone with high blood pressure, a hypersensitivity to cold, or frostbite should not use cryotherapy unless under close supervision of a health professional, he says.

"Most people already know if they have an odd reaction to ice," says Dr. Waters. "If the skin quickly blanches and goes white, that's a bad sign."

"We know that cold helps release the body's own painkillers. If you release endorphins, the effect can go on for some time," says Robert Kennedy, M.D., director of geriatric medicine at Maimonides Medical Center in Brooklyn, New York. "And if a muscle spasm is the root of the problem, cold could certainly relieve that."

Cold can also speed healing and decrease the need for medication. In Canada, researchers studied 45 people who had undergone minor arthroscopic knee surgery. In the first week after surgery, some people performed a therapy of exercise and cryotherapy. Others did a regimen of exercise only. Researchers found that the group using ice took less medication for pain and were better able to bear weight on their knees.

Ice may be the simplest and safest of all pain therapies. It can be done at home using nothing more than a bag of ice chips and common sense, says Dr. Waters.

WHAT RESULTS CAN YOU EXPECT?

Because of its numbing effects, cold tends to have an immediate impact on pain. And in some cases, pain relief from cold may be longer-lasting than the effects of heat.

WHAT DOES IT COST?

A 16-ounce bag of frozen peas runs about $1.50. Cold packs used by sports trainers sell for about $25. Freezing ice cubes in your refrigerator takes about 2 hours and costs just pennies in electricity.

Companionship

Friends, family, some health-care professionals, even a faithful pet can all provide companionship. They can be with you when you really need them, meeting at least some of your needs, whether it's a laugh, a back rub, a distracting game of checkers, a shared moment of silence, a pleasant memory, a soft shoulder, or a contented purr. They remind you what life is about. And they get as much out of being there as you do.

And though providing companionship for someone who is ill or in pain can be challenging, it is vitally important, says Maggie McKivergin, R.N., a certified holistic nursing specialist and the nurse coordinator for the Center for Alternative Health in Charleston, West Virginia. In addition to the usual family and friends, companions can include support groups, volunteers who provide respite care for the caregivers, and members of a spiritual community.

"For family members, especially, it's both a burden and a joy to care for someone who is ill," McKivergin says. "The caregivers suffer seeing their loved ones in pain, and so they need a team of support to help diffuse the requirements for care in every way."

Heck, even Florence Nightingale needed a night out on the town now and then.

HOW DOES IT EASE PAIN?

When caring for a loved one who is in pain, it helps to remember that humans are pack animals; that is, they tend to do better as part of a group than alone. Social isolation is a risk factor for heart disease, cancer, and depression. But if we have what's called psychosocial connections—friends, family, church, someone we can lean on—we live longer and healthier lives, says David Spiegel, M.D., medical director of the Complementary Medicine Clinic at Stanford University School of Medicine and author of *Living beyond Limits: New Hope and Help for Facing Life-Threatening Illness.*

"One's ability to have intimate and satisfying relationships actually predicts longevity," he says. And medical literature is full of studies that document this.

The positive emotions generated by supportive, loving relationships and the opportunity these relationships can provide to let us express *all* emotions make us more resilient to stress, Dr. Spiegel says. One study, done at the Institute of HeartMath in Boulder Creek, California, showed that as individuals focused on feelings of compassion and caring, they showed a marked improvement in their immune systems. And Dr. Spiegel found that in a study of 86 women diagnosed with late-stage breast cancer, the 50 women who met once a week to share their emotions and deepest fears lived significantly longer—an average of 18 months longer—than those who didn't participate in such a support group.

"Psychological support is so valuable that it should be an essential component of medical treatment," he says. And support groups can be a way to allow people to stop putting up a front that is draining and isolating. "These groups can provide a stable and deep sense of connection at a time when friends, fearful of illness, may fade out of the picture," he adds.

How Is It Done?

Whether you're visiting someone sick, helping out, or caring full-time for someone, try to stay in your heart, McKivergin says. "Heart-centered care is just the best; it's very healing. Whatever else you are doing for that person or talking about with that person, you still feel like you are connected."

To offer heart-based caring, you need to be "present" for the other person, McKivergin says. Being present means truly listening to a person, being mindful, offering unconditional love—not judging or criticizing. "The essence of presence is nurturing the essence of another, really tuning in on an intuitive level to the core of that person, recognizing the special soul this person represents," she says.

Taking a moment to focus your intentions on the person you're offering companionship to is something hospital volunteers and nurses may do and something that family and friends can also benefit from doing, says Charlotte Eliopoulos, R.N., Ph.D., a specialist in holistic geriatric and chronic-care nursing and author of *Integrating Conventional and Alternative Therapies*. "Before you meet with the person, pause, take a deep breath, center yourself, and clear away the trivia that's floating around in your mind. You might even say a little prayer asking that you be guided to meet this person's needs or to recognize what this person needs and be able to serve to the best of your capacity."

On a more practical level for visitors, once you've established a connection and shown that you care, distraction can be a welcome thing, Dr. Eliopoulos says. If you're not much of a talker, offer to read or to play a game, bring along a magazine for the person, or photographs. "Even if it's just a 5- to 10-minute conversation to get your friend outside of his circle of pain and illness, that can really be a big service," she says. And don't be afraid to simply share some silence.

If you are able to offer help, let your friend and the family know. Make a specific offer of something you are willing to do or ask what you can do. "Knowing there is someone who can be called on to help when needed is really important," she says.

WHAT DOES IT FEEL LIKE?

Sharing companionship can produce a deep sense of connection and validation. It can produce trust and calmness.

WHAT RESULTS CAN YOU EXPECT?

Offering companionship to someone who needs it can make their difficult circumstances easier to endure, increase their trust, improve their coping strength and self-esteem, decrease their isolation and alienation, increase their sense of being heard and understood, and help meet their needs.

Anyone can offer companionship. If you want to support a friend or family member, call and ask to stop by, or invite the person to meet you somewhere. And while they may express strong emotions in your presence, it is not your role—nor is it possible—for you to take on their emotional burdens. The intention of offering a heart-centered presence is often the key in helping a person to heal.

If you are concerned about soaking up negative energy, try this visualization technique, McKivergin suggests. "Put yourself in a bubble of light, which protects you from absorbing some of the negative stuff, the sad and painful stuff, and set for yourself the intention of giving and receiving only love."

If you're interested in joining a support group, you can contact the American Self-Help Clearinghouse, 25 Pocono Road, Denville, NJ 07834-2954. They maintain a database of more than 800 national and international support groups and can provide information on starting new groups. Or look in your local library for a copy of *The Self-Help Sourcebook*

(sixth edition), which includes contacts for hundreds of groups.

WHAT DOES IT COST?

Support groups are often free; if they're run by a therapist, there may be a modest fee. For more information about groups for seniors, call your local YMCA. At Jewish community centers, the average cost for senior citizens is $227 a year, or $350 per couple. Dues at social clubs such as the Odd Fellows vary from region to region and can cost from $10 to $100 a year. And don't forget—churches or synagogues are pay-what-you-can.

Exercise

When you consider that pain frequently is a product of chronic diseases like osteoporosis, arthritis, and heart disease, exercise is perhaps the single most important thing you can do to avoid pain.

Physical exercise, at its most basic, is nothing more than physical activity. You can exercise by raking the leaves, cleaning the house, line dancing, or walking. You can also participate in more organized activities: water aerobics, weight lifting, or a three-times-a-week workout on a treadmill.

How Does It Ease Pain?

Exercise is so good for your mind and body that it's hard to know where to begin. By helping to reverse the aging process of muscles, bones, and joints, exercise is a natural antidote to the painful effects of osteoarthritis and osteoporosis, says Robert Kennedy, M.D., director of geriatric medicine at Maimonides Medical Center in Brooklyn, New York.

Osteoarthritis, a degenerative joint disease, affects the knees, hips, shoulders, and neck. It can make it difficult to take a walk around the neighborhood or reach up and take something off a shelf in the kitchen. And it's a condition made worse by a lack of exercise. "Because it hurts, you avoid taking that walk or going up the stairs. And soon, you can't do those things at all," says Dr. Kennedy. "Your joints stiffen up from disuse, and you lose that range of motion. Exercise can prevent that from happening."

Exercise won't be your only therapy for arthritis pain and stiffness, but it can help a great deal. Walking or swimming, for instance, increases the production of synovial fluid, the natural lubricant in your joints. Exercising with light hand weights or elastic bands—this is called resistance training—can build up the muscle structures around your joints and take pressure off bones.

Resistance training also builds or maintains bone density. It may be one of the most important things that a woman can do to avoid osteoporosis. Research shows that athletic women have higher bone density than nonathletic women. It's not a stretch to say that physically active people may be less susceptible to bone loss due to osteoporosis.

Many types of exercise, when done with some vigor, increase blood circulation in your body, lower cholesterol and blood pressure levels, strengthen your immune system, help you maintain a healthy weight, and improve your cardiovascular health.

Researchers at the University of Colorado Health Sciences Center in Denver found that exercise rehabilitation was especially effective for claudication—painful plaque blockages and a narrowing of the blood vessels of the legs. People with this condition experience severe pain while walking. Programs of regulated exercise were found to help study participants increase both their speed by 65 percent and their distances walked by 44 percent.

The psychological benefits of exercise may be as great as the physical. Exercise spurs your body to release endorphins, those natural opiates that give you a feeling of well-being. It also may reduce the production of nasty stress hormones.

No doubt, exercise is a stress buster, a simple way to relieve the tension that builds up and accentuates pain, says Beth Fisher, R.N., a health fitness instructor certified by the American College of Sports Medicine. "When you feel better, your perception of pain decreases. When pain is part of what is causing you stress, it's a vicious circle. Stress accentuates pain, and pain causes stress," says Fisher, who coordinates exercise programs for senior citizens and cardiac patients at Memorial Hospital of Towanda, Pennsylvania.

How Is It Done?

Exercise should be pleasurable. It should be an activity you like to do and are willing to do regularly, says Dr. Kennedy.

Take the dog for a brisk walk. Exercise with a partner. Join a class where you can get instruction—and motivation—from a group leader and other participants. Turn on the radio and do a soft-shoe routine as you clean the house. If it has been years since you've ridden a bike, try out one of the new mountain bikes, with their wide tires and comfortable seats.

"What you don't have to do is go to a gym, put on a pair of sneakers and stretch pants, and start bouncing around and pumping weights," Dr. Kennedy says. "That notion of exercise turns off a lot of people."

Of course, if you're trying to relieve a particular pain—say, in your lower back or an arthritic joint—you may need to focus on specific exercises. Pelvic tilts can loosen and strengthen lower-back muscles. Stretches can increase range of motion in stiff joints, and weight or resistance training builds stronger muscles.

Although many people associate resistance training with young people who pump iron in a gym, it doesn't have to involve barbells or weight machines, says Fisher. Resistance exercise can be climbing steps and doing arm curls with soup cans (each can weighs about 1 pound), leg lifts while watching television, or pushups against the wall.

they can't work out. Soon, they get disgusted and quit. If you haven't been active, start slowly. Exercise just 5 minutes the first day. Perhaps just walk down the block and back. Then try to go a little farther the next day.

Eventually, you should work up to 30 minutes a day three to five times a week. You can meet that minimum goal by doing an activity for 30 minutes. Or, you can break that 30 minutes into three 10-minute periods and still reap much of the same benefits, she says.

When you exercise, you shouldn't become so breathless that you can't carry on a conversation. Also, you should be able to repeat the same activity the next day, says Fisher. "If you walked ½ mile yesterday, you ought to be able to do the same today. You should not be so exhausted that it takes you a whole day to recover."

The only downside to exercise is the narrow risk of injury. Minor muscle pulls and strains aren't uncommon, but even these can be reduced by avoiding high-impact sports like jogging, cautions Fisher.

WHAT DOES IT FEEL LIKE?

Forget that no-pain, no-gain stuff. Exercise will tire you, but it shouldn't hurt or make you really sore afterward, says Fisher.

Too often, people get rambunctious, throw themselves into an exercise program, and end up so stiff the following day that

WHAT RESULTS CAN YOU EXPECT?

To really reap the benefits of exercise, you need to do more than just get into shape—you have to stay in shape and exercise regularly. Even an athlete who falls out of condition quickly loses all benefits of physical fitness. You simply can't bank exercise.

Although 30 minutes per day three to five times a week is the recommended minimum amount of activity, there are benefits to doing more, like adding an extra bike ride or strength-training session once or twice a week. A regular program of exercise can reverse many of the pains and frailty of old age, such as poor balance, joint stiffness, and lack of wind, says Dr. Kennedy.

That's because physical decline is mostly related to disuse. If you don't use it, you lose it, says Dr. Kennedy. "You can really turn around that decline by exercising. The people who have the most to gain are people who have not been exercising at all. They will see the biggest improvements."

In a study conducted over the course of 18 months at Wake Forest University in Winston-Salem, North Carolina, medical researchers studied the exercise habits of three groups of older adults with osteoarthritis of the knee. The study's aim was to determine if aerobic exercise or resistance training had any positive effect on their abilities to climb stairs and their perceptions of pain. During the study period, one group did aerobic exercise, another did resistance training. The remainder received health-education information but did not exercise. At the end of 18 months, the exercise groups had greater capacities to climb stairs and lowered perceptions of pain as compared with the group that did not exercise. Not surprisingly, the researchers found that the exercisers were getting around better and felt better, too.

WHO'S QUALIFIED TO DO IT?

You can certainly get started on your own. If you need motivation or instruction, however, join an exercise group at the local college, enroll in a health club, see a physical therapist, or even hire a personal trainer. Ultimately, if you are to make exercise a part of your life, the desire has to come from within. You have to want to do it, says Fisher.

WHAT DOES IT COST?

The price of a treadmill runs from a few hundred dollars to $8,000. A beginner set of cast-iron barbells costs less than $100.

On the other hand, you can take a walk outside for free. And you could begin a weight-lifting program with soup cans and do leg lifts while watching television.

Guided Imagery

Actors use guided imagery to rehearse their lines. High jumpers, in the moment before they run to the bar, visualize the execution of a perfect leap. Cancer patients conjure up images of white blood cells roving through their bodies like sharks, devouring wayward malignant cells.

When you use guided imagery as a therapy, you consciously create mental pictures in your mind to distract yourself from pain, rally your body's defenses, or calm down an overactive nervous system and tense muscles.

"You can open the deep levels of the mind to the influence of images. When you do, beliefs and images can become actual events in the body," says Emmett Miller, M.D., author of *Deep Healing: The Essence of Mind/Body Medicine.* Dr. Miller practices in Los Altos and Nevada City, California.

The history of imagery probably goes back to a time when humans first sat around a fire, chanted, danced, and imagined the success of the hunt in the coming day. In primitive societies across the world, shamans (tribal healers) advocated the use of dreams and images to heal.

Aristotle, Hippocrates, and Galen—ancient Greek physicians and philosophers— were great believers in the power of images to manage disease. But as Western medicine emerged as the dominant form of medical care, imagery fell out of favor as a treatment.

The mind/body connection has undergone a renaissance, however, and many scientific studies now show its effectiveness, particularly in pain management, says Dr. Miller.

HOW DOES IT EASE PAIN?

The way that imagery relieves pain isn't entirely understood. Clearly, there is an element of distraction at work. If you're able to conjure up a rich, sensation-laden image that fully engages your mind, you'll distract yourself from pain— at least temporarily, says Roy Grzesiak, Ph.D., a psychologist at the New Jersey Pain Institute and the Robert Wood Johnson Medical School in New Brunswick.

Because relaxation is the foundation of guided imagery—you have to reach a near-meditative state before you can begin to visualize—the relaxation response alone may be enough to cause pain reduction, he says.

"Whenever you relax, you quiet down the nervous system. You dampen and mute pain signals traveling down the line," says Dr. Grzesiak. "Tight muscles relax and let go of all that tension that makes pain that much worse."

Imagery may also be a form of self-hypnosis, a way to take control and will away the pain. You can imagine giving yourself an injection of morphine or novocaine. Some folks picture the level of their pain as a needle on a meter, then they concentrate on the needle and move it back several notches, explains Dr. Miller.

No matter the image, the important thing is that it gives you some personal control over your pain, says Dr. Miller. "You take the physical pain and transfer it into an entity you can control. When you feel you have control over it, you have less pain."

There's speculation that guided imagery may prompt the body to release endorphins, a natural, narcotic-like painkiller. Another theory hypothesizes that the mind increases circulation, literally flushing out waste products from muscles and bringing oxygen-rich blood into aching areas.

"It's very hard to determine the mechanisms. It seems incredible that these work, but they do," concedes Dr. Grzesiak. "I believe it is a true mind/body connection. The psychological triggers a physical response."

HOW IS IT DONE?

Opening your mind's eye requires focus and relaxation and quiet. You can get in the mood by using several techniques: biofeedback, meditation, self-hypnosis, breathing techniques, or whatever works for you. Some people create their own cue words, such as *beach, relax,* or *breeze,* that recall the scene or sensation they are trying to visualize, says Dr. Grzesiak.

"When you repeat a cue word over

and over, it helps you get into a relaxed state more quickly. You get conditioned to relax whenever you use the word," he explains.

Most people begin with breathing exercises while sitting in comfortable chairs. You may take several deep breaths. Using your diaphragm or belly, inhale through your nose and then exhale through your mouth.

At the same time, you might tense and relax muscles in your body. Each time you tense and then relax, the muscle tends to revert to a looser state, says Dr. Grzesiak. You might begin at your toes and slowly work your way toward your head. Or, you can concentrate on the muscle group nearest the site of the pain.

During guided imagery sessions with patients, Dr. Grzesiak uses autogenic phrases, words that are suggestive and help bring on relaxation. "I might say over and over again, 'Your neck muscles are becoming warm and heavy. Your jaw feels slack and loose.' Autogenic therapy is simply a technique of muscle relaxation."

Once relaxed, many people choose to visualize a favorite place: a beach, a cabin in the woods, or a boat floating in the water. The place or image is highly personal, but it should be a place where you feel safe, calm, and comfortable, says Dr. Miller.

WHAT DOES IT FEEL LIKE?

Although vision is the dominant framework, imagery isn't just imagining pictures in your head. Imagery may also have a sound, taste, and smell, says Dr. Miller. You might imagine waves hitting the shore or wind rustling leaves in the forest. You might imagine the feeling of the sun on your face.

There's also what Dr. Miller calls feeling, or kinesthetic, imagery, where you imagine yourself doing an activity. Perhaps it's dancing in a ballroom, skiing down a hill, or having sex in a Jacuzzi.

Although pastoral settings and kinetic images probably work best as distractions, there are other visualizations that allow you to face your pain more directly. In a session with a therapist, you may be asked to describe your pain: What does it look like? Does it have a color, a smell, a sound, or a taste? Is it hot or cold? Maybe your pain is like a roaring bonfire or a tidal wave that threatens to wash you out to sea.

Once you decide what your pain looks like, you then conjure up images that negate or jettison this pain, explains Dr. Miller. Maybe it's a fire hose putting out the fire or an ice-cold mountain stream into which you lower your pain. If you see your pain as red, the therapist may coach you to think of blue.

"You might image yourself breathing in

a cool, blue healing liquid and exhaling the red painful image," says Dr. Miller. "With each breath, the pain subsides."

WHAT RESULTS CAN YOU EXPECT?

The benefits are both short-term and long-term, says Dr. Grzesiak. Obviously, if you're able to tune out the pain, you can get immediate relief. Even the residual relaxation of tight muscles and an overwrought nervous system may be enough to keep pain at bay for hours.

Guided imagery may also be very effective at reducing the anxiety that accompanies pain and surgery.

A research study done at the Cleveland Clinic examined 130 patients who had colorectal surgery. Half the group received routine care after the operation. The other half listened to guided imagery tapes before the operation, during anesthesia, and for several days in recovery. The patients in the guided imagery group had considerably less anxiety and pain and required 50 percent less narcotic pain medication than the control group.

Whether it be increased endorphin activity or blood circulation, or simply a break from stress, guided imagery isn't just good for pain. It's good for your overall health, says Dr. Grzesiak. "Even if you look at imagery just as a form of meditation, it has a lot of terrific benefits."

WHO'S QUALIFIED TO DO IT?

You can certainly do guided imagery on your own. For some—maybe the daydreamers among us—guided imagery isn't all that difficult. For others, it's unfamiliar territory. We're accustomed to having our thoughts and attention directed by outside influences—a movie, television, our families, our work. Reaching into our own heads requires some practice.

It may be best to start out by getting some help from a professional. Psychologists, hypnotists, and psychiatrists certainly are familiar with the techniques and probably use them regularly in their practices. Some medical doctors and dentists use guided imagery as a way to calm patients down for procedures or to give them healing therapy—as a supplement to medications.

Dr. Grzesiak tends to see pain patients for just a few sessions, then they are on their own. "I get them started, teach them techniques, and encourage them to practice it," he says. "After that, it's really up to them."

Usually, people need help learning how to focus, choosing an appropriate image that will relieve the pain, and then linking that meditative state and image to a cue word, says Dr. Grzesiak.

Dr. Grzesiak also records one or two office sessions so that the patients have him on tape talking in his soothing, hypnotic voice and using the autogenic phrases that bring on a meditative state. They use these personalized tapes at home for self-therapy.

You can also buy more generic visualization tapes in many bookstores. These can be equally valuable and an inexpensive and effective way to learn imagery techniques, says Dr. Miller. Tapes can set the proper mood, take you to a relaxed state in a step-by-step process, and then allow you to form your healing images.

WHAT DOES IT COST?

Guided imagery tapes run as little as $10. Sessions with psychologists run on average between $40 to $150 per session.

Heat

Using heat to relieve pain falls under a type of physical therapy known as thermotherapy. There are four types of therapeutic heat: conduction, radiation, conversion, and convection. Conduction involves dry heat, usually from a chemical instant-warm hot pack. Radiation uses infrared or ultraviolet lamps. Conversion is a method of heating fluids beneath a surface, usually accomplished by ultrasound. Convection transmits heat from a liquid, as in a wet towel, a soaking bath, or a pool of water (hydrotherapy).

HOW DOES IT EASE PAIN?

Heat is an analgesic. After an afternoon of working in the garden or a 30-minute bout of shoveling snow, you know that resting your aching limbs in a hot bath feels good.

Here's why: Heat disrupts muscle spasms, relaxes tight connective tissues and ligaments, opens up blood vessels, increases bloodflow, and accelerates the metabolism of tissues, explains Lawrence Miller, M.D., of the Coast Pain Management Center at the Orange Coast Memorial Medical Center in Fountain Valley, California. "It's not only going to make the pain lessen, it will help with the healing, too."

Increased circulation brings in fresh blood brimming with oxygen and nutrients that are essential for healing. It also takes out waste products and by-products of inflammation. This metabolic refuse, when allowed to build up in tissues, may by itself be enough to cause pain as well as delay healing.

Heat would not be your first choice after an acute injury, however, such as a twisted knee. Cold is best for killing the pain immediately and keeping down swelling. But after a few days, it's heat you want. Heat not only accelerates healing but also loosens up ligaments and muscles so that you can move the injured part more freely. When combined with massage or gentle stretching, heat's pain-relieving effect can be magnified.

This analgesic effect is what makes heat well-suited for the chronic pain of osteoarthritis and bursitis. When joints are involved, for example, heat increases the viscosity, or slipperiness, of synovial fluid—the "grease" that makes joints move freely, says Patrick Waters, D.C., a chiropractor at the Waters Chiropractic Clinic in Dallas.

Heat may also reduce swelling in the joint itself that can be a source of sharp, irritating pain.

"All of this frees up pressures in the joint and the surrounding muscle structures," says Dr. Waters. "You'll have more free movement—and probably less pain when you try to walk and move."

Although it's not clear why, just slightly raising the temperature of the tissues may be enough to soothe irritated nerve fibers.

That mechanism may be tied to the release of endorphins and enkephalins, the body's own painkillers, says Dr. Waters.

HOW IS IT DONE?

The idea is to get the heat where you need it, which is usually down below your skin and into the belly of your muscle or your joint itself, says Dr. Miller.

If recommended by your doctor, a therapist in a pain-management facility may use an infrared lamp to generate deep heat. Skin is a poor heat conductor, so infrared waves through the skin are absorbed in the lower tissues and instantaneously turned into heat energy. Typically, an infrared treatment lasts no more than 30 minutes.

Diathermy is a technology that uses high-frequency electrical current and waves to create heat below the skin surface. There are three types of diathermy: short wave, microwave, and ultrasound. Each treatment lasts about 20 minutes and must be done by a medical professional. Diathermy is very effective in opening up capillaries, increasing bloodflow in a specialized area, and raising the pain threshold of the surrounding area. It can actually warm up the capsule of a joint, while the surrounding tissues remain normal body temperature.

At home, you can reach the deeper tissues by using moist heat. There's no clear reason why moist is better than dry heat, but moist heat may be a little hotter, a little more penetrating than dry heat, says Dr. Waters. Also, it won't dry out your skin.

Moist heat is just like it sounds—wet. Therapists may use a specialized heating pad that generates its own moisture. You can take a warm shower, plunge an arm or leg into a warm bath or whirlpool, place a hot-water bottle wrapped in a thin towel on your pain, or wet some towels with warm water, says Dr. Miller. You can even wrap an aching joint with plastic sandwich wrap to retain body heat and moisture.

No matter what method you use, realize that the heat does not have to be hot to be effective.

Warm, yes; hot, no, says Dr. Miller, who has seen people come into his office with skin burns from applying hot compresses for too long a period. One of the most common mistakes people make is falling asleep with a heating pad, he says. The problem comes from nerve endings acclimating to the heat. It's like putting your big toe into a hot bath. What first seems extremely hot becomes tolerable as you lower yourself in.

That does not mean that you're not getting burned, however. Older people, especially those with circulatory problems, may not be able to feel the heat as well, so it's always recommended that you check with your physician before starting heat therapy, reminds Dr. Waters. Heat should be applied to the skin for no more than 20 minutes at a time. Ten minutes may be plenty. Placing a thin towel between your skin and the heating pad is an added precaution.

WHAT RESULTS CAN YOU EXPECT?

Because heat breaks muscle spasms and, generally, just loosens up a stiff, aching body, most of its pain-relieving qualities are short-term and fairly immediate, says Robert Kennedy, M.D., director of geriatric medicine at Maimonides Medical Center in Brooklyn, New York. "Muscles spasms really accentuate pain. Relieve those cramps, and you're going to have less pain."

When heat is able to significantly increase the production of endorphins and enkephalins, the painkilling effects can last in the body for many hours. In these cases, heat can be a real alternative to pain medication, he says.

Less dramatically, heat may simply give you enough relief to move about with less stiffness or to relax and get a good night's sleep, says Dr. Kennedy. "There is no standard prescription for everybody. I would try it and see if it works. If makes you feel better, use it."

There are some cautions. If your pain is due to an inflammatory condition, such as rheumatoid arthritis, you may want to avoid heat. It can actually irritate and accelerate the inflammatory process and the degeneration of the joints.

Because heat acts as a vasodilator, causing blood vessels to expand, it can lower blood pressure. If you have a heart condition, you should be careful with heat and check with your doctor before using heat to relieve pain, especially when you're immersing your entire body in warm water.

WHO'S QUALIFIED TO DO IT?

The more complicated forms of thermotherapy should be performed by a doctor, chiropractor, physical therapist, or other professional familiar with the technology.

WHAT DOES IT COST?

A warm bath or shower costs just pennies; a chemical instant-warm hot pack, $1 to $2. Professional thermotherapy shouldn't cost much more than a typical doctor's office visit.

Homeopathy

Homeopathy is a holistic practice of healing based on the premise that like cures like. Homeopathic practitioners believe that tiny doses of substances that when given to a healthy person cause a particular set of symptoms to appear can cure those same symptoms in someone who is ill.

For example, when belladonna is taken internally, it produces restlessness, throbbing pains, and a sensitivity to light—symptoms that are similar to those of scarlet fever. Consequently, homeopaths may use a very dilute solution containing belladonna to treat scarlet fever.

The premise of like cures like is also known as the law of similars. It goes back some 5,000 years to the medical beliefs of ancient China and India.

Samuel Hahnemann, a German physician, founded modern homeopathy in the late eighteenth century. Hahnemann was disgusted with the poisonous doses of mercury and the bloodletting practices that doctors of the day used to treat patients. Homeopathy, he declared, was a way to use natural, gentle substances to stimulate the body's own defenses or vital force.

How Does It Ease Pain?

Homeopathy raises the level of a person's health, explains Laura Sholtz, a registered homeopath who practices in Exeter, Maine, and teaches courses in homeopathy at the University of Maine in Orono. "When the level of health is raised, a person is better able to deal with their pain, and the pain might even diminish or disappear."

How Is It Done?

Although you can buy homeopathic remedies in health food stores and treat yourself for an acute condition, the best way to introduce yourself to this healing art is to visit a practitioner of classical homeopathy, says Sandra Wyner, a registered homeopathic consultant practicing in Amherst, Northampton, and Williamstown, Massachusetts.

At your first office visit or interview, the homeopath may spend up to 2 hours (sometimes more) talking with you about yourself, including your complaints or pain, Wyner says.

The conversation will be wide-ranging, encompassing your emotional and spiritual health as well as physical condition, Sholtz adds.

A homeopath doesn't treat just a medical condition or a disease, but treats the entire person in order to improve the patient's level of health and strengthen the constitution, explains Wyner. "My job is to get a picture of the whole person, to really understand the state he is in. It's a very individual way of treating someone."

The interview is designed to help the homeopath determine which remedy is right for that particular person at that particular time. If the remedy is not correct, the patient may feel no benefit at all.

Homeopaths work mainly with about 50 commonly used homeopathic medicines, but theoretically, remedies can be made from any substance in nature. At present, remedies derived from about 3,000 substances are available, Wyner says. The medicines are diluted with alcohol or water into microdoses and then shaken vigorously (a process known as succusion). A potency of 6X indicates a 1-in-1,000,000 dilution. (The six indicates the number of zeros in the dilution.)

Most acute homeopathic medicines used in the United States have a dilution ranging from 6X to 30X. Professionally trained homeopaths use higher dilutions as well, says Wyner.

As you can imagine, these are extremely dilute solutions, so much so that most homeopathic remedies contain none of the original material. That's why a highly toxic substance such as mercury can be rendered harmless by dilution but can still be used as a remedy.

Finally, these prepared substances are made into tiny pills or pellets that are designed to be taken under the tongue. Homeopathic remedies also include creams, tinctures (highly concentrated herbal extracts), ointments, and lotions. One of the most popular creams is Arnica, used to treat muscle soreness, bruising, and trauma from surgery.

WHAT DOES IT FEEL LIKE?

The effects of a homeopathic medicine can be subtle. You may feel immediate relief of pain. But if your pain is related to a chronic condition, such as diabetes or arthritis, it's unlikely that you'll have an instant recovery, although alleviation of symptoms may take place over time as your body's own healing forces are activated, says Wyner.

"What you will feel is increased energy, and some people experience a feeling of protection," she says. "You will be in much better shape to deal with your pain,

which can be diminished." Homeopaths believe that the remedies stimulate the inner natural defenses of the body, what they call the vital force. Disease and pain, they believe, result from an imbalance of the vital force.

That's why the focus of the remedies is not to eliminate a particular complaint or pain, but to bolster the vital force, says Sholtz.

WHAT RESULTS CAN YOU EXPECT?

Although some studies suggest that homeopathy may be effective, most medical doctors argue that positive results are caused by the placebo effect. In other words, there's a 30 percent chance that any given remedy will work, even if the remedy is an inactive substance, according to at least one medical report.

Regardless of the reason, if you do experience a favorable reaction from a homeopathic remedy, it can be months before another treatment is necessary. If you do not experience a beneficial effect, the homeopath will reevaluate your condition and perhaps try a different remedy, Wyner adds.

WHO'S QUALIFIED TO DO IT?

Homeopathy is practiced by many different healers, although some may not have professional training.

If you want to visit someone trained in and practicing classical homeopathy, you should ask the practitioner if he is registered with the North American Society of Homeopaths (NASH) or certified by the Council for Homeopathic Certification. You can also write to the National Center for Homeopathy, 801 North Fairfax Street, Suite 306, Alexandria, VA 22314-1757 for general information on homeopathy and for a referral to a trained homeopath near you.

WHAT DOES IT COST?

The initial visit and 2-hour interview with a homeopath costs between $150 and $250. Follow-up visits are briefer and less costly. The homeopathic remedies themselves tend to be relatively inexpensive—just a few dollars in the health food store or drugstore or via the mail.

Hydrotherapy

Hydrotherapy, not surprisingly, involves healing with water. It can range from taking a whirlpool bath to help loosen up an arthritic joint to enrolling in an organized program of water aerobics to build muscle strength and flexibility. More loosely, it includes sitz baths, ice and hot packs, saunas, steam baths, and hot tubs.

As a pain reliever, hydrotherapy has a long history. Native Americans cleansed themselves both spiritually and physically by gathering in sweat lodges. Romans and Turks frolicked in mineral hot springs. And Scandinavians steamed away their rheumatic complaints in saunas. Even today, hot tubs and whirlpools dot residential backyards and are a feature of health clubs.

HOW DOES IT EASE PAIN?

Water has two main benefits: temperature and buoyancy.

Although ice and cold water can be therapeutic (cold has the capacity to break muscle spasms and relieve painful inflammation), hydrotherapy usually involves the use of warm water.

Wet heat seems to be therapeutically superior to dry heat, such as that delivered by a heating pad, says Robert Kennedy, M.D., director of geriatric medicine at Maimonides Medical Center in Brooklyn, New York.

"Moist heat seems to get deeper into the tissues," he says. "It may be better at relaxing the muscles and providing a soothing sort of warmth."

You can apply moist heat with compresses, such as towels soaked in warm water. Or you can simply immerse your body or aching arm or leg into a bath or pool of warm water.

Warm water dilates blood vessels and increases circulation. Fresh blood pulsing into a painful, inflamed area removes waste products and brings in nutrients and oxygen. Improved circulation can beat infections, ease pain, and generally improve body function. Heat also relaxes tight muscles and limbers stiff and sore joints.

"Generally, it just feels good," says Dr. Kennedy.

For many people, especially those folks hobbled by arthritis or excess body weight, the other benefit of water is buoyancy. Water has the capacity to make an aching body or body part essentially weightless, says Andrew Spitzer, M.D., associate surgeon at the Kerlan-Jobe Orthopaedic Clinic in Los Angeles. "Buoyancy neutralizes all those gravitational forces across the joint. When that happens, you can immediately eliminate some, or perhaps all, of the pain."

Buoyancy also enables overweight folks to exercise safely. Water aerobics, sometimes called aquacizing, is fast becoming a popular form of hydrotherapy in many clinical settings. It's not unusual to see it offered as part of YMCA or community pool programs.

"This kind of pool work is an opportunity for people with joint pain to exercise in a weightless environment," says Dr. Spitzer. "For people in pain or folks who are overweight, even simple exercise on land—like walking or stretching—may be too much."

Water aerobics helps maintain range of motion, increase circulation, and, in particular, build muscle strength, says Dr. Spitzer. That's important because strong muscles help support and take stress off painful joints. Exercise also releases endorphins, the body's own painkillers.

A study done of 139 people with chronic rheumatoid arthritis found that those who participated in 30-minute group hydrotherapy exercise sessions two times a week for 4 weeks experienced significant improvement in their conditions. They had greater knee movement, less pain, and less tenderness in their joints than others who did land-based exercises or simply immersed themselves in warm water.

How Is It Done?

Most hydrotherapy pool work involves a lot of stretching and bending of the joints, says Denise De Lorenzo, P.T., a physical therapist at the Kessler Institute in West Orange, New Jersey.

"There's not a lot of jumping or bouncing around," she explains. "We usually start with the large muscle groups and then work on particular areas like the knees or the arms."

Starting off gently, you may hold on to a railing or the side of the pool and move your legs, bend your knees, or do ankle circles. In waist-deep water, you may be asked to walk forward, sideways, and backward, says De Lorenzo. If people have good balance or coordination, they can work out in deeper water, which is more buoyant but also more resistant to movement.

WHAT DOES IT FEEL LIKE?

A therapeutic pool isn't nearly as warm as a steam bath or a hot tub. The water temperature hovers between 80° and 92°F, and the air temperature is kept a bit cooler than the water. When you enter the water, it feels pleasantly warm.

Even though the pool is well below body temperature, it's still plenty warm enough for heat to penetrate muscles and joints, says De Lorenzo. "Water doesn't have to be hot to be therapeutic," she adds.

Even at moderate heat, the combination of warm water and exertion can drive up blood pressure. Hydrotherapy—at least pool therapy—may not be advisable for anyone with high blood pressure or a heart or lung condition, she cautions.

WHAT RESULTS CAN YOU EXPECT?

Besides it's more immediate, feel-good effects, hydrotherapy simply makes it easier to move, says Dr. Spitzer.

The pulse and movement of water in a whirlpool applies gentle pressure to a joint. The water's motion may allow you to more easily bend a stiff knee or stretch a spasming back muscle. Cold water or ice can stop swelling and bleeding in tissues. Warm water can speed up the healing process and reduce inflammation.

Sometimes, it's a combination of hot, cold, and wet that works wonders, says Dr. Spitzer. After a therapy session in the pool, he tells his patients with arthritis to apply ice packs to their sore joints.

"Exercise causes irritation and may actually cause more pain later," he says. "Icing the joint right after a workout keeps inflammation from flaring up. You can head off the problem."

WHO'S QUALIFIED TO DO IT?

If you like to swim and you feel comfortable in water, you can certainly go to a pool and practice your own program of hydrotherapy, suggests De Lorenzo. If you've been looking for an excuse to put a hot tub in the backyard, here it is. And, of course, putting ice and heat on pain or taking a soaking, relaxing bath have long been do-it-yourself home remedies for pain.

If water aerobics in a pool sounds appealing, you may want to start out taking a class led by a physical therapist or aerobics instructor. That way, you'll learn proper technique and the routines that are right for you.

WHAT DOES IT COST?

You can get started by joining one of the aquatics classes offered at many YMCAs and community pools. Classes usually run less than $100 for 10 sessions. Many health clubs also offer whirlpools and other forms of hydrotherapy with the price of membership.

Hypnosis

Officially, hypnosis is "a state of highly focused internal concentration, coupled with a reduction in peripheral awareness," says Stephen Lankton, president of the American Hypnosis Board for Clinical Social Workers in Pensacola, Florida. More simply, it's a bit like looking through a microscope. Your range of vision is narrow, but the details within that range are sharp and have your full attention. The narrow focus also helps you pay less attention to unwelcome thoughts, feelings, and perceptions—such as pain. And it lets your imagination work better, without judgments from your critical mind.

A hypnotist may initially help you into a state of hypnosis, but ultimately all hypnosis is self-hypnosis, says Lankton. "The imagination is controlled by the individual being hypnotized, not the hypnotist. It is not projected on the subject." So even if you want an excuse to act silly, you can't blame the hypnotist. "You really won't do anything you don't want to, including shifting your focus away from your pain," he says. By the end of the first session, he says, most people *do* believe that they can shift their focus away from their pain—because they have done it.

HOW DOES IT EASE PAIN?

Hypnosis actually has a fairly good and long track record when it comes to pain relief of all sorts, including chronic pain and cancer pain, says Jose R. Maldonado, M.D., assistant professor and medical director of consultation/liaison service for the department of psychiatry and behavioral sciences at Stanford University School of Medicine. In fact, a National Institutes of Health technology assessment panel found strong clinical evidence for the use of hypnosis in alleviating cancer pain.

In one study, a 10-year follow-up of 86 people with cancer, those who received self-hypnosis training along with group therapy had 50 percent less pain and survived 1½ years longer than did those who had routine medical care.

Because it helps people put aside their conscious awareness of things they would ordinarily be focusing on, hypnosis can help reduce pain and anxiety during medical and dental procedures, Dr. Maldonado says. In one study, self-hypnosis was taught to half of a group of people who were undergoing invasive medical procedures such as cardiac catheterization. Everyone was given access to extra medication if they wanted it. Those who were taught self-hypnosis used a fraction of the medication used by those who weren't taught hypnosis. And yet they had significantly less pain, less anxiety, and less instability of their heart rates and blood pressures, and they got out of the recovery room sooner than those who were not taught self-hypnosis.

"There are two components to pain: the physical sensation itself and the amount of attention you pay to it," Dr. Maldonado says. "And you can think of the brain as kind of an amplifier. It gets turned down when your attention is focused on other competing thoughts." Hypnosis is very good at reducing the amount of attention your brain pays to the stimulus of pain. "You literally hurt less," he says

After training in self-hypnosis, you learn to condition your response to pain, explains Dr. Maldonado. Instead of the usual reactions to pain, perhaps tensing up and focusing on your pain, you learn to modify your body's reactions. "Self-hypnosis allows for dissociation, or distancing, from the painful stimulus," he says. "Thus, your body remains comfortably relaxed. Highly hypnotizable individuals may master self-hypnotic techniques to the point of being able to enjoy their everyday activities without discomfort or only with minimal discomfort." With practice, patients may learn to use self-hypnotic techniques to create alternative sensations or mind states rather than pain.

How Is It Done?

Hypnosis has been called effortless experiencing, and the nice thing about hypnosis is that you don't have to try very hard to notice some results, Dr. Maldonado says.

Every practitioner has his own way of inducing a hypnotic state, and the steps often vary for each client. "It's difficult to explain in all its complexities without experiencing it yourself," Lankton says. "You certainly can't lull yourself off into pain-free land simply by saying, 'I feel no pain. . . . I feel no pain.'"

You first learn a few things with the aid of the hypnotist, then you do it on your own. "I also tell people that they will respond only to suggestions that are relevant to them, or if they hear something they can use by modifying, then they modify it," Lankton says. "The intent is that they use suggestions in the sessions to come up with a technique that works for them."

Some hypnotists initially help their patients induce a state of body-wide relaxation by helping them feel very light and buoyant. Others, such as Lankton, initially induce a state of heightened internal awareness, coupled with a pleasant feeling, sensations that are incompatible with feeling pain. "I ask people to try to find the pleasant little pulsations that go on all the time, all over their bodies," he says. Once they can find the pulsations in their fingertips, he asks them to extend the sensations up their fingers, into their hands, arms, shoulders, chest, head, and ultimately their whole bodies.

When your brain is processing this pleasant whole-body sensation, "you have kind of a bulletproof vest, so that any pain signals trying to get to the brain dissipate," Lankton says.

Once that's done, Lankton asks patients to focus their attention on the spots where they thought the pain sensations *were* going to be. "I am very careful about the use of my verbs at this point. I don't want to say, 'Go where the pain *is*,' because I want them to be making the connection that the sensation they are feeling no longer is pain. I want them to hold on to the pleasant sensation that they were able to extend throughout their bodies and now use it as a kind of sensory 'filter' to filter the hurt out of the pain." Other people may learn to use warmth, coolness, tingling, or numbness as a way to "filter the hurt out of the pain."

WHAT DOES IT FEEL LIKE?

When you watch a movie that has your total attention, you are, in effect, in a trance. That's what hypnosis is like. You feel focused and free of distractions. But you also often experience time distortions and amnesia, Lankton says. "Some people feel like nothing happened, but they also wonder what they were doing for 40 minutes."

WHAT RESULTS CAN YOU EXPECT?

Most people can be hypnotized and realize during their first session that they can reduce their pain, Lankton says. "So they are really very excited about the possibility that it works." Lankton asks them to put in ½ hour a day using the pulsation-sensing exercise to induce a state of self-hypnosis. "The induction exercise stimulates the whole process because it is all hooked together. It's like a special song that gives you the feeling of being there and recreates a whole mental environment," he says. So even though people may not ever understand the mechanics of the process, they can do it.

About half the people who try can do self-hypnosis at home after one session, but even they and most others need three to five sessions to really get it down right, Lankton says. Some rare people have instant pain relief after one session and have no further need for hypnosis, and a few people just never do get it.

Hypnosis should reduce your need for medications, even for bad pain, Dr. Maldonado says. "Here, we tell people, try the hypnosis first, and if it works for you,

fine. If it doesn't work, then we'll use drugs." People who are taking morphine or other sedating drugs have great difficulty using hypnosis, he says. "The two are not compatible, so sometimes you have to make a choice."

WHO'S QUALIFIED TO DO IT?

In most states, anyone can set himself up as a hypnotist, so it's best to look for one who is licensed in your state, Lankton says. To be licensed, a hypnotist must have an M.D., a Ph.D., or a master's degree in psychology or social work from an accredited university, and must have training in hypnosis. Two societies offer free lists of appropriate hypnotists: the Society for Clinical and Experimental Hypnosis, 2201 Haeder Road, Suite 1, Pullman, WA 99163-8619; and the American Society of Clinical Hypnosis, 2200 East Devon Avenue, Suite 291, Des Plaines, IL 60018-4534.

WHAT DOES IT COST?

Hypnosis costs from $100 to $150 a session and is usually covered by medical insurance and workers' compensation.

Massage

Massage is a form of healing and relaxation that has been around for centuries. It's officially defined as "the systematic and purposeful manipulation of the soft tissues of the body," which include muscles, connective tissues, even organs—just about everything but bone, says Janet Kahn, Ph.D., a licensed massage therapist and senior research scientist at Wellsley College Center for Research on Women in Takoma Park, Maryland.

The manipulation can include gentle and stimulating motions: kneading, pressing, rubbing, rolling, tapping, featherlight stroking, even just touch—the laying on of hands, if you will.

There are many different schools or traditions of massage: Swedish, Shiatsu (meaning "finger pressure"), and sports massage, just to name some of the more popular types.

"Most massage therapists pick and choose from a variety of forms during a session, depending on their clients' needs and preferences," Dr. Kahn says. Massage has proven benefits for people with arthritis, fibromyalgia, chronic fatigue syndrome, back pain, diabetes, cancer, high blood pressure, and carpal tunnel syndrome.

HOW DOES IT EASE PAIN?

Massage, even just simple touch, can produce a relaxation response in the body, Dr. Kahn says. "And when people relax, they experience less pain."

A study of people with fibromyalgia, done by the Touch Research Institute at the University of Miami School of Medicine, found that people with fibromyalgia who got 30 minutes of massage two times a week for 5 weeks had less anxiety and lower levels of stress hormones. Over time, they reported less pain and stiffness, less fatigue and depression, and less trouble sleeping.

Other studies have shown that massage can reduce stress hormone levels, reduce anxiety, even increase the number of immune cells circulating in the bloodstreams of patients with HIV.

Massage can also act as a mechanical cleaner, hastening the elimination of waste and toxic debris, such as lactic acid and uric acid, that are stored in your muscles, especially after exercise, Dr. Kahn says. "If you get a massage soon after your workout, your muscles get less achy and stiff," she adds.

A specific form of gentle massage called manual lymph drainage is used to help reduce swelling, especially swelling that occurs in a woman's arm if lymph nodes are removed during surgery for breast cancer, says Arline Reinking-Hanf, R.N., a massage therapist for the Complementary Care Service Center at the New York Presbyterian Hospital in New York City.

Massage can also improve range of motion in joints and help seniors regain a sense of balance, Dr. Kahn says.

And massage can improve the quality of your sleep, studies confirm. "A back rub before bedtime used to be standard care for hospital patients, and it really did help people to relax and sleep better," Reinking-Hanf says. Massage can be especially helpful for older people, who might have trouble falling asleep or staying asleep and who often become confused and disoriented if they take sleeping pills. "Simply massaging their feet and hands upon waking up or when agitated can be a good way to help them fall back to sleep," she says.

How Is It Done?

Initially, your massage therapist should ask you some questions, including whether this is your first massage, what your reasons are for wanting a massage, and if you have any health problems.

Then, you'll be asked to take off whatever clothes you feel comfortable removing and to climb under a sheet or large towel draped over a comfortable, padded massage table. If you're getting shiatsu, you

(continued on page 131)

RUBBING OUT PAIN

While it's pure luxury to have professional pampering, there's something to be said for massaging yourself. For one thing, it's always instantly available, and you know exactly where it hurts—and what feels good. Here are some ways to get started.

Head and face #1. Place the inner sides of your thumbs against the bony socket surrounding your eyes, by the bridge of your nose. Put your forefingers on top of the edge of the socket, on your eyebrow. Lightly press against the bone with your thumbs, holding for 5 to 10 seconds. Release the pressure and move your fingers a bit, slowly working your way to the outside corner of the socket. Don't drag your fingers along the skin around your eyes.

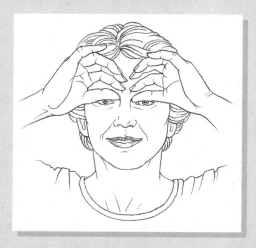

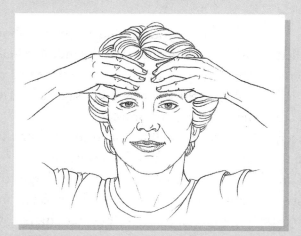

Head and face #2. Place all your fingers together in two side-by-side vertical lines on the middle of your forehead, letting your thumbs rest on your temples. Press lightly with your fingers for 5 to 10 seconds and release. Move your fingers about 1 inch apart and repeat. Continue until you cover your entire forehead. Don't press too hard.

Head and face #3. Place your middle fingers on your temples and your thumbs on your jawbone for support. Gently massage your temples on both sides of your head by rotating your middle fingers upward and backward, away from your eyes, for 15 seconds. Use the same movement to massage just above your ears on either side of your head. You can also massage your jaws and around your ears this way.

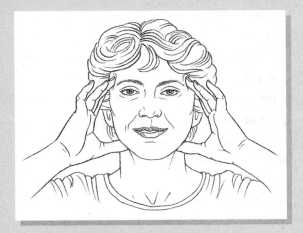

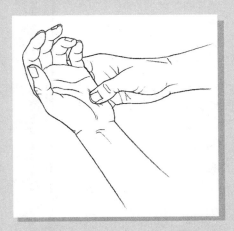

Hands. Press with your right thumb into the lower part of the palm of your left hand, in line with your little finger, making small rotations with firm pressure. Then, going clockwise, use your thumb to massage around your palm in a circle. When you reach the top of your palm, concentrate on the fleshy spaces in between the bones. Repeat on your right hand.

(continued)

RUBBING OUT PAIN—CONTINUED

Back. Sit on a sturdy straight-back, armless chair with your feet more than shoulder-width apart. Put a tennis ball in the toe end of a long sock. Hold the sock by the other end and, reaching over your shoulder, drop the tennis ball between your back and the chair. Position the ball to the side of your spine. Pull up and down on the sock to work it up and down your back. Then reposition the ball to work the other side of your spine.

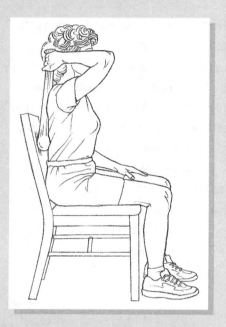

Feet. Sitting on a sturdy armless chair, rest your right ankle on your left thigh, and with lengthwise or circular motions, use your thumbs to work all over the sole of your foot. Then massage all across the top of your foot with your thumbs, working from your ankle down to your toes and up the side of your foot, from your big toe to your inner ankle. Repeat on your left foot.

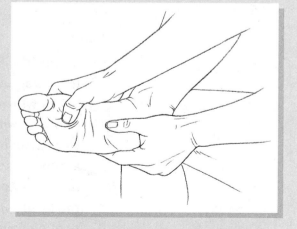

might not remove any clothes, and you may be asked to lie on a mat on the floor. Proper massage etiquette requires that only the part of your body being massaged be exposed. Most therapists use oil or lotion. They may start anywhere on your body, but they are more likely to start on your back, head, or feet. They may work over your whole body or may concentrate on certain parts, depending on what you want. "It's important to communicate with your massage therapist about what you want and what feels good or bad," Dr. Kahn says.

A typical session may last 45 minutes to an hour. People who are very frail or sick, though, may do better with shorter, more frequent sessions of 20 to 30 minutes, Dr. Kahn says.

WHAT DOES IT FEEL LIKE?

Most forms of massage are extremely pleasant and relaxing. Sometimes, a massage therapist will apply pressure over a knotted muscle and produce what is called good pain, which quickly fades as the muscle relaxes. But older people, and especially people who are frail or immobilized, don't need this deeper kind of work, Dr. Kahn says. During your massage, you should feel calm and nurtured. Afterward, you should feel calm and energized.

WHAT RESULTS CAN YOU EXPECT?

One massage session may reduce your pain for a few hours or days, and regular massage sessions may help keep certain types of pain at bay for long periods of time and even improve your ability to function, Dr. Kahn says. One study conducted by researchers at the Group Health Center for Health Studies and the University of Washington, both in Seattle, and the Center for Alternative Medicine Research in Boston found that people with lower-back pain who got up to 10 massages had less pain and improved ability to function compared with people who got acupuncture or just educational materials after 10 weeks of treatment.

Regular massage sessions should help you feel less stiff and sore after exercise and should help you stay more mobile, with more range of motion in your joints and better balance. Regular massage sessions should also help you to sleep better and, if you are immobile, to be less likely to develop sore spots or tissue breakdown due to impaired circulation, says Dr. Kahn.

WHO'S QUALIFIED TO DO IT?

Roughly 29 states and the District of Columbia regulate massage therapists, and all of those states have a minimum training requirement. To find out if your state has licensing requirements, call your state regulatory office or contact the American Massage Therapy Association (AMTA) at 820 Davis Street, Suite 100, Evanston, IL 60201-4400. This organization can also provide the names of AMTA members near you.

Massage therapists can also be nationally certified. As a member of AMTA, a massage therapist has a minimum of 500 hours of training (from a school accredited by the Commission on Massage Therapy Accreditation or a member of the AMTA Council of Schools), plus continuing education, and carries malpractice liability insurance.

WHAT DOES IT COST?

Self-massage is free. For a professional massage, prices range from $45 to $100-plus for a 60-minute session. Prices are higher in urban areas and on the East and West coasts, lower in the rural Midwest.

Meditation

In Sanskrit, the language of the culture that originated meditation, the word for the practice is *bhavana*, which means "being" or "becoming." That meaning reflects the purpose of meditation—to become more aware of yourself, observing thoughts and feelings, seeing what is really going on in your mind.

There are many different forms of meditation. Some of them involve sitting still, sometimes for hours. Some involve walking, chanting, yoga poses, or breathing exercises. Some involve repeating a phrase, or mantra, or focusing on an object such as a flower or flame. Every religion has some form of meditative practice—even Judaism and Catholicism.

What does all this have to do with the fact that you hurt? "Painful experience is given meaning and value in meditative traditions," says Joseph Loizzo, M.D., Ph.D., director of the Center for Meditation and Healing at Columbia-Presbyterian Medical Center in New York City. "It is thought that from pain one can learn and change and grow, and that it can be used as an opportunity and a motivation to learn to gain more understanding and control of your mind." The potential benefit of that mind control is less pain.

A form of meditation popular in the United States and proved effective for pain and stress management is called mindfulness meditation. The heart of Buddhist meditation, mindfulness meditation is also the base for many other forms of meditation. It's taught at the Center for Mindfulness in Medicine, Health Care, and Society at the University of Massachusetts Medical Center in Amherst, directed by Jon Kabat-Zinn, Ph.D. Meditation teachers trained at the center teach at about 200 places in the United States, including dozens of multi-disciplinary pain centers.

"Meditation is really about paying attention," says Dr. Kabat-Zinn. "And that's all it is: paying attention to what is happening in your mind and body." Mindfulness meditation, he adds, "is a particular way of paying attention in the present moment, intentionally and without judging."

HOW DOES IT EASE PAIN?

Meditation works at several different levels, says Patrick Randolph, Ph.D., director of psychological services at Texas Tech University Medical Center in Lubbock. "You start to watch your thoughts and feelings and start to realize that you're actually inflaming the sensation—the 'real' pain, so to speak—by your thoughts and feelings about it. The thoughts and feelings are your reactions to the pain, and they are something you can control. So you learn to separate the pain sensations themselves from your reactions to the pain. And you can modify those reactions."

Instead of trying to distract yourself from your pain or running away from it, "we are actually suggesting that people bring mindfulness to the body," Dr. Kabat-Zinn says. That might seem counterintuitive, he says, but "in laboratory studies, results show that up to a certain point, as the pain gets more intense, distraction is a good strategy. But beyond a certain point, attention actually becomes a more powerful strategy for managing pain."

"When we develop the capacity for being with our pain as it is, the threat of pain becomes lessened, which decreases the sympathetic (automatic) nervous system response to it," Dr. Randolph says. "Whenever the sympathetic nervous system is turned on, it is like a switch to pain. It actually increases the subjective perception of pain. So reducing its reaction is very useful in pain management." Reducing stress also decreases blood pressure and muscle tension and may improve bloodflow in the body. All those things can help reduce pain.

HOW IS IT DONE?

There are many different ways to get to the same point in meditation, Dr. Loizzo says. "And they all involve using your mind to change the way you experience things and to change the way your body is working. They are all self-healing or self-regulating, and they all involve paying attention to what might otherwise be automatic processes."

In mindfulness meditation, people may start out focusing on their breath, or they may start by focusing on eating, Dr. Kabat-Zinn says. "Sometimes, we give people a raisin to eat and spend 10 minutes eating it, so we really begin to see how little we pay attention in our daily lives to anything. During this exercise, you see that you can shift the level of awareness that you bring to the raisin in your mouth."

Simply pay attention and bring your attention back again and again as needed, being with whatever is happening in the present moment as best you can, nonjudgmentally. That's meditating.

WHAT DOES IT FEEL LIKE?

Every time you meditate can feel different. You can feel frustrated, impatient, calm, alert, and often, you go through all of these feelings during a meditation session.

"The most important feeling is that you are present and paying attention," Dr.

Loizzo says. "It's a kind of alert, clear relaxation." You are paying attention to what is really going on—at the same time, you're maintaining a certain level of calm and relaxation. Over time, this state becomes one that you spend more time in, even when you're not meditating.

WHAT RESULTS CAN YOU EXPECT?

You may not expect meditation to have a lot of proof to back it up, but in fact, Dr. Kabat-Zinn says, "people do get results, and we spend a lot of our time documenting them and publishing them." In one study of people treated at the University of Massachusetts Pain Clinic, he compared patients who received meditation training as adjunct treatment to those who received regular medical treatment. The meditators were able to use less pain medication and said their pain was much less likely to stop them from doing things as compared with the nonmeditators. The people who meditated also reported less anxiety and depression. Most of the meditators said that they considered the meditation a very significant component of pain control.

In another study, people with psoriasis who meditated while undergoing ultraviolet light treatment cleared up their skin about four times faster than nonmeditators. "So we showed that the mind can influence a healing process and speed it up," Dr. Kabat Zinn says.

WHO'S QUALIFIED TO DO IT?

Most people can learn to meditate, but they need instruction to learn the skill. At some multidisciplinary pain centers, meditation is taught as part of an 8-week program that includes weekly 2-hour classes, daily ½-hour practice, and a daylong retreat toward the end of the program. People can also learn from tapes.

You don't have to believe that your pain has meaning to benefit from meditation, Dr. Loizzo says. "But, instead of trying to kill and fight the pain, you have to be willing to experience it objectively, without distress or judgment, and to see whether that changes the quality of the pain, which, in fact, it does. It is very a dramatic response."

To learn meditation for pain relief, you can contact the Center for Mindfulness in Medicine, Health Care, and Society at the University of Massachusetts Medical Center, 55 Lake Avenue North, Worcester,

MA 01655-0267. They can give you a free referral to a mindfulness-based stress-reduction teacher near you. Or call a nearby chronic pain center, teaching hospital, or yoga center. "A good teacher makes a big difference," Dr. Loizzo says.

If you can't find one, Dr. Kabat-Zinn offers instructional tapes that you can obtain by contacting the Center for Mindfulness in Medicine, Health Care, and Society.

WHAT DOES IT COST?

At the University of Massachusetts Medical Center, meditation costs about $670 for a 10-week program that has 28 hours of contact time. At other places, the cost is about the same as seeing a psychologist, generally from $60 to $80 an hour. Health insurance is most likely to pay for instruction in meditation if you go to a multidisciplinary pain center and if you have a medical diagnosis. Your pastor or rabbi may also be able to point you in the right direction for free instruction in the meditative practices associated with your religion.

Music

We all know how certain pieces of music affect us. One melody may help us relax and drift off to sleep, another has us tapping our feet and feeling energized, while yet another moves us to tears. Music therapy takes advantage of music's ability to affect us physically, emotionally, and spiritually and uses it to promote healing, reduce stress and anxiety, and promote an overall sense of well-being.

How Does It Ease Pain?

"Stress is a large component of pain, so simply being able to relax can do a lot to reduce pain," says Joanne Loewy, M.T.-B.C. (board-certified music therapist), director of music therapy at Beth Israel Medical Center in New York City and editor of the book *Music Therapy and Pediatric Pain*. And music can induce relaxation, resulting in lower heart rate and blood pressure levels, slower breathing, reduced muscle tension, and increased production of endorphins, the body's own feel-good chemicals, she says.

Music also has the ability to coax out emotions, allowing people to express anger, fear, joy, and sorrow, Loewy says. "Expressing emotions helps to reduce the psychological discomfort that is a part of many health problems." Music also has the ability to stir long-lost recollections and can spur new levels of awareness.

Certain kinds of music also transmit vibrations through the air and into objects. Witness the opera singer shattering a crystal goblet with her high C. Some music therapists use this vibrational quality to help "break up" areas of muscle tension and pain in the body. They may use large gongs, chimes, or tone bars, which vibrate strongly.

Music with a clear, pronounced beat, such as marching music, can stimulate and arouse the motor system, says Michael Thaut, Ph.D., professor of music and bio-medical engineering at Colorado State University in Fort Collins. While that might help soldiers keep moving long after they would have otherwise pooped out, in terms of music therapy it also helps people who have trouble walking because of strokes or motor-skill conditions like Parkinson's disease. The strong rhythm of marching music, he says, "helps the brain to control and stabilize—and, if necessary, speed up—the movements of walking." In Dr. Thaut's studies, virtually everyone who used strong rhythmical music as part of their physical therapy programs improved their walking speeds and stability, in some cases by as much as 50 percent.

Research confirms music's usefulness in reducing anxiety and pain. In one study, music helped burn victims experience less pain while undergoing debridement, an excruciating procedure that involves removing damaged skin until healthy tissue is exposed. And another study found that half of the women who went through a program of music therapy–assisted child-birth needed no medication during labor and delivery.

How Is It Done?

You're feeling like a complete slug, so you crank up a jazzy number on the radio to get you moving. Well, music therapy is a more refined version of the same process. It includes an initial assessment that covers your musical likes and dislikes; it takes into consideration your age, ethnic background, level of pain, and need for medications; and it sets goals for what is to be achieved.

It may be done one-on-one or in a group. You may simply listen to music, and the therapist may help you focus your attention on a particular instrument at a time. You may participate in creating the music, playing an instrument, singing, improvising, or even writing lyrics. You may move with the music or use the music as a means of learning relaxation techniques such as imagery or progressive muscle relaxation, which also help reduce pain.

"We might just ask someone to tone, to vocalize as loud as he can, an 'Ahhh,'" Loewy says. "There might be so much anger attached to this pain that he just needs to release." The music therapist may also use African drumming techniques "to pull all the tension out" or use Suzuki Tone Bars, long-resonating chimes, along with breathing techniques to help people breathe easier and reduce anxiety and muscle tension.

One axiom of music therapy is that people respond best to music they like, says Paul Nolan, M.T.-B.C. (board-certified music therapist), associate professor of mental health sciences and director of music therapy education at MCP–Hahnemann University in Philadelphia. "One study even found that heavy metal music was relaxing to the people who preferred it," he says. "So some people can use rock and roll to relax, absolutely."

What Does It Feel Like?

Music can be anything from a pleasant distraction to transportation into a world of your own. And music helps you express your emotions—positive or negative—in a way you couldn't otherwise, Loewy says.

What Results Can You Expect?

You should expect to feel less pain and anxiety. You should expect the pain to have less impact on your life and your ability to function.

Who's Qualified to Do It?

Many music therapists are certified, which means they have degrees in music therapy, supervised clinical experience, and have passed a national certifying exam. For a referral to a qualified music therapist, write to the American Music Therapy Association, 8455 Colesville Road, Suite 1000, Silver Spring, MD 20910-3392.

What Does It Cost?

Music therapy costs an average of $40 to $50 a session. Medical insurance will sometimes cover costs, so it's best to check with your insurer.

Physical Therapy

Physical therapy is really a catchall term to describe the many treatments you might do in a clinic with a licensed physical therapist or at home by yourself. These include the uses of heat and cold, mobilization (which is the movement of a joint to relieve pain) and massage, whirlpools and stretching, ultrasound and electrical stimulation, aerobic exercise, and strength training.

Physical therapists may also educate you in ways to avoid pain, showing you a more ergonomic way to lift, recommending a brace or device to assist movement, or designing a daily program of exercise.

Perhaps the most important thing you may gain from physical therapy, however, is a sense that it's up to you to manage your own pain, says Patti Winchester, P.T., Ph.D., a physical therapist and chairperson of the department of physical therapy at the University of Texas Southwestern Medical Center at Dallas. Because once all the evaluations, therapies, and recommendations in the clinic are complete, you're really left on your own.

"The work we do in a clinic may get the pain under control," she says. "Then, my challenge is to teach people exercises and positioning they can do at home or at work to avoid pain and injury."

HOW DOES IT EASE PAIN?

Exercise is the cornerstone of physical therapy, but initially some people may be in too much pain to exercise, says Karen Mohr, P.T., a physical therapist and research director at the Kerlan-Jobe Orthopaedic Clinic in Los Angeles.

The first step is addressing the pain. This is done in a number of ways. The therapist may use hydrotherapy, getting the patients into a warm pool of water where the buoyancy and heat relieve stiffness and stress on the joints. Hot packs and ultrasound can warm up deep tissues and reduce inflammation. Cold packs may interrupt the cycle of muscle spasms. A therapist also may use electrical stimulation to block pain signals or may do mobilization and massage to relieve back pain.

Depending on your problem, the therapist may use several of these modalities in combination, says Dr. Winchester. "There are no panaceas for pain. You never use just one approach. You do what works, and then follow up with the appropriate exercise and positioning."

How Is It Done?

When you first visit a physical therapist, you will go through a physical evaluation and a personal interview. The therapist wants to know not only where it hurts but also what activities cause your pain.

The therapist will look at the function and strength of your muscles and skeletal system. He might observe how you get out of a chair and the way you walk. He might ask, "Can you reach around and remove your wallet from your back pocket?" Or "Can you unhook your bra by yourself?" Or "Can you walk up a staircase?"

During the interview, a therapist asks questions designed to set some goals for recovery, says Mohr. For example: "What would you like to do that you can't do today because of your limitations?" A very active 70-year-old may want to be able to play golf every other day without pain. Another person may want nothing more than to be able to go shopping at the grocery store and to walk across the parking lot without assistance, she says. Because goals are very individual, the therapies and exercises for each patient will differ.

"My job is to put together individual programs that will help them reach their goals," says Mohr. "It may be that they want to be able to walk up and down stairs without pain—not run a road race."

What Does It Feel Like?

Physical therapy requires active participation from the patient, so be prepared to do some work during your clinical sessions.

Typically, a patient will be scheduled for two or three visits per week for perhaps a 4- to 6-week period. It really depends on your injury or condition, but under managed-care insurance, most people get only a few visits. Then you're on your own at home.

That may be enough time, however, for a therapist to teach you an exercise program, demonstrate how to use an electronic nerve-stimulating pain-blocking machine, or give you the motivation to join a water aerobics class down at the YMCA.

If you haven't been physically active for some time, you may consider exercise therapy a cure worse than the disease or pain. But the therapist's goal is to make you better, and in time, exercise may reduce inflammation, ease your pain, and very likely, build up muscles. Weak muscles are often at the heart of many pain syndromes, particularly osteoarthritis, says Mohr.

Many older people have lost much of the cartilage that works as a shock absorber in their joints, and their bones virtually rub together. Stronger muscles, however, act as shock absorbers and take up some of the shock once mitigated by cartilage. If you've been inactive physically, your muscles aren't giving your joints much support, says Mohr.

What Results Can You Expect?

Research and personal experiences show that the multiple methods and therapies used by physical therapists do help with a wide range of pain.

Research at the University of Minnesota in Minneapolis found that physical therapy may play a significant role in the reduction of pain in many injuries and chronic orthopedic problems, including rotator cuff injury, lower-back pain, knee pain, neck pain, and sacroiliac pain. Sometimes, patients did not show much improvement in function after physical therapy, but most experienced a reduction in pain between the initial assessment of the injury and discharge from physical therapy.

Who's Qualified to Do It?

Physical therapists go through rigorous training programs to become certified, as do chiropractors, osteopathic physicians, and other doctors who use or recommend physical therapy. In some states, patients can seek out physical therapy on their own, but most people see a doctor first. Usually, insurance companies and HMOs require that you be referred by a physician.

Seeing a doctor first is a good idea, especially if your ache is something new and not an old injury or a familiar ache, says Robert Kennedy, M.D., director of geriatric medicine at Maimonides Medical Center in Brooklyn, New York. "You need to find out why you're having this pain in the first place. Pain is a symptom, and the underlying cause of pain needs to be determined, especially if the pain is severe or new. A good diagnosis and perhaps some tests by a physician will do that."

WHAT DOES IT COST?

The cost of a short course of clinical outpatient physical therapy is almost always covered by insurance, workers' compensation, and Medicare. The kinds of exercises and advice gleaned from a therapist may be invaluable in your own efforts to manage pain.

Prayer

No one knows where or when prayer began, but it likely was the world's first pain reliever.

"Early man probably had little else he could turn to for relieving pain, so rituals and prayers were essentially medicine," says Harold Koenig, M.D., associate professor of psychiatry and behavioral sciences at Duke University Medical Center in Durham, North Carolina, and author of *Is Religion Good for Your Health?* "People prayed. That was their only alternative."

In many ancient cultures, pain was considered to be a punishment from the gods. In fact, the word *pain* is derived from the Latin *poena*, which means punishment. So it wasn't uncommon for priests, sorceresses, and medicine men to use charms and other religious sacraments to ward off pain. Prayers, exorcisms, and incantations for the relief of pain, for instance, have been found on clay tablets dating back to the ancient Babylonians, at least 12 centuries before the birth of Christ.

To this day, prayer has a fundamental role in spiritual and physical healing in virtually every religion in the world, says the Reverend Ralph Ciampa, director of pastoral care at the University of Pennsylvania Health System in Philadelphia. So no matter if you are Christian, Jewish, Muslim, Buddhist, or a follower of one the world's other faiths, prayer is likely to be at the core of your beliefs.

In the United States alone, there are more than 500,000 churches, temples, and other places of worship, representing more than 2,000 denominations, according to the Princeton Religion Research Center in New Jersey. Nine out of every 10 Americans say that they pray regularly, and more than 50 percent say they do it daily. About 75 percent of us pray to a supreme being, such as God.

"Prayer really does mean different things to different people. It can be individual, communal, private, or public. It may be offered in words, sighs, gestures, or silence. But it does have to come from the heart and must be sincere," says Larry Dossey, M.D., executive editor of the bimonthly journal *Alternative Therapies* and author of *Prayer Is Good Medicine*. "I prefer this broad definition: 'Prayer is a communication with the Absolute.' That's a definition that affirms religious tolerance, and it invites people to define what for themselves is 'communication' and who or what 'the Absolute' may be."

How Does It Ease Pain?

Researchers are still sorting out exactly how prayer helps relieve pain, but even Hippocrates, the father of medicine, acknowledged its effectiveness when he wrote, "Divine is the work to subdue pain."

"In medicine, we often know something works long before we understand how. So I would urge people not to dismiss the power of prayer just because we don't have the explanation for it yet," Dr. Dossey says. "Religious devotion, which almost always includes prayer, is associated with lowered incidence of practically every disease that has been examined. Many of these diseases are painful, so it is not a stretch to view prayer as a potent tool in preventing pain."

In fact, evidence from many studies suggests that prayer can have effects on nearly every system in the body, presumably including the parts of the brain that regulate pain, Dr. Koenig says. "Prayer affects your mental state, your physiological being, and many of the senses. And for all of those reasons, it can have a powerful impact on how you think and feel."

Physically, prayer's effects on the body are similar to those of relaxation techniques. Studies have shown that it can elevate your mood, lower your blood pressure and heart rate, and relieve muscle tension, all of which can help diminish your perception of pain, Dr. Koenig says. Psychologically, prayer eases anxiety, depression, and other emotions that can intensify pain.

"People pray to God for help and strength," Dr. Koenig says. "This belief that God is listening to you and cares about you can give you a sense of control that can help relieve much of the suffering and anguish that pain causes."

THE FAITH FACTOR

Nobel Prize–winning physicist Albert Einstein found common ground between science and prayer. "Science without religion is lame," he once said. "Religion without science is blind."

And now, nearly a half-century after his death, medical researchers are discovering he was right. In fact, far from being incompatible, science and religion can be a potent one-two punch in your effort to relieve pain, says Herbert Benson, M.D., associate professor of medicine at Harvard Medical School and president of the Mind/Body Medical Institute in Boston.

Researchers have discovered that prayer and scientifically based mind/body techniques have similar effects on the body. Doing any such technique can elicit the relaxation response, an altered physical and emotional state that can lower blood pressure, relieve muscle tension, curb anxiety, and trigger other physiological changes that can diminish your perception of pain, Dr. Benson says.

But if you are religious and pray to elicit the relaxation response, you may enhance these physiological changes and dampen your pain even further, Dr. Benson says. He calls this combination the faith factor.

HOW IS IT DONE?

Prayer can be done in all the ways you can imagine—standing, kneeling, bowing, crouching, or lying down. Your hands can be raised, outstretched, folded, crossed, or clasped. Prayer also has many voices. It can be "Lord, Jesus Christ, relieve my misery,"

When you're in pain, he suggests practicing the following technique for 10 to 20 minutes twice a day.

1. Sit in a comfortable position with your eyes closed. Relax your muscles, starting in your toes and progressing upward through your body. Stretch and relax your hands and arms. Gently roll your head from side to side. Shrug and relax your shoulders.

2. As you slowly inhale and exhale, begin to focus your mind on your breathing. Each time you breathe, silently repeat the same word or phrase. A neutral word like *peace* or *love* will work fine. But to trigger the faith factor, try choosing a word or short phrase that reflects your personal beliefs. Christians, for instance, might choose a phrase such as "I am the way, the truth, and the life." If you are Jewish, perhaps "Shalom," "*Echod*," or reciting a line from a psalm will help you. Try "*Inshallah*" if you're Muslim.

3. Don't fret if your thoughts wander or worries pop into your head. Simply let them drift away as you refocus your attention on your repetitive word or phrase. Disregard judgmental questions like "Am I doing this right?" or "Is it working?" Just go with the flow and let it happen. Don't force yourself to relax; it will happen naturally. As you do relax and the faith factor kicks in, you could notice that your pain is ebbing and find yourself feeling more spiritual.

"Hail Mary, full of grace," "*Sh'ma Yisrael*," "*Inshallah*," or just a simple "Om." It can be shouted from the rooftops, sung in a hymn, or spoken silently to yourself. It can be used to thank a deity, speak with a supernatural power, or make a direct appeal to the universe, Dr. Dossey says.

But no matter the language or religion,

most prayers fit into four basic categories, according to Dale Matthews, M.D., associate professor of medicine at Georgetown University School of Medicine in Washington, D.C., and author of *The Faith Factor*. Here are the categories, developed by sociologist Margaret Poloma.

Colloquial prayer: speaking with God as if you were talking with your best friend in an informal, intimate way

Petitional prayer: asking God for specific things for yourself by making requests such as "Please, God, ease my pain"

Ritual prayer: a more formal, structured invocation or rite such as a rosary, the Lord's Prayer, or a prayer from a prayer book

Meditative or contemplative prayer: spending time just quietly thinking about God or the universe, or reflecting upon the teachings of your faith

The type of prayer that works best varies from person to person. But more than likely when you are in intense pain, a prayer of some type will naturally seep out, Reverend Ciampa says.

"There is no one right way to pray," Reverend Ciampa says. "When people cry out in pain, they're not thinking about which is the best prayer to pray. They're just doing a natural human thing. They're in pain, and they're praying for relief. And sometimes, people experience relief when they do that."

When you are in pain, pray as often as needed to ease your suffering. But at the very least, Dr. Dossey suggests praying when you first awaken each day. "That's a great way to start your day," he says. "Give thanks in your own way for a pain-free night and pray for the best of days ahead."

WHAT DOES IT FEEL LIKE?

If you've prayed seldom or never, you'll likely feel awkward at first. But the more you try it, you'll notice the same effects felt by people who've prayed all their lives. As you pray, you will likely feel a sense of calm, peace, and serenity envelop you, Reverend Ciampa says. Eventually, you'll feel a sense of comfort, an easing of your burden—and an easing of your pain.

Reflexology

Reflexology is a technique of pressure-point therapy used on the feet, and sometimes on the hands or ears, to affect your entire body. The practice of working these areas of your body to affect other parts of your body is not new—it's been done for centuries. But the specific technique of reflexology is relatively new.

It was developed in the 1930s by an American woman, Eunice Ingham, who went on to write the book *Stories the Feet Can Tell*. Ingham taped cotton balls to people's feet, then had them walk around with the cotton balls in place, creating pressure, to determine if certain parts of the feet seemed to have some sort of connection with other parts of the body. She found that they did. Pressing the big toes seemed to affect the head and brain, for instance, while pressing the arches of the feet seemed to affect the lower back. A similar theory about such connections exists in oriental medicine.

It may sound incredible, but some studies bear out the effects of this practice. Zang-Hee Cho, Ph.D., a pioneer researcher in brain imaging, did a brain scan on a man while a point on the man's small toe was stimulated by an acupuncture needle. The point is traditionally selected for vision problems. Dr. Cho, professor in the department of radiology at the University of California, Irvine, found that when the toe point was stimulated, the part of the man's brain called the visual cortex "lit up just as it would if you had shone a light in his eyes."

149

GAINING A FOOTHOLD ON PAIN

This reflexology "road map" of your feet will help orient you on your way to better health. This hands-on healing method postulates that certain areas of the feet correspond to organs in the body.

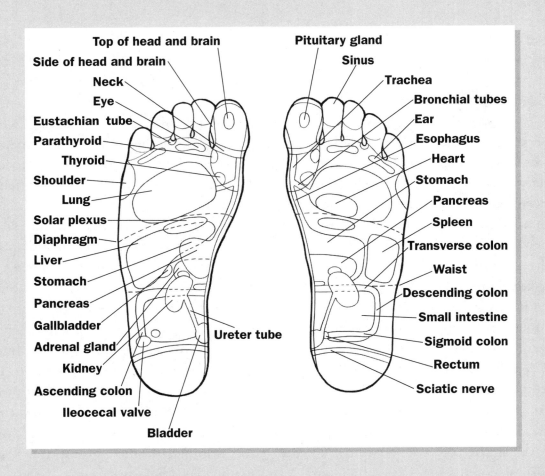

Top of head and brain
Side of head and brain
Neck
Eye
Eustachian tube
Parathyroid
Thyroid
Shoulder
Lung
Solar plexus
Diaphragm
Liver
Stomach
Pancreas
Gallbladder
Adrenal gland
Kidney
Ascending colon
Ileocecal valve
Bladder
Ureter tube

Pituitary gland
Sinus
Trachea
Bronchial tubes
Ear
Esophagus
Heart
Stomach
Pancreas
Spleen
Transverse colon
Waist
Descending colon
Small intestine
Sigmoid colon
Rectum
Sciatic nerve

How Does It Ease Pain?

The theory behind reflexology is that pressing on particular parts of the feet stimulates reflex reactions in the corresponding body parts, which somehow promotes healing and balance in the body, says Terry Oleson, Ph.D., chairperson of the department of psychology and director of behavioral medicine at the California Graduate Institute in Los Angeles. "There's a lot of anecdotal evidence and case reports that it works for conditions all over the body," he says. It's been said to help relieve constipation, dizziness, circulation problems in the legs, even to help people pass kidney stones.

Dr. Oleson and his colleagues have done the only "scientific" study of reflexology to date. The study involved 35 women with symptoms of premenstrual syndrome (PMS). Half the women were treated with reflexology. The others received simple massage. Those who received the reflexology treatments reported a 46 percent reduction in PMS symptoms, compared with 19 percent for the women who simply got massages.

"Some people contend that the only reason reflexology helps people feel better is because it can be relaxing, but this disputes that argument," Dr. Oleson says.

How Is It Done?

You usually lie in a recliner or on your back on a padded massage table, with the reflexologist sitting in front of your clean, bare feet. He'll first do a foot inspection, something that's especially helpful for people with diabetic neuropathy, who sometimes have unnoticed foot problems. Then, he will work over each foot, using his thumbs to press in. "I feel people's feet, and I can tell where knots and blocks are, and I apply gentle pressure until the flow of energy is restored," explains Larry Clemmons, a certified reflexologist practicing in Chicago. As with massage, there are several different types of hand movements that might be used, including "walking" the thumbs along the feet, both gentle and deep pressure, brisk taps, vibrating pressure, and circular rubbing.

No oils or creams are used, except perhaps at the end, when the therapist may finish off with some kneading and sweeping strokes. A session may be as short as 20 minutes, but most are about 45 minutes, Clemmons says.

Most reflexologists also encourage their patients to work their own feet at home between sessions. It's easy enough to do, provided you can reach your feet. If you have trouble with that, you can roll your feet around on a medium-hard rubber ball about the same size as a golf ball, Clemmons says. (A golf ball is a bit too hard for this.) Do this for less than 10 minutes a day.

WHAT DOES IT FEEL LIKE?

Real reflexology looks a lot like massage but is more akin to acupressure, Clemmons says. And since attention is concentrated on the areas that are hard, sensitive, or "blocked," there can be at times so-called good pain, which usually eases quickly and results in a release of blocked or congested energy in the feet or in other areas of the body.

WHAT RESULTS CAN YOU EXPECT?

Practitioners say that you should feel a reduction in pain by the end of your first session, although if you have chronic pain problems, you may need five or six sessions before the pain starts to feel manageable. "You should feel more relaxed by the end of a session, and if you have pain, especially in your legs and feet, it should feel better for at least a few hours," Clemmons

says. Stress reduction is the prime focus of this healing modality. As reflexology relieves stress, your body can gradually rebuild, repair, and regenerate itself. After a session, drink plenty of water and give your body time to heal.

WHO'S QUALIFIED TO DO IT?

Look for someone who is nationally certified. To locate a certified reflexologist in your area, contact the American Reflexology Certification Board, P.O. Box 620607, Littleton, CO 80162-0607; or the International Institute of Reflexology, P.O. Box 12642, St. Petersburg, FL 33733-2642. Include your name, phone number (including area code), city, state, and ZIP code when you make your request.

WHAT DOES IT COST?

Expect to pay $30 to $60 per session. Medical insurance does not usually cover reflexology treatments.

Relaxation Response

The relaxation response isn't a pain-relieving treatment; it is a physiologic response by your body that can be brought about by multiple techniques: prayer, yoga, forms of meditation, self-hypnosis. It's a natural response, something everyone can elicit. It's not mystical or magical, but it's not something you do automatically.

The relaxation response is often paired with a meditation technique of focused concentration and repetition of a neutral word, such as *one*. The term *relaxation response* was coined by Herbert Benson, M.D., president of the Mind/Body Medical Institute at Beth Israel Deaconess Medical Center in Boston, and was popularized in the book *The Relaxation Response* in the 1970s. Dr. Benson explained that most religions and philosophies have some sort of "meditative prescription" that induces the relaxation response, and that all these meditations have two things in common: focusing on a repetitive word, phrase, breath, or object; and disregarding thoughts as they come into your mind.

"They are all attempts to get the mind quiet and focused," says Margaret A. Caudill, M.D., Ph.D., codirector of the department of pain medicine at the Dartmouth-Hitchcock Medical Center in Manchester, New Hampshire, and author of *Managing Pain Before It Manages You*. "It doesn't matter what technique you use, the relaxation response is quite adaptable to various belief systems and practices." In fact, if you are someone who can't sit still, you can incorporate it into exercise. Some forms of yoga do this, as does walking meditation.

HOW DOES IT EASE PAIN?

The relaxation response is the opposite of the stress response. While you're doing it, your metabolism and blood pressure decrease, your muscles relax, and your brain waves are slower.

And it's not just when you're meditating that the benefits exist, Dr. Caudill says. One study done in the 1980s found that after 4 weeks of daily meditation to induce the relaxation response, people seemed to develop some protection against stress. "Their bodies had changed so that it took more adrenaline to raise their heart rates and breathing than it did before they began meditating—and more than it took people who were simply relaxing and reading a book," she says. "That carryover in between sessions is what's responsible for its stress-management benefits."

Pain creates stress, and stress is often a major component of most people's experience with pain, so people can get caught in a vicious cycle, Dr. Caudill says. If muscle tension is a major component of a person's pain, then inducing the relaxation response may help to reduce the pain. "But it's al-ways helpful to people in managing the stress that the pain brings," she says. "Even if people continue to have pain, they start to sleep better, have fewer digestive problems, and feel like they have more control over things."

The relaxation response is often part of other stress-management techniques used for pain. It is especially effective for pain relief used in conjunction with self-hypnosis or visualization, Dr. Caudill says. It is rarely used on its own for the treatment of pain.

HOW IS IT DONE?

If you are practicing Dr. Benson's method of inducing the relaxation response, you might find a quiet spot, sit comfortably, loosen your clothes, close your eyes, and take a few nice relaxing breaths. Then, for about 20 minutes, repeat a word or phrase you have picked to focus your attention on. When your mind wanders, gently bring it back again and again to the focus word or phrase.

Some people use a word or phrase that has religious meaning, such as *shalom*, which in Hebrew means "peace." And there may be a certain advantage in that, Dr. Benson says. "If you're focusing on the words 'The Lord is my shepherd,' repeated over and over again, it's almost impossible to be thinking about credit card bills," he explains. "Religious convictions or life philosophy can enhance the relaxation response. Survey results indicate that a subjective feeling of spirituality is linked to better psychological and physical health."

If you're using some other method of inducing the relaxation response, you'll want to focus on your breath, the cadence of your step as you walk, the ripples in a stream of water, or the flicker of a flame, and again, let your thoughts simply come and go.

WHAT DOES IT FEEL LIKE?

People's initial experience of the relaxation response varies, Dr. Caudill says. "After a period of time, they will feel a letting go—letting go of the tensions, letting go of the worries, those kinds of things."

People in chronic pain, however, especially women, may initially feel anxious. "They close their eyes, they start letting go and relaxing, and they find themselves having panic attacks," she says. If that's your experience, you may want to include a visualization technique that allows you to go to a safe place in your mind first. Some people also find that they have less anxiety

if they keep their eyes open and simply stare at a candle flame or a point on the wall, she says. Some women find that being in a room where they can lock the door is also helpful.

For some people, pain comes to the forefront when they begin to try to relax. If that happens to you, get as comfortable as you can before you try to relax, Dr. Caudill says. Most meditative techniques involve upright sitting, but in this case you may want to use a recliner, lie down, or get into a warm tub of water. Also, pick times when your pain has lessened, not increased, to do your practice. It's possible to learn to focus intensely on your pain. "People are often afraid to focus on their pain because they are afraid it will get worse, and in fact, it never does," she says. "Like everything else that your brain tries to pay attention to, it gets bored after 30 seconds, and the pain subsides again."

WHAT RESULTS CAN YOU EXPECT?

The more immediate changes include a lowering of blood pressure, heart rate, breath rate, and oxygen consumption, which is a measure of metabolic rate. The long-term results include less anxiety and depression, better sleep, better digestion, less muscle tension, and, perhaps, less pain, Dr. Benson says. Regularly inducing the relaxation response can reduce insulin requirements in people with diabetes and can allow people with high blood pressure to reduce their dosage of medications, with their doctor's guidance.

WHO'S QUALIFIED TO DO IT?

Anyone can learn to induce the relaxation response in one way or another. "The biggest stumbling block for the people I see is that they don't feel like they deserve to take the time, because it looks like they are doing nothing," says Dr. Caudill. Another problem is that the effects are subtle. Inducing the relaxation response helps you to manage your pain, but it may not take it away.

You can use a variety of tapes to induce the relaxation response. In fact, you can buy the same tapes developed by Dr. Benson and used in the pain program at Deaconess Hospital in Boston. To get a list of the tapes available, write to the Mind/Body Medical Institute, Beth Israel Deaconess Medical Center, 110 Francis Street, Suite 1A, Boston, MA 02215-5501.

Look for a practitioner certified in biofeedback and hypnosis, Dr. Caudill says. Nurses, psychologists, and physician's assistants as well as traditional medical doctors may all receive training and certification in the relaxation response, she adds.

You can learn meditation, yoga, or even healing prayer techniques at places around your community. If you're in severe or chronic pain, though, your best bet for help in learning a relaxation response technique may well be a nearby multidisciplinary pain center. The psychologist there can help you learn a variety of stress-management techniques.

WHAT DOES IT COST?

Tapes from the Mind/Body Institute cost $10 each. To work with a psychologist may cost $50 to $150 a session, but this is generally covered by health insurance.

Rest

It used to be that when your back got sore, the doctor recommended a couple of days of complete bed rest. Or, after surgery, you'd lie beneath the sheets, eat bad hospital food for a day or two, and buzz the nurses for your every need.

No more. Now, you're up and walking the corridors, sutures and all, within a few hours of leaving the operating room. And lying around the house with a strained back is no longer always a prescription for healing.

It's not that rest and relaxation aren't good for you. It's just that rest is a medicine to be taken in small doses and only as one part of a therapy designed to speed healing and reduce pain, says Karen Mohr, P.T., a physical therapist and research director at the Kerlan-Jobe Orthopaedic Clinic in Los Angeles.

"When a doctor or physical therapist tells you to rest, they're not suggesting that you sit in front of the TV for days and be a couch potato," she says. "We recommend *active* rest. In other words, you rest from the thing that hurts you, but otherwise, you stay active. Activity increases circulation and, therefore, bloodflow, which can help the healing process."

How Does It Ease Pain?

Stress and fatigue make pain worse, and people often increase their pain by overdoing it and not paying attention to their bodies' pain signals, says Robert Kennedy, M.D., director of geriatric medicine at Maimonides Medical Center in Brooklyn, New York.

157

Denise De Lorenzo, P.T., a physical therapist at the Kessler Institute in West Orange, New Jersey, counsels chronic-pain patients to practice *energy conservation*, a term that essentially means "knowing your limits." When you have a chronic condition or disease, you're not necessarily going to be able to work through the pain.

"We want people to stop an activity before they enter that pain territory," she says. "You have to recognize when the pain is about to come on, and then rest."

What Does It Feel Like?

Rest feels, well, restful. When you stop using an injured part of your body, in most cases, the pain diminishes or even vanishes. Sometimes during rest, an injured limb or muscle may feel stiff or swollen, but there are ways to combat these sensations while resting the injured part, says Dr. Kennedy.

How Is It Done?

Passive rest is easy to do: Simply do nothing. Active rest, which seems contradictory, can be trickier but in its own way just as healing and restful.

Let's say that you're a walker with a bruised heel or a bad case of shinsplints. Even a stroll on a hard sidewalk is going to be painful and not conducive to healing. But to do nothing wouldn't be beneficial either. The solution is cross-training, doing several different kinds of activities or exercises to work your body, says De Lorenzo. For a walker, an alternative could be lap swimming, stationary bicycling, and striding on a low-impact gliding machine. Even though you're active, you're still "resting" yourself by doing less strenuous activities.

In another example, let's suppose you're a 75-year-old man or woman with angina pectoris and arthritic knees. You need to exercise daily to strengthen your heart muscle and retard the progress of heart disease, but your knees may make walking painful and limited. The alternative may be to swim or use one of those exercise machines that requires only the use of your arms.

"There's usually some kind of alternative that still allows you to use your muscles and rest what's hurting," says Dr. Kennedy.

What Results Can You Expect?

Rest in moderation will ease pain slowly and naturally. Your body has a chance to heal itself better and faster if you rest. In active rest, you can expect to keep a certain level of mobility even as you minimize the workload on your injuries.

Who's Qualified to Do It?

You're probably the best person to determine when you need a break. It's your body. A doctor or therapist, however, may give you a good idea of how to pursue active rest and do it safely.

What Does It Cost?

If you need to rest but still be active, look into community resources, such as a local pool or health club. For a nominal membership or use fee (prices range widely), you can have access to such restful resources as saunas, whirlpools, or just a large body of water in which to float and rest your aching parts.

If you need total rest and relaxation—perhaps a little snooze after your 3-mile afternoon walk—you might consider flopping into a rocker recliner that has radiant heat and a 12-motor device that gives you warm, wavelike massage. One of these contraptions runs about $600. Maybe R and R in the Caribbean is more your style. A weeklong cruise can go for as little as $1,000. Even on the boat, you can go to the gym, massage room, Jacuzzi, or pool for a little workout or soothing.

Of course, you can stay home and just take it easy. That doesn't cost anything.

Sex

Seems like it might depend on what generation you ask, but people middle-aged or older tend to take a wide view on what they regard as sex. Anything that involves cuddling, heavy petting, or intercourse fits the bill.

As we age, we begin to enjoy intimacy more. Our sexual needs are less geared toward orgasm, says Jean D. Miller, D.O., medical director of BodyCentered in New York City.

HOW DOES IT EASE PAIN?

Well, sex can definitely be a distraction, a way to divert your gray matter away from pain. It helps people remember what is normal and pleasant about their lives. But the biggest way sexual intimacy eases pain is by releasing endorphins, the body's own feel-good chemicals, Dr. Miller says. In fact, you don't even have to have an orgasm for an endorphin release. "Just gently touching is enough to release the same endorphins and to mitigate pain," she says.

Along another line, having sex seems to help some people with migraine headaches relieve their pain. Researchers say that one possible reason is that orgasms short-circuit the nervous system activity that's causing the pain.

And research suggests that women who are sexually active have less vaginal atrophy than women of the same age who are celibate. One theory is that sexual arousal improves blood circulation to vaginal tissues, helping them stay healthy. The same may go for men. Nourishing the tissue of the

160

penis with richly oxygenated blood—which happens every time a man gets an erection—is good for the penis.

How Is It Done?

When you're in pain, you may need to make some adaptations so that sex doesn't aggravate or increase your pain, and there are many ways you can do that. One of the most comfortable positions for people with back pain or arthritis is spooning. Both lie on their sides facing the same direction, the woman in front of the man. This position also is easy on knees and elbows, Dr. Miller says.

Because women past menopause often suffer from vaginal dryness, which can make intercourse painful, they should use a good, water-soluble lubricant such as K-Y jelly or Astroglide, suggests Larry Grunfeld, M.D., clinical associate professor of obstetrics and gynecology at Mount Sinai Medical Center in New York City. The advantage of Astroglide is its staying power. It doesn't dry out or become tacky as quickly when exposed to air. Or you can try a vaginal moisturizer that contains polycarbophil, such as Replens. This lubricant lasts longer and balances vaginal pH.

And since one application works for several days, you don't need to reapply it as often.

What Does It Feel Like?

Expect sex to feel pretty much like any other very pleasant activity. If you can really get into it, you might feel a sense of euphoria and comfort. Afterward, you might have a bit of afterglow. If you have any kind of pain during sex, stop and change positions or change the type of sexual activity you're doing, Dr. Miller says.

What Results Can You Expect?

The trick to enjoying and getting the most out of sexual intimacy is to not have expectations of some payoff, says Dr. Miller. "You enjoy the process instead of the results." But in doing so, you actually increase your chances of receiving something from the experience—an increased sense of aliveness and awareness and less focus on your aches and pains.

"If you had an active sex life before you had pain, don't assume that it can't still be active," says Judy Paice, R.N., Ph.D., a clinical nurse specialist in pain management in the department of neurosurgery at Rush Medical Center in Chicago. You may need to do some troubleshooting, however, if your sex life seems offtrack.

Many of the drugs used to treat pain affect both libido and performance, Dr. Paice says. "Antidepressants, often used to treat pain, can have a major impact on sexual desire." Your doctor may be able to switch you to a different type of antidepressant.

Opioids (morphine and codeine) lower testosterone and other sex hormone levels as well, reducing desire and performance. If your problem is lack of libido, or desire, hormone supplements are a better choice than a drug like sildenafil (Viagra), the popular anti-impotence drug for men, Dr. Paice says. "Viagra may help performance, but it does little to enhance libido." The appropriate hormone in this case is testosterone, and both men and women can take forms of supplemental testosterone to kindle desire.

Strength Training

Strength training is exercise that is designed to build or maintain muscles. It involves the use of a force that resists the muscle (such as a weighted dumbbell), which is why it is also called resistance training.

Weight lifting is the most popular form of strength training. But the force can also include your body's own weight—pushups are a good example of this, and tai chi and yoga also strengthen the same way. It can involve what we normally think of as aerobic exercise if it works muscles hard, as when biking uphill. And it can involve all sorts of resistance-producing gadgets—rubber exercise bands, squeeze balls, and of course, exercise machines, which still let you do all the work.

"Strength training is high-intensity, low-repetition exercise," says Kristin Baker, Ph.D., a researcher at Tufts University USDA Human Nutrition Research Laboratory on Aging in Boston, which investigates the effects of exercise on aging and chronic diseases.

How Does It Ease Pain?

You need strong muscles to help keep your joints stable and properly aligned. Unstable or injured joints are more likely to develop painful wear-and-tear osteoarthritis, says Tina Allen, P.T., a physical therapist at the Exercise Training Center at the University of Washington in Seattle, who sees many patients from the university's large chronic-pain center.

"If you have adequate muscle mass, you

(continued on page 167)

STRONG HEALING MEASURES

Maintaining strong muscles, especially around your joints, can help reduce pain from osteoarthritis and preserve bone mass, says Kristin Baker, Ph.D., a researcher at Tufts University USDA Human Nutrition Research Laboratory on Aging in Boston. Here's one way to get started on regaining muscle strength. Do 12 repetitions of each exercise three times a week, and make sure that you always do both sides of your body. If you're a beginner, do the exercises without weights until you are comfortable with the exercise.

Knee flexion. Wrap an ankle weight around each ankle. While standing behind and holding on to the back of a chair, bend your right knee, bringing your heel toward your buttocks. Then, slowly lower your lower leg. Try not to move your upper leg—your knees and thighs should stay together. Repeat with your left leg.

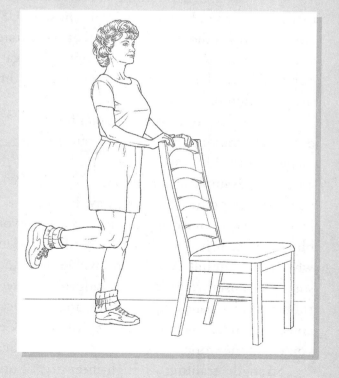

Knee extension. Wrap an ankle weight around each ankle. Sit in a sturdy chair that supports your entire thighs, from your hips to your knees. With your left foot on the floor, slowly extend your right leg until it is straight but not locked, then slowly lower it. Repeat with your left leg.

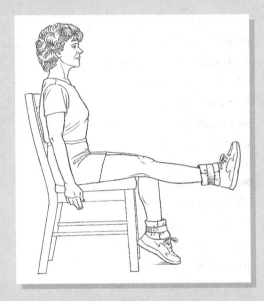

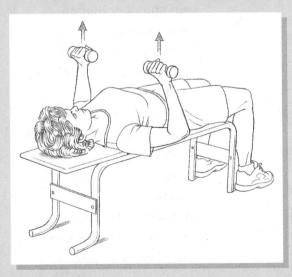

Chest press. Lying on an exercise bench, hold dumbbells end to end at about chest height, with your knuckles facing the ceiling and your elbows pointing toward the floor. Press the dumbbells up, extending your arms. Don't lock your elbows. Keep your wrists in line with your forearms. Hold, then lower to chest height again.

(continued)

Strong Healing Measures—Continued

Seated lateral row. Sit on the floor with your back straight and your legs out in front of you. Bend your knees slightly. Loop an exercise band around your feet at the arches. Hold an end in each hand, with your palms facing each other. Your hands should be on either side of your knees, with your arms relaxed and the exercise band taut.

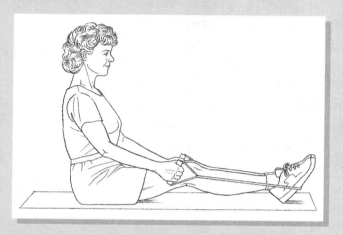

Slowly pull your arms back toward your chest, feeling your shoulder blades squeezing together. Continue until your hands are just below and to the sides of your chest. Hold, then slowly return to start. Keep your back straight. Don't wear smooth-soled shoes when doing this exercise; the band may slip and fly back at you.

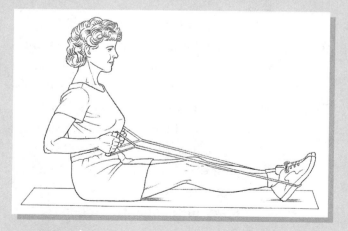

put less stress on your joints," Allen says. "We can help people with arthritis to develop more muscle strength around joints, which makes the joints more stable and may reduce pain because it also makes the joints work better."

Strength training also helps to maintain bone density, Dr. Baker says. In one study of postmenopausal women, those who lifted weights to build major muscle groups such as those of their hips, shoulders, backs, and abdomens had increases in bone mass in the upper parts of their thighbones and lumbar spines, both places prone to fractures from osteoporosis. A comparable group of women who didn't exercise actually lost bone density, setting the stage for osteoporosis.

Studies also show that strength training helps people to sleep better and improves mood, which can make a big difference in quality of life, Dr. Baker says.

How Is It Done?

You don't need to strength train at a gym or physical rehab center. But if you are learning it for the first time, it's best to get help right from the start so that you don't hurt yourself. After you learn how to do it right, there's no reason not to do it at home if you prefer.

If you haven't exercised in a long time, first get your doctor's okay, Dr. Baker says. Your doctor may give you some suggestions for limitations and can write you a prescription for physical therapy, which will give you the advantage of learning strength training under professional guidance. That's a good idea when you're older. You can also learn at a gym, with a certified trainer, then continue to do the exercises at home, or you can hire a personal trainer.

As a beginner, you should work without weights until you are comfortable with the exercise. Then, you'll slowly increase the weight, a method called progressive resistance training. As the weight you're lifting becomes easy to lift, you'll add on a bit more to once again challenge your muscles. To do this, Dr. Baker says, pick a weight that you can easily lift for 12 repetitions. After 1 to 2 weeks, slowly add weight by 1 to 2 pounds until you reach a weight that fatigues your working muscle in 12 repetitions. Start with one set and progress to two sets with 1 to 2 minutes of rest between sets.

You may have only four different exercises to begin with, two for your upper body and two for your lower body. Over time, you may add more if you like. Initially, you'll see fast gains in strength, but eventually, you'll get to the point where you will plateau and mostly maintain your strength. "That's okay. It happens to everyone," Dr. Baker says. That's when it may be time to start adding some more variety to your routine to keep your muscles fresh and to help maintain your interest in exercise.

a little sore and stiff—you'll know you used them—but they should never hurt so badly that you can't move. By the second day or so after your workout, your muscles should feel ready for another workout. It's important to have at least one full day of rest between workouts to allow your body to recover.

What Does It Feel Like?

When you are actually lifting weights or doing some other form of strength training, you can feel your muscles engage and work. "It should not hurt, but it should feel hard at the end of a set," Dr. Baker says. "If it doesn't feel at all like you are working your muscle, you aren't getting enough resistance to build muscle." As you near the end of your set, your muscles will begin to fatigue and might shake a little. That's fine. But you should never be lifting so much weight that your joints hurt or that you arch your back or start using other parts of your body to help you move the weight. If you are holding hand weights, they should be light enough for you to be able to keep your wrists straight as you lift them.

The next day, your muscles might feel

What Results Can You Expect?

Strength training builds muscles, no doubt about it. "And research confirms that it can build muscle mass even in very old people," Dr. Baker says. It will make it easier for you to continue to do the things that allow you to live independently, like get up and down stairs, in and out of the car, and on and off the toilet; carry groceries and laundry; hoist pots and pans; mop floors; and even walk the dog.

"One important thing we have found is that older people who do strength training become more active throughout their day because things become easier to do," Dr. Baker says. "They are more likely to spend time playing with grandchildren, walking, or taking part in other recreational activities."

Who's Qualified to Do It?

If you're just starting out, it's best to work with a trainer, perhaps someone at your local YMCA. If you really want to develop a regular strength-training routine, it's best to work with a trainer certified by the American College of Sports Medicine or the National Strength and Conditioning Association. That certification means the trainer has some knowledge of working with older people and with people with chronic diseases.

Your doctor, a local rheumatologist (a doctor who specializes in arthritis), or workers at a nearby senior center or nursing home may all be able to suggest a good physical therapist or trainer.

What Does It Cost?

To get started, a few sessions with a personal trainer or physical therapist can cost from $30 to $50 an hour, or more. Health insurance usually pays for physical therapy.

At home, costs can be fairly minimal. A set of hand weights from 1 to 12 pounds might be appropriate for starters. Costs range from 44 to 99 cents per pound for hand weights.

Stretching

We all know what it is to stretch. We tend to do it instinctively when we wake up in the morning, when we get up after sitting for a while, or if we develop muscle cramps. A nice big inhale, a nice big exhale, and a nice big head-to-toe s-t-r-e-t-c-h.

"Muscles have the ability to contract, but they also have the ability to lengthen greatly under certain conditions, and that's what a stretch is," says Herbert DeVries, Ph.D., professor emeritus of exercise physiology at the University of Southern California in Los Angeles and author of *Fitness after 50*.

Muscles stretch and contract naturally as you move. But you also stretch them deliberately, mostly because it just plain feels so good. And stretching also provides important stimulus to muscles. "It makes the muscles supple and allows them to maintain or regain their original length. If a muscle remains in a contracted state, it interferes with bloodflow, and you get sore muscles," explains Dr. DeVries. Over time, muscles that aren't stretched shorten up, so you get stiffer and stiffer.

How Does It Ease Pain?

When you stretch regularly, your muscles retain their ability to lengthen, Dr. DeVries says. That improves your body's flexibility and mobility. It makes it easier to do things such as bending over to pick something up, scratching your back, or twisting to get into or out of a car. It also makes it less likely that your muscles will tear if you make a sudden movement—for instance, if you slip in the shower. Keeping the muscles that surround and support your back strong and flexible is a good way to help prevent painful muscle spasms from strains or injury.

Muscles that are regularly stretched also sustain less injury during vigorous exercise that can cause tiny tears called micro-injuries, he says. These tiny tears do heal fairly quickly, but in the meantime, they can make muscles swell and become stiff and sore.

Proper stretching—not overstretching—also reduces muscle tension because it signals your muscle fibers to reduce their electrical activity and to relax even more. "That's why stretching routines such as yoga are so relaxing," explains Dr. DeVries.

People can tune in to this sensation of relaxation to learn how to maximize a stretch without overdoing it, says Bob Anderson, owner of Stretching, Inc., in Palmer Lake, Colorado, and author of the now-classic *Stretching*.

How Is It Done?

You want to relax, melt into a stretch, move slowly, and never force your body or push it until it hurts. In fact, if you push too far or try to bounce yourself farther in a stretch, it becomes counterproductive because your muscle starts to contract against the movement, Anderson says. "Stretching is not a contest. What someone else can do has nothing to do with you. You don't want to strain or tear tissue, trying to be like someone else."

Before you start stretching, you'll want to warm up by doing some easy movements like walking and swinging your arms for circulation enhancement. "If you're really stiff in the morning, do some easy stretches before you get out of bed," Anderson says. Or you may want to take a 20-minute stroll before you start to stretch.

You'll want to do a series of stretches that target your whole body and that hit your tightest muscles, Anderson says. Most people are tight in the backs of their upper thighs and in their lower backs, necks, and shoulders. So those are areas that you'll want to focus on.

Staying relaxed is very important. "Keep your jaw and shoulders relaxed, let your shoulders relax downward, and keep your hands and feet relaxed as you stretch," Anderson says. "Make your breathing slow, deep, and rhythmic."

PAIN-STOPPING STRETCHES

This series of gentle stretches targets your whole body, says stretching guru Bob Anderson, owner of Stretching, Inc., in Palmer Lake, Colorado, and author of the now-classic *Stretching*. If you have had a hip or knee replacement or have hip or knee problems, check with your doctor before trying any stretches that work those joints.

Shoulder shrug. Stand with your feet shoulder-width apart, or sit in a sturdy armless chair with your back resting against the back of the chair. Raise the tops of your shoulders toward your ears until you feel slight tension in your neck and shoulders. Hold this feeling of tension for 3 to 5 seconds, then let your shoulders drop down into their normal position. Repeat two or three times.

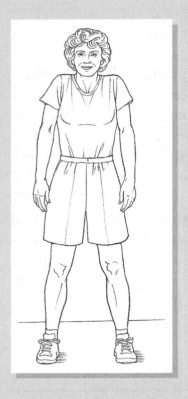

Inner-arm stretch. Stand with your feet shoulder-width apart, or sit in a sturdy armless chair with your back resting against the back of the chair. Interlace your fingers above your head. Then, with your palms facing upward, push your arms slightly back and up, straightening your arms but not locking your elbows. Feel the stretch in your arms, shoulders, and upper back. Hold for 15 seconds, and remember to breathe.

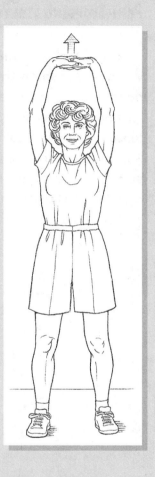

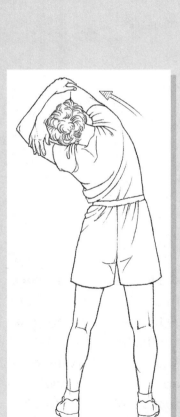

Side stretch. Stand with your feet shoulder-width apart and your arms overhead. Bend your right arm and hold the elbow with your left hand. Pull your elbow behind your head as you bend left at your hips. Don't nod your head; keep it in line with your arms. Hold for 10 seconds, then switch sides.

(continued)

PAIN-STOPPING STRETCHES—CONTINUED

Calf stretch. Stand 3 to 4 feet from a wall and lean on it with your forearms, your head resting on your hands. Bend your left leg and plant your foot in front of you, leaving your right foot straight behind you. Slowly move your hips forward until you stretch the calf of your right leg. Keep your right heel on the floor, toes forward. Hold for 30 seconds, then switch sides.

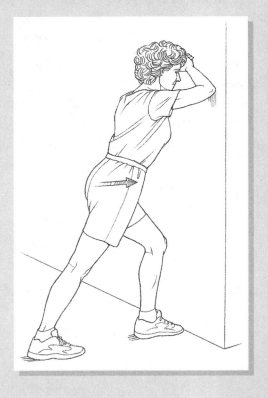

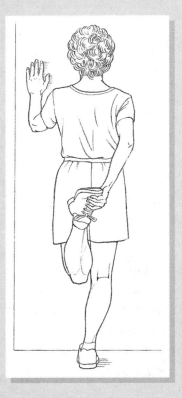

Quads stretch. Stand a foot away from a wall, facing it. Steady yourself by placing your left hand on the wall at shoulder height. Shift your weight to your right foot. Keeping your thighs together, lift your left foot behind you. Grab the top of your left foot with your right hand and gently pull, drawing your heel toward your buttocks. Hold for 15 to 20 seconds, then repeat with your right leg.

Hip stretch #1. Stand with your feet shoulder-width apart. Move your left leg forward until your left knee is directly over your left ankle. Bend your right leg and lower your body until your right knee is resting on the floor with your foot extended so that the top of it is on the ground.

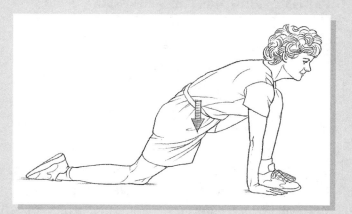

Rest your palms on the floor on either side of your left foot for balance. Your chest should rest on your left knee. Without changing the position of your right knee on the floor or your left foot, lower the front of your right hip downward to create an easy stretch. You should feel this stretch in the front of your hip and possibly in your hamstrings and groin. Hold for 20 to 30 seconds, then switch sides.

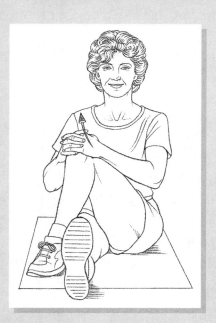

Hip stretch #2. Sit on the floor with your legs extended in front of you. Cross your left leg over your right. Rest your left foot on the outside of your right knee. Interlace your fingers around your left knee. Pull your knee across your body toward your right shoulder until you feel an easy stretch on the side of your hip. Hold for 20 seconds, then repeat with your right leg.

(continued)

PAIN-STOPPING STRETCHES—CONTINUED

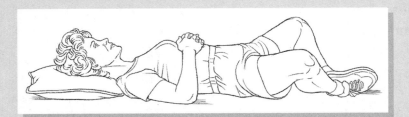

Groin stretch. Lie on your back on the floor. Bending your knees, let your legs fall open, and touch the soles of your feet together. This comfortable position will stretch your groin. Hold this stretch for 30 seconds. If necessary, place a small pillow under your neck and head for more comfort.

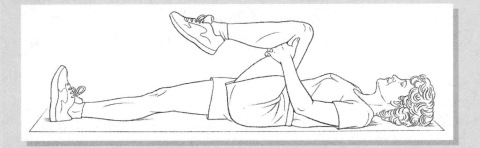

Hamstring stretch. Lie on your back on the floor, with both legs straight. Relax, interlace your fingers underneath your left thigh, then pull your left leg toward your chest. Keep the back of your head on the floor, but don't strain. Keep your lower back flat, pressed against the floor. Hold a comfortable stretch for 30 seconds, then repeat with your right leg.

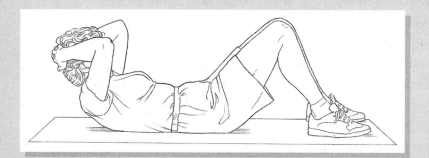

Upper-back stretch. Lie on your back on the floor, with your knees bent. Interlace your fingers behind your head, and rest your arms on the floor. Using the power of your arms, slowly bring your head, neck, and shoulders forward until you feel a slight stretch. Hold an easy stretch for 5 seconds. Repeat three times. Do not overstretch; you should not feel pain in your head, neck, or shoulders.

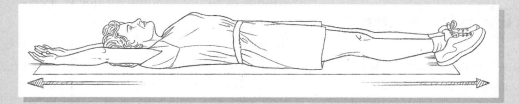

Torso stretch. Lie on your back on the floor, with your legs straight. Straighten out your arms over your head, with your palms up. Point your fingers and toes as you stretch as far as you can. Hold this stretch for 5 seconds, then relax.

WHAT DOES IT FEEL LIKE?

When you stretch, you'll want to slowly and carefully move your body in a way that stretches the muscles you're targeting, paying attention to how each muscle feels as it stretches. As you hold the stretch for 10 to 20 seconds, the feeling of tension should somewhat subside, and your muscle should relax. You may feel a pleasant unwinding sensation as you stretch. Sometimes, though, you may feel stiffness or resistance as you stretch, but you should never feel any real pain. If you feel pain or the stretching sensation becomes more intense, you may be overdoing it. Back off from that point a bit, relax, and hold it. Remember to stretch according to how the stretch feels, not how far you are stretching.

WHAT RESULTS CAN YOU EXPECT?

Over time, you should be able to move more easily and feel less stiff when you get up in morning or after sitting for a while. You should have more range of motion in your joints, including your back. But older people need to be patient about improving flexibility, Dr. DeVries says. Real improvement could take a few months.

WHO'S QUALIFIED TO DO IT?

The best teachers for stretching are certified trainers, yoga instructors, or physical therapists. It's also possible to learn proper technique from a book or videotape, Anderson says.

WHAT DOES IT COST?

Since stretching can involve just you and your body, it's ultimately free. But if you want to learn how to stretch, it's a good idea to invest some money in a class at your local YMCA or even a video or book of stretches. In that case, costs could be anywhere from $15 to $60. For additional information and a free catalog of stretching products and publications, contact Stretching, Inc., at P.O. Box 767, Palmer Lake, CO 80133-0767.

Tai Chi

Perhaps you've seen photographs or video of thousands of people going through methodic moves—as if they were dancing in slow motion—in Tiananmen Square in Beijing, China. In fact, in the public parks of many cities with reasonably sized Chinese populations, most mornings you'll find people gathering to do exactly the same thing, starting as early as 5:30 A.M. What they're doing is tai chi, a centuries-old Chinese discipline for health, relaxation, self-defense, and self-discipline.

Tai chi is a series of continuous and slow exercises that get the body moving in all directions and that have poetic counterparts in real life. The movements represent such activities as "Carrying the Tiger to the Mountain," "Parting the Mane of the Wild Horse," and "White Stork Beats Its Wings." Usually, about 24 of these "forms" are strung together in a 5-minute routine, but it's possible to do routines as short as 2 minutes.

"Tai chi requires a willingness to focus on what you're doing and to practice regularly," says Jin H. Yan, Ph.D., assistant professor of motor behavior/sports physiology in the department of exercise, sport, and health studies at the University of Texas at Arlington. In exchange, it offers physical and mental benefits, including relief from pain and chronic disease. It improves balance and increases range of motion in joints. It's said to cultivate inner metaphysical energy, called *qi* (pronounced "chee"). This is the same energy that gets moved around or unblocked during acupuncture treatments. "And tai chi gives you inner strength and calm, balance, and clarity of thought," says Aihan Kuhn, O.M.D., a doctor of oriental medicine and director of the Chinese Medicine for Health and Tai Chi Healing Center in Holliston, Massachusetts.

HOW DOES IT EASE PAIN?

Tai chi has a longtime reputation for alleviating many ailments such as high blood pressure, stomach problems, arthritis, hip and back pain, and heart disease. Studies and observations from China do suggest that tai chi is helpful for these conditions, Dr. Yan says.

In the United States, not much research has been done, but one study does confirm that tai chi can definitely improve balance, preventing falls. Older people who practiced tai chi for 15 weeks were able to hold off falls 50 percent more than people using a high-tech computer system to help them improve balance. "Over time, people can lose sense of the kinds of adjustments they need to make to maintain balance," Dr. Yan says. "Tai chi actually helps people relearn how to control balance. They experience so many different body positions that, when something really happens to get them off balance, they can respond faster."

Tai chi has been used to help people who are recovering from strokes and those who have multiple sclerosis. It is being evaluated to see if it can help people with Parkinson's disease as well, says Steven Wolf, P.T., Ph.D., a physical therapist and professor of rehabilitation medicine at Emory University School of Medicine in Atlanta.

It make sense that tai chi would also help people with arthritis and improve blood circulation, since these stretching movements make the body limber, tone up muscles, and help release tension, Dr. Yan says. In fact, a study of people with rheumatoid arthritis who did tai chi found that they reported less pain and more mobility.

HOW IS IT DONE?

To do tai chi, you first learn some basic positions and movements, such as shifting your weight from one leg to another with your knees straight or bent, legs spread or together. Then you learn some forms, such as "Move Hands like Cloud" or "Grasp the Bird's Tail." Eventually, you learn a group of forms and the transition movements between the forms that weave them into a seamless whole. The patterns and movements, in subtle succession, activate different parts of your body.

"You work to maintain a consistently slow tempo and even quality over a long period of time, and this requires inner control," Dr. Kuhn says. Like ballet, the actions are supposed to look weightless, airy, and easy. But here's where the yin/yang comes in. What seems effortless really isn't. "The movements feel natural, but there is a lot of mind focus involved," Dr. Kuhn says. "It's energy flow, not physical force."

Tai chi is usually taught in hour-long group classes. It may take older people 40 to 60 hours of instruction (plus daily practice at home) to learn an initial 24-form routine, Dr. Yan says. Beginners are taught without music, which would be distracting. In China, though, advanced students do their movements to music played on ancient Chinese instruments.

WHAT DOES IT FEEL LIKE?

While you're doing tai chi, you can feel the warm flow of energy throughout your body, Dr. Kuhn says. "You feel full of energy, like you have absolute power inside of you, like you can do anything you want, solve any problem. You feel like nothing will be in your way." That feeling continues during your day, giving you a sense of balance and focus.

And since you need to concentrate fully on what you're doing, you tend to have peace of mind, Dr. Yan says. "You don't think about anything else."

WHAT RESULTS CAN YOU EXPECT?

You can expect to have a better sense of balance and feel more confident when moving around. You may feel more flexible, with better range of motion in your joints. And you should have a sense of clarity and feel less confused, Dr. Yan says. "You gain confidence in virtually everything you are doing, both physically and mentally." People simply begin to enjoy life more, which sometimes translates into less pain and better health.

WHO'S QUALIFIED TO DO IT?

Tai chi classes are offered at YMCAs, health clubs, and martial arts schools, but generic classes are not typically geared toward special medical problems. And some forms are more strenuous than others. So it's best to find an instructor who has worked with older people and who approaches tai chi from an exercise point of view, not a martial arts point of view. There is no certification required in the United States to teach tai chi. Some people who are "tai chi masters" have received certificates from martial arts schools in China. You may try calling the physical therapy department of your local hospital to find a reputable instructor.

WHAT DOES IT COST?

Class prices run about $10 and up.

Touch

People tend to use the healing power of touch instinctively. When someone they care about is in pain, physically or emotionally, they reach out—to touch an arm or hand, squeeze a shoulder, or enfold the wounded in their embrace.

There are several types of touch, or hands-on, therapies, including massage, acupressure, and reflexology. Massage and acupressure are forms of touch that have confirmed physical benefits, says Tiffany Field, Ph.D., director of the Touch Research Institute at the University of Miami School of Medicine and author of *Touch Therapy*.

Just plain touch itself, the kind of spontaneous, untrained gesture we all make, has also been shown to make a psychological impact, says Dr. Field. For example,

people are more likely to prefer a library where the librarian has touched their hands as she gives them their books, and waitresses get bigger tips if they touch customers on the hands as the customers pay the bills. Women who are touched by the nurses who explain procedures prior to surgery regain normal blood pressure more quickly after surgery.

How Does It Ease Pain?

"A calming touch can reduce stress hormones, strengthen immunity, reduce pain, and normalize heart rate and breathing," Dr. Field says.

Studies done on massage show that it

Touch without Touching

Some touch therapies take a more hands-off approach. Take Therapeutic Touch, which doesn't actually involve touching the body. Instead, Therapeutic Touch involves simply using the hands *close* to the body to help enhance someone's energy flow. In Chinese medicine, flow of energy, or *qi*, is health. Therefore, blocked energy leads to illness or disease.

Therapeutic Touch is a contemporary integration of Eastern and Western approaches to healing, says Francelyn Reeder, R.N., Ph.D., associate professor at the University of Colorado School of Nursing in Denver. Practitioners believe that they can use their hands, almost like magnets, to move and restore *qi*, or vital energy. Therapeutic Touch really shines in situations where you don't want to directly touch someone, such as a person in a burn unit or someone in extreme pain, she says.

People who receive Therapeutic Touch also feel rested and may have less pain for a period of time afterward, Dr. Reeder says. "They report feeling cooler when they have been burning up. And if they've been cold, they say they feel warmer," she says. " To sum it up, after Therapeutic Touch, persons express feeling like they're moving toward well-being."

If you're interested in learning more about this mode of healing or you want to find someone in your area who practices Therapeutic Touch, you can contact Nurse Healers Professional Associates, 1211 Locust Street, Philadelphia, PA 19107-5409.

causes a decrease in cortisol, a potent stress hormone. It also helps to normalize heart rate and breathing, inducing relaxation. In people who are HIV-positive or who have cancer, massage can cause an increase in natural killer cells that ward off viruses and kill cancer cells. And studies have confirmed that massage can reduce pain for people with fibromyalgia, chronic fatigue syndrome, lower-back pain, migraine headaches, and juvenile rheumatoid arthritis, she says.

Emotions play a large part in people's perception of pain, and "the touch that tells them someone cares about them can send a flood of positive emotions," says Stanley E. Jones, Ph.D., professor of communication at the University of Colorado in Boulder and author of *The Right Touch: Understanding and Using the Language of Physical Contact.* "We talk about tactile experiences the same way we talk about emotional experiences, because touch is one of the most emotionally affecting kinds of behaviors," he says. "'I was touched by that' is a synonym for being emotionally influenced. Touch can generate positive emotions."

Back rubs used to be a pleasant bedtime routine for people in the hospital, and they not only reduced the incidence of bedsores, they helped people relax and sleep better, Dr. Field says. Even premature babies have better growth and development if they are massaged regularly, she says.

How Is It Done?

If you're simply looking to comfort someone in pain, use your instincts and be sincere, Dr. Jones advises. He tells the story of a nurse's first meeting with a suicidal female patient who had recently tried to slash her wrists. "The nurse took one look at the sad expression on the woman's face and immediately embraced her," he says. "No one had come near the woman since her suicide attempt, and the uncalculated and spontaneous touch was exactly what was needed. It said not only 'I care' but also 'You are touchable, someone I want to reach out to.' That hug was the first step in establishing a relationship in which the nurse could guide the woman back to physical and emotional health."

This is just one example of a "support touch," which is done when someone expresses some kind of concern. It is intended to comfort and is given to the shoulder, upper-middle back, elbow, and occasionally the hand, or, if the person is lying down, to the hand or forearm, explains Dr. Jones.

"It is usually just a subtle touch that

says, 'I'm sorry you are feeling bad' or 'I care, and I want to comfort you,' and it tends to convey the message more fully than saying it with words," Dr. Jones says. If you're big on hugs, you should know that many people, especially older people, prefer to reserve hugs as major ammo, to be employed only when people are feeling really sad and in need of comforting of a very strong kind.

With any kind of touch, look for a re-action to see whether your touch is wel-come—or ask first. If someone is in extreme pain, touch might not be what he needs or wants. A firm touch usually elicits the best response, Dr. Field says. But be careful about squeezing, even a hand. It might hurt. And also avoid light stroking, which people, including prema-ture babies, often find aversive. Also avoid pats, tickling, or interrupting or startling someone with a touch.

Your touch may say it all, or you may feel compelled to convey its meaning ver-bally. "I'm here for you." "I care about you." "I'm sorry you're feeling that."

WHAT DOES IT FEEL LIKE?

If you are being touched in a sup-portive, appropriate way, you should feel calmer almost immediately. "Sometimes, it takes more than one touch, as someone needs to continue expressing the feelings that are concerning them," Dr. Jones says.

WHAT RESULTS CAN YOU EXPECT?

Don't underestimate the power of touch to calm, to help someone sleep, or to draw their attention away from their pain, Dr. Jones says. "Part of pain is how you re-spond psychologically. And if someone comforts you, it takes your mind away from the pain. It may replace the pain with pleasurable thoughts and feelings."

Even people who have lost some sensory perception—sight or hearing, for instance— still often have the full ability to sense touch. So it's a good way to get through to people in varying states of awareness, he says.

Transcutaneous Electrical Nerve Stimulation (TENS)

Zapping pain with electricity goes back thousands of years. Ancient Egyptian physicians shocked their pharaohs with electric catfish native to the Nile River. Greeks and Romans applied the torpedo ray of the Mediterranean Sea to lessen "unbearable headache and gout." These electric fishes delivered jolts between 40 and 50 volts. Exactly how a fish killed pain wasn't clear. Nowadays, we know the answer: electricity.

Transcutaneous electrical nerve stimulation (TENS) works on the same basic principle as those ancient fish. TENS sends small charges of electricity through nerves to block pain signals before they reach the brain. A TENS unit consists of an electronic stimulus generator and two electrode wires that attach to electrodes applied to the skin. The generator is small, portable (about the size of a tape player worn on the belt), and operates on rechargeable batteries.

"The beauty of TENS is that you can do it by yourself at home," says Lawrence Miller, M.D., of the Coast Pain Management Center at Orange Coast Memorial Medical Center in Fountain Valley, California. "It's convenient and completely safe."

HOW DOES IT EASE PAIN?

It wasn't until the mid-twentieth century that scientists began to understand how electricity acts as an analgesic. The breakthrough came with the gate theory of pain. It states that if you vigorously stimulate large nerves, the brain will ignore messages sent by smaller nerves, which carry pain signals.

The pain messages from the small nerves don't travel as quickly to the brain as the touch signals from the large nerve fibers. If you barrage the brain with touch signals—in a sense, keep the brain busy—it ignores messages sent by small nerve fibers. In other words, it slams the gate shut on pain. The gate theory explains why rubbing a painful area of the body makes the hurt feel better.

Electrical stimulation from TENS is akin to continuous rubbing. TENS comes in two forms: conventional TENS and acupuncture-like TENS. Each relieves pain in a unique way. With conventional TENS, pain relief is temporary but usually immediate, says Patti Winchester, P.T., Ph.D., a physical therapist and chairperson of the department of physical therapy at the University of Texas Southwestern Medical Center at Dallas.

To ease more severe or chronic pain, you may have to turn to acupuncture-like TENS (also called motor TENS). The electrical charges are much stronger, able to produce twitches or contractions in mus-cles. The idea is not so much to close down pain pathways, but to stimulate the release of enkephalins and endorphins, the body's natural opiate-like painkillers. Acupuncture-like TENS works well for deep pain such as sciatica or myalgia.

Motor stimulation also increases blood circulation. Increased bloodflow relieves inflammation and speeds healing, says Dr. Winchester.

Although it works with many pain syndromes, Dr. Winchester warns that TENS is no panacea. "TENS is just one tool that we have. We always use it along with other therapies," she adds. "But it does give some people some control over their pain. And you can do it almost anywhere."

HOW IS IT DONE?

With a TENS unit, you typically place electrodes on either side of the painful area—astride the spine in the case of a back injury, or above and below an aching joint when treating osteoarthritis. The idea is to "bracket" the pain.

In motor TENS, the electrodes are frequently placed on trigger, or acupressure, points. A bit of gel rubbed on the skin increases electrical conductivity.

No one charge of electricity fits all pain.

You adjust the unit—change the strength of the signal and the pulse of the frequency—to find the right stimulation. It takes less current, for example, to reach the surface nerves in your face than it does to activate deeply buried nerve bundles, such as the sciatic nerves in your buttocks.

Regardless of electrode placement, a TENS treatment lasts between 20 and 30 minutes. After a rest period of about 2 hours, it may be repeated. There aren't any significant side effects with TENS. Sometimes, you get skin irritation from the electrodes or you experience muscle fatigue and soreness after the first few treatments.

What Does It Feel Like?

During conventional TENS, you feel a mild tingling sensation on and near the skin surface, explains Dr. Miller. In conventional TENS, the unit produces a strong sensory response without activating the muscle's motor response.

In acupuncture-like TENS, the aim is to turn up the current enough to cause muscle twitching. The strength of the current and the muscle contractions can be uncomfortable. Many patients tolerate it better by setting their TENS units for shorter pulses or higher frequencies. The current is more intense, but the bursts are short.

What Results Can You Expect?

When it works, TENS works immediately. Electricity races down the nerve, the brain slams the pain gate closed, and you feel better.

"Conventional TENS works best for mild pain, like an old back injury that aches occasionally, or when you're healing up from surgery or an injury," says Dr. Miller. "With more severe pain, it may just diminish it some and make it more tolerable."

With conventional TENS, pain usually returns when you turn the current off, says Dr. Winchester. But that temporary relief may be enough to get you through a situation that exacerbates pain.

"I had one patient, a businessman, with ruptured disks and chronic lower-back pain. It was very uncomfortable for him to sit on an airplane," she recalls. "He used his TENS unit during the flight to block the pain. That enabled him to travel."

The analgesic effects of acupuncture-like TENS tend to be more long-lasting due to the body's release of natural opiates. In a study done in the late 1970s, Scandinavian researchers found that patients had higher endorphin activity after TENS treatments.

"The effect may last for hours after you turn off the electrical stimulation," Dr. Winchester adds. In fact, several studies have shown that the use of TENS may reduce the amount of drugs that people need to relieve their pain.

trical stimulation by your therapist, who will show you how to place the electrodes and modulate the frequency. Then, the practitioner will experiment with electrode settings and frequencies to help you find the right combination. Once you're familiar with the basic workings, you may be given the option to do the therapy at home.

WHO'S QUALIFIED TO DO IT?

You can be your own TENS therapist after you've gotten instructions from your doctor, physical therapist, or chiropractor. Traditional TENS units are designed to be used at home or on the road.

Typically, you'll be introduced to elec-

WHAT DOES IT COST?

Traditional TENS units, available by prescription only, cost between $200 and $500. Sometimes, a pain or physical therapy clinic will rent TENS units to their patients. Medicare and health insurance may cover the cost.

Walking

Long before automatic transmission, remote controls, and home-delivery pizza, there was walking. People walked to get somewhere and to do things—around their houses, land, and towns. Even if you don't have to walk much in day-to-day activities, it's a good thing to do anyway, a skill you don't want to lose.

"Walking is one of the best ways to ease into a regular exercise program, to keep moving even when you're older or overweight, and to stay fit," says Suki Munsell, Ph.D., director of the Dynamic Health and Fitness Institute in Corte Madera, California. "A daily walking program is the cornerstone of a healthy lifestyle for many people, young and old."

How Does It Ease Pain?

Our bodies are meant to move, no matter what our age. When we are sedentary, we slowly lose muscle and gain fat, setting the stage for diabetes, high cholesterol and blood pressure, and heart disease. We also lose bone mass, which can eventually develop into osteoporosis.

"But when we stay active, we counteract all these effects, so we are more likely to be spared the painful consequences of living—perhaps for many years—with a debilitating chronic disease," says Linn Goldberg, M.D., director of the human-performance laboratory and head of the division of health promotion at Oregon Health Sciences University in Portland.

191

"Studies show that walking can help to reduce high blood pressure, and it is a good way to help manage diseases like type 2 diabetes." Walking increases insulin sensitivity, improving the cells' ability to take up sugar, which reduces the high blood sugar levels that are one of the more dangerous symptoms of diabetes.

You don't have to put in long hours of high-intensity exercise either. "In one study, a group of women with high blood pressure had their pressures reduced as much by low-intensity exercise as by high levels of exertion after 3 months of training," Dr. Goldberg says.

Walking has proven better than rest at relieving lower-back pain. It also helps us sleep better, makes our bowels function properly, clears our heads, improves moods, and reduces anxiety by reducing blood levels of stress hormones.

How Is It Done?

Walking for exercise is easy and convenient for most people, which makes excuses hard to come by. But if you haven't exercised in years, you'll want to underdo it at first, Dr. Munsell says. "Ten minutes a day may be all you should do for the first week or so." Then, you can add about 10 percent more each week in distance, time, or speed.

For cardiovascular health, you'll want to work up to a minimum of 30 minutes four times a week. Don't get too hung up about how much you're exercising or how well you're doing it, Dr. Goldberg says. "Just do *something*. You don't have to be gung ho to reap substantial benefits."

If the world outside seems full of mean dogs and high curbs, try doing a few laps around your local mall. "Many malls open early in the morning just for this," he says. It's a safe, controlled, friendly environment, where chances are good you'll meet other walkers. Plus, you get to see what's on sale before everyone else does.

Treadmills are safe if you have good balance and know how to use one, Dr. Munsell says. But if you're not as steady as you'd like to be, it's better to walk on terra firma.

You can set a time aside specifically for walking exercise, or you can catch it in bits and pieces during the day by parking a few blocks away from your destination, strolling around the block, or walking to the store. If you need to carry things, consider using a small backpack, which is easier on your body than a shopping bag or a large purse. Or use a cart, Dr. Munsell suggests. In either case, maintain body balance by using both arms or by alternating between your left and right arms.

Get walking or running shoes that offer good support and cushioning, Dr. Munsell says. If you go to a running store that's been around awhile, you're most likely to find salespeople who can steer you in the right direction on selection and fit. Plan on replacing your shoes at least yearly.

When you walk, pay particular attention to heel-toe roll, Dr. Munsell says. "Seniors tend to walk flat-footed and widen their stance, so they roll from side to side like a drunken sailor." Instead, imagine your foot as the bottom of a rocking chair, curved. "Plant your foot at the heel, slightly on the outside of the heel, and roll down the footprint and off between the big toe and first toe," she says. Until you get the feel of it, you may need to do this slowly a few times each time you start out. Keep your knees relaxed, not locked. Let your arms and legs swing like pendulums, and let their weight help propel you forward. Don't pump your arms until you are warmed up and you really need them to add to your push-off.

After you've walked for about 10 minutes, stop and stretch your arms overhead, twist gently at the waist, and shake it out. "Stretching rebalances your body and maximizes the rest of your walk," Dr. Munsell says. "Walking works a lot better with stretching." You should also stretch after your walk.

WHAT DOES IT FEEL LIKE?

You should never push yourself so hard that walking doesn't feel good. "The point is to build up over time, keeping yourself within what you perceive as a mild effort," Dr. Goldberg says. It takes about 6 weeks for walking to become a habit, but by 6 months, the people who are still at it begin to enjoy walking. "They feel better when they do it than when they don't do it. And that's a big motivator," he says.

"If you are walking properly, it should feel delightful. It should feel like a glide," Dr. Munsell says. Poor posture and stiffness can contribute to aches and pains when you walk. It's possible to find a walking coach to troubleshoot your stance and show you ways to improve.

WHAT RESULTS CAN YOU EXPECT?

Over time, walking should produce stronger muscles in your lower body, less lower-back pain, more flexible joints, improved mood, better sleep, improved immunity, and better overall health. You can't get all that in a bottle at any price.

WHO'S QUALIFIED TO DO IT?

Just about anyone can walk, although some may need help at first, Dr. Goldberg says. If you haven't exercised in years, it's wise to first see your doctor to see what he recommends and any limitations he may suggest. If you have risk factors for or symptoms of coronary disease, such as chest pain or shortness of breath when you walk, an exercise stress test is in order. If you're more than 50 pounds overweight, to spare your joints, Dr. Goldberg suggests that you use an exercise bike, rather than walk, until your weight is within 30 pounds of normal.

You may be able to get into a doctor-prescribed exercise program if you have risk factors, such as high blood pressure, high cholesterol, diabetes, or being overweight. Such a program can get you off safely. Lots of community centers have programs for seniors, so you might check at your local YMCA or Jewish community center.

WHAT DOES IT COST?

Walking will cost you the price of a pair of decent sneakers—$55 to $75. If you decide on a treadmill, it's worth investing in a good one, which you can get for about $600 if you weigh less than 200 pounds. (Heavier people will need to pay more for sturdier models.) If you decide on instruction, you can find a walking coach by contacting the North American Racewalking Foundation, P.O. Box 50312, Pasadena, CA 91115-0312.

Yoga

If you've seen photographs of its poses, you might think that yoga is a form of torture only a pretzel could love—something more likely to *cause* pain than to relieve it.

It's true that some of the more advanced poses—feet behind the head, balancing on one arm—require great strength and flexibility. But yoga actually builds strength and flexibility. And yoga poses can be adapted to anyone's limitations. Even people who have to stay in bed or who can't get out of a chair can do yoga. What's more, yoga has been proven to relieve certain types of pain, including osteoarthritis. Its less extreme forms are an ideal choice when the prescription calls for exercise.

The word *yoga* means "union," and yoga teachers talk of yoga as a practice, or system, of poses and movements that helps people to unify and balance the body and mind, says Amy Kline Gage, a yoga instructor who works with the Preventive Medicine Research Institute founded by healthy-heart guru Dean Ornish, M.D., in Sausalito, California. "Yoga was developed centuries ago specifically to make the body healthy," she says. "The asanas, or poses, were designed to take the distractions the body has—the sore muscles, the twitches and itches and aches—and get rid of them so that a person could sit still and meditate."

The practice of yoga also quiets the mind, says Julie Lawrence, a certified Iyengar yoga instructor in Portland, Oregon, and former chairperson of the medical research and yoga therapeutics committee of the B. K. S. Iyengar Yoga National Association of the United States.

"An important component of yoga is

195

(continued on page 202)

Yoga: The Ahhhh Routine

Here's a sampler of extra-gentle yoga poses. It's always best to do yoga in a quiet, warm setting. Breathe naturally in and out through your nose instead of through your mouth. This encourages relaxation.

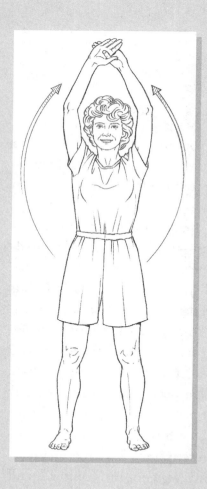

Standing reach. Stand firmly with your feet shoulder-width apart and your arms at your sides. Breathe out completely and fix your gaze on a spot on the floor or wall to help you keep your balance. Then, as you breathe in, bring your arms up in a wide circle to the sides and over your head. Hold your breath for just a second as you clasp your hands and stretch a bit higher. Then breathe out while returning your straight arms to the sides and down. Repeat three times.

Tree pose. With your feet together, stand with the right side of your body to the back of a sturdy chair. Position yourself about a foot away from the chair, and hold the back of the chair for support. Steady yourself by fixing your gaze on a spot on the wall or floor in front of you. Shift your weight to your right foot. Pick up your left foot and place the sole of your foot against your right inner thigh as high as possible, with the toes of your left foot pointed toward the floor. If at first your foot will not go high enough to rest on your inner thigh, just brace it below your knee. Try to breathe steadily. Consciously relax your breath by relaxing your abdominal muscles. Hold for about 10 seconds at first, working up to 30 seconds or more. Then repeat, standing on your left foot. After awhile, if you feel that your balance is steady enough, raise one arm straight up. The final, full position is both arms overhead, palms together.

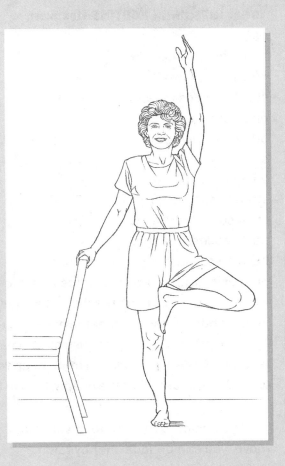

(continued)

YOGA: THE AHHHH ROUTINE—CONTINUED

Child's pose in a chair. Place two sturdy, armless chairs, one in front of the other and facing the same direction, about 2 feet apart. Sit up straight on the rear chair so that your lower back touches the chair back. Rest your hands 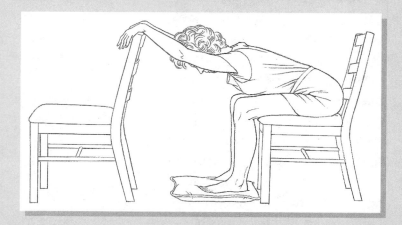 on your legs, just above your knees. Your feet should be firmly on the floor and hip-width apart. If they don't reach the floor, put a block or firm pillow under them. Draw in your abdomen as you breathe out and sit up tall. Then, lengthen your spine forward by bending forward at your waist, almost resting your chest on your thighs, in order to rest your wrists on the chair in front. Keep your neck in line with your spine and look toward the ground. Breathe deeply. Rest in this position for as long as you like.

If you want to try a more advanced move, you can bend farther by taking your hands down toward your feet. Keep your hips firmly in place on the chair. Lean forward at your waist, resting your chest on your thighs. Gently, let your head drop so that your ears are close to your shoulders and you are looking at your knees. Breathe deeply. Rest in this position for as long as you like.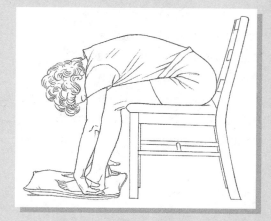

Downward-facing dog.

Stand in front of a chair and bend at your hips, with your back, neck, and head aligned. Put your palms flat on the front edge of the seat, about shoulder-width apart. Spread your fingers so that your middle fingers are parallel and are in line with your wrists. Move your

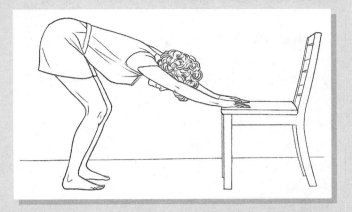

feet backward until they're under your hips and your arms are straight. Bend your knees and point your tailbone toward the ceiling, creating a gentle arch in your back. Lower your head so that your ears are between your upper arms.

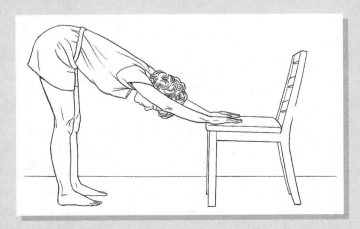

Keep your hands parallel as you slide them away from your body, toward the back of the chair. Straighten your knees, but don't lock them, and balance your weight between your upper and lower body. You will feel a lengthening stretch extend from your shoulders to your wrists. Breathe evenly and naturally. Repeat 3 to 10 times a day.

(continued)

YOGA: THE AHHHH ROUTINE—CONTINUED

Chair twist. Sit up straight in a sturdy, armless chair with your feet flat on the floor. Breathe out and slowly turn your trunk to the right, keeping your head and neck even with your shoulders and moving your right arm behind the chair back, until your shoulders are in line with your right thigh. Keep your hips facing forward. Turn your head gently a bit more so that you are looking over your right shoulder. Hold for as long as is comfortable, breathing normally, then slowly come back to center. Take a deep breath in, then breathe out and slowly turn to your left. Do each side three times.

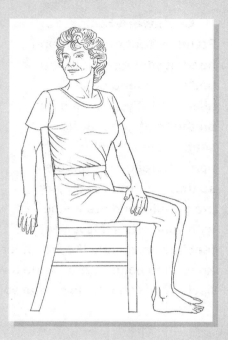

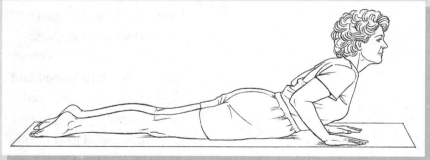

Cobra. Lie facedown with your hands under your shoulders, palms on the floor. Keep your legs slightly apart, with the tops of your feet on the floor. Press toward the floor with your pubic bone. Then slowly raise your upper body 3 to 6 inches, without pushing yourself up with your arms. Breathe out, drop your hips, and lengthen forward as you come up. Keep your elbows close to your body. Repeat twice.

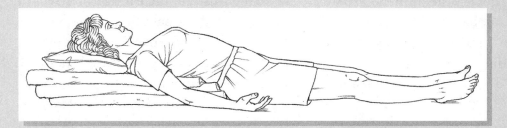

Supported corpse pose. Use two or three blankets, folded lengthwise, to support your back and shoulders. Lie down with your legs slightly apart and your feet dropping to the sides. Keep your neck in line with your spine. Allow your chest to open and your arms to drop away from your body, palms up. Relax. Each time you breathe out, let your weight drop down so that your body feels fully supported by the floor beneath you. Lie quietly for at least 5 minutes at the end of your yoga practice.

Modified corpse pose. Lie on the floor a few inches from the front legs of a chair. Put your legs on the chair. The chair height should allow your lower back to rest on the floor and your calves and heels to rest flat on the chair seat. Allow your chest to open and your arms to drop away from your body, palms up. Relax. Each time you breathe out, let your weight drop down so that your body feels fully supported by the floor beneath you. Lie quietly for at least 5 minutes at the end of your yoga practice.

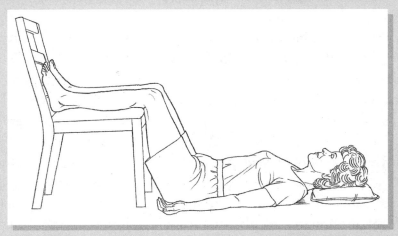

that it asks us to concentrate on what is going on in the present moment, and that relaxes and quiets the mind," explains Lawrence. And, like meditation, that quieting of the mind allows people to put things, including pain, into perspective and perceive the deeper meaning of their lives.

HOW DOES IT EASE PAIN?

"Yoga's combination of stretching tight areas and strengthening weak areas of the body brings a sense of balance to the body, and that in itself relieves pain," Lawrence says.

People who do yoga over a lifetime don't develop nearly as much stiffness as they age, and people who start yoga at an older age can reverse some of the stiffness that they might attribute to old age but which is really a consequence of inactivity, Kline Gage says. "By stretching muscles regularly, you maintain range of motion in joints, which helps to keep joints healthy and pain-free."

In fact, a study from the University of Pennsylvania School of Medicine in Philadelphia found that an 8-week yoga routine reduced pain and tenderness and improved range of motion in people with osteoarthritis of the hands. A similar study by the some of the same researchers found that yoga worked better than wrist splinting for reducing pain and increasing grip strength in people with carpal tunnel syndrome.

Studies also show that 70 percent of people with lower-back pain can substantially reduce their pain if they do yoga regularly.

And since stretching and greater flexibility can ease bursitis and tendinitis pain as well, yoga may be the best cure for these nagging pain problems. Using yoga, you can push your body enough that you increase your range of motion, but not so hard that you irritate your joints, says Larry Payne, Ph.D., director of the International Association of Yoga Therapists and coauthor of *Yoga for Dummies*.

Plus, yoga improves your balance tremendously, reducing your chances of taking a tumble. "You become more aware of your body in space and how you're moving, so you might take a little bigger step so that you're not shuffling, or you might make sure your feet are positioned under your hips so that your balance is a little more stable," Kline Gage says.

Yoga is also very relaxing, the ultimate stress-management system, says Barbara Lang, director of the yoga program at the Center for Living at Duke University in Chapel Hill, North Carolina. "It spills over into the rest of your life. People really learn how to pay attention to what's going on in their bodies, to listen in a way we don't often tend to because we are in such a hurried pace in our lives." Such listening helps people recognize the early symptoms of stress and pain, allowing them to reduce stress and pain before they become incapacitated.

How Is It Done?

You wear clothes that allow your body to move freely. You work on a relatively hard floor or on a thin mat that keeps your feet and hands from sliding. If you can't get down on the floor, you can work from a chair or even from a bed. Some people even do yoga in water.

A yoga class generally runs an hour, sometimes more. It may include warmup poses to get loosened up, more vigorous poses for strengthening and stretching, and a cooldown, often a period of deep relaxation.

A typical 1-hour class may have students warm up with a sun salute, a series of moving poses that include stretching overhead, forward bends, and upward and downward bends. Someone needing to adapt to a less vigorous style for a warmup may simply move and stretch their arms and legs. The class may include a series of standing, sitting, or lying poses, such as a triangle pose, which is a standing side stretch; balancing poses, which you can do with a chair or against a wall; forward and backward bends; a twist pose; and then, end with a period of flat-on-your-back relaxation, where people simply melt into the floor in deep relaxation.

But a class always depends on the teacher, and even on the style of yoga being taught, Lawrence says. Some styles, such as Ashtanga (Power), Choudhury, and Iyengar yoga, can be much more vigorous than others, such as Kripalu or Integral/Sivananda yoga.

Among the styles Dr. Payne recommends are Vini yoga, which takes into account each student's capability, as well as the Easy Does It or User-Friendly yoga classes, which are trademarked styles.

But most styles of yoga can offer gentle or restorative classes that are most appropriate for beginning older students.

If you are doing yoga at home, you can devise your own routine or use a videotape, which generally follows the same format as a class.

What Does It Feel Like?

Know how you feel when you stretch in bed before you get up in the morning? Like you are getting things moving, working the kinks out, waking up your whole body? That's what yoga can feel like, Kline Gage says.

"After a yoga class, people say they feel great, and it's a glorious thing to feel so rejuvenated and refreshed, cheerful and at peace with yourself," she says. If you're in pain when you start a yoga session, you will need to take it slow and easy, but you should have less pain at the end of a session.

"Even if you work only on your breath during a session, sometimes that can help stop a cycle of pain," Kline Gage explains. Meanwhile, some poses—known as restorative poses—require little or no effort and appear to do the most for a system overtaxed by disease or stress. Restorative poses are held by using the support of props, such as blankets, belts, and pillows, allowing the muscles to be quiet and sink into deep relaxation.

What Results Can You Expect?

Over time, you will begin to feel more mobile, less stiff and creaky, and stronger, with a better sense of balance, Kline Gage says. "I've worked with people in nursing homes, and by the third class, they are sitting up straighter, walking better, more cheerful, and—the nurses tell me—less likely to be constipated."

Who's Qualified to Do It?

Many people teach yoga, but several membership organizations offer training that lead to certification as a yoga instructor. Some yoga techniques, such as Iyengar, require years of training; others, only a few months. To make sure that your instructor knows how to adapt poses to fit your limitations and steer you away from poses that could aggravate your pain, it's best to stick with a certified instructor with several years' experience working with older people. Your local YMCA, senior center, or health club should be able to refer you to a reputable instructor.

What Does It Cost?

Yoga classes are offered free of charge at some churches and schools. In general, though, group classes range in price from $5 to $15. Private classes average about $50 an hour. "Working with a good yoga teacher can make the difference between learning yoga safely and correctly or getting hurt," Lawrence says. "There is no substitute for the attention to detail and individual guidance a good teacher can offer you."

You can do yoga without props, but most people get a mat, which can cost about $20.

PART THREE

Pain Makers— The Top 20

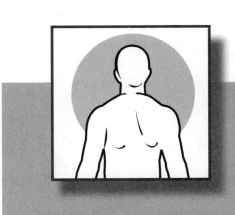

Erasing the Worst Pains

Jack Benny knew how to make people laugh. His secret weapon was simple: Mix an ounce of droll wit with a pound of truth. So predictably, one time when he was giving an acceptance speech at an awards ceremony, the comic legend quipped, "I don't deserve this, but I have arthritis, and I don't deserve that either."

Like Benny, we all get aches and pains we don't deserve—a toothache here, a backache there, a twinge of arthritis everywhere. And like this great jester, hopefully we can joke about our discomforts occasionally. But often, aches and pains aren't funny. They just hurt. And just as often, the natural inclination is to blame these pains on aging and conclude that nothing can be done.

But our message here is a different one. Most of the pains that you experience actually have little to do with the process of aging. What's more, in reality, there are plenty of things that you can do to relieve even the most intractable discomforts at ages 60, 70, 80, and beyond.

That's what the following section is all about. The next several chapters offer an in-depth look at the causes of and the treatments for the 20 worst pains affecting older Americans.

How do we know these are the nastiest? These pains were selected for special emphasis in this book based on surveys and interviews with hundreds of seniors just like you. In addition, we spoke with a multitude of physicians, chiropractors, physical therapists, and other health-care professionals who, every day, see and treat older Americans who are in pain. At the end of this process, the consensus was clear. Overwhelmingly, your fellow older Americans and the health-care professionals who treat your pains mentioned the same problems over and over again.

So in the pages that follow, you'll discover a comprehensive guide to alleviating your most nagging, lingering, and debilitating pains, including those associated with arthritis, cancer, and your joints. And by the end of this section, we hope that you will emerge with the knowledge that you need to get what you really deserve—a pain-free life.

Angina

Short-lived but severely painful, angina comes from a Greek word meaning "a strangling." If you've ever had angina pain, you certainly understand the analogy. The heaviness in your chest—sometimes described as the mass of an elephant pressing down—comes from a sudden constriction of blood vessels around your heart.

When angina occurs, you're usually under a lot of physical or emotional stress—perhaps climbing a set of stairs or swearing at that reckless driver who just cut you off on the interstate. In response to the stress, your coronary arteries may go into spasm, says Bernard Clark, M.D., director of noninvasive cardiology at the Hoffman Heart Institute at St. Francis Hospital and Medical Center in Hartford, Connecticut. Your heart muscle needs more blood and oxygen but can't get

enough because the pipelines are narrowed with plaque and scarring.

Perhaps you haven't felt the classic symptom of angina but have experienced a sense of fullness or indigestion, perhaps a burning in your upper chest and esophagus, says Dr. Clark. These, too, can be manifestations of angina and heart disease.

"Seniors may not have symptoms that are as overwhelming, as heavy, or as painful. Their angina may be more subtle," he warns. "Still, it's not something you should ignore. Angina is a very clear sign that you may have heart disease."

High cholesterol, smoking, excess weight, lack of exercise, and poor diet all contribute to angina and heart disease. First, you'll need to get a proper diagnosis from your doctor, then, you usually can manage angina with medication, exercise, and stress management and by changing lifestyle habits, says Dr. Clark.

When an angina attack hits, the most immediate remedy is to take the nitroglycerin your doctor has prescribed for you. Here are some other things you can do in addition to taking your medication.

For Fast Relief

Come to a complete stop. After you've taken your medication, you can help yourself even more by stopping whatever it is you're doing. If it's physical exertion like climbing a hill, you should sit down and rest. If it's emotional stress, such as an encounter with a rude cashier in the grocery store, you need to pull back from the conflict and remove yourself from the situation.

"Whenever your blood pressure and heart rate go up, you put more demand on your heart for oxygen," says Dr. Clark. "Once your blood pressure drops and your heart slows down, the heart will be able to reestablish its oxygen balance. The pain will ease."

To help this happen, he recommends that you close your eyes and visualize a pleasant scene, such as floating on a lazy river in a rowboat, and slow your breathing down by taking air in through your nose and exhaling through your mouth.

"Relaxation is very important. You can teach yourself to change the way your body reacts to stressful situations," he says.

For Lasting Relief

Don't smoke. This is hardly startling news, but dropping the habit is a must if you want to lessen your chance of angina pain. "Smoking fuels the underlying fire of heart disease. It stokes the furnace," says Dr. Clark.

Smoking is a major cause of arteriosclerosis, or plaque buildup, in your arteries. It also increases blood pressure, constricts blood vessels, and lessens bloodflow in the coronary arteries of your heart—the very mechanisms that lead to angina pain.

Cigarette smoke also contains carbon monoxide, which inhibits your body's ability to use oxygen effectively. The more you smoke, the more you rob your body and, especially, your heart of the capacity to get oxygen, Dr. Clark says.

Don't eat that burger. Some studies show that you can stop—and maybe even reverse—plaque deposits with an extremely low fat diet, one where fat makes up less than 10 percent of daily calories. Talk with your doctor or a nutritionist, suggests Michele Clark, a cardiac rehabilitative specialist and manager of Cardiac and Pulmonary Rehabilitation Services at Crouse Hospital in Syracuse, New York. Then, change your diet. Eat less red meat and more fish. Strongly consider a vegetarian diet. Stay away from processed foods. Add more whole grains and vegetables to your diet. Choose low-fat over high-fat items.

"Even if you're older and have already had a heart attack, it's not too late to make lifestyle changes to reduce your risk of a second heart attack or worsening of your heart disease," she says.

Get a tune-up. Increase your physical activity, and you'll improve the ability of your body to tolerate work, leisure, and recreational interests. There are several benefits to regular exercise and increased physical activity. Even by adding a little activity at a time, you may enjoy improvements in muscular strength, endurance, joint flexibility, cardiovascular endurance, and body composition. Increased physical activity improves oxygen use and your body's ability to move blood through your arteries, says Michele Clark.

"I compare it to getting better gas mileage after you tune up your car," she explains. "Tune up your body, and it works more efficiently. You won't need to use as much fuel— in this case, oxygen—to climb those stairs as you did before. You'll be a more efficient machine. This is important to people who may

experience symptoms with activity, such as shortness of breath or fatigue. Regular exercise, designed with your individual needs in mind, may lessen these symptoms."

There's no lack of scientific evidence showing the benefits of exercise. The more you exercise, the less likely you'll have heart problems. Even if you're already getting angina attacks or recovering from a first heart attack, it's never too late to start, says Dr. Clark.

"I recommend walking. It's easy to do. You can start slowly and gradually build up how long and how far you walk," he adds.

Put on your hat. Going outside on a cold or windy day can trigger an angina attack. The cold air on your skin causes blood vessels to constrict, which may in turn increase oxygen demand on your heart, says Dr. Clark.

"We always tell patients to dress properly in cold weather. Wear a hat, mittens, and a scarf. Don't expose a lot of skin to the cold," he says.

Take a swim. If walking hurts because you have arthritis or you're overweight, try swimming or water aerobics, suggests Michele Clark. The buoyancy of the water takes pressure off your joints and makes you essentially weightless.

"Swimming and water exercise are really outstanding forms of exercise for your cardiovascular system," she says. "They're fun, too." Most YMCAs and community swim programs offer some type of water aerobics and swimming classes for older adults. Be sure to contact a physician for clearance to participate before starting a new exercise program.

Relax and chill out. Any way you can, you should reduce stress in your life. Take up yoga, go for a walk, pray, smell the flowers, try biofeedback, sew a quilt or take up another relaxing hobby, use guided imagery and self-hypnosis, or practice progressive relaxation techniques, in which you tense and relax various muscle groups in your body, says Michele Clark. "What exactly relieves stress is really very individual. Do what works for you."

Stress directly influences angina discomfort. When you're really stressed, your body releases catecholamines, substances that increase, among other things, the rate and force of your heart's pumping. Catecholamines also constrict blood vessels, which is the last thing you need to happen when your heart is pumping harder and demanding more blood and oxygen, she says.

"Immediately, you have a supply-and-demand mismatch. Your heart needs more blood, but the flow is reduced because the stress is increasing vessel constriction," she explains. "That's why mental stress all by itself may bring on an angina attack or make it more likely to occur."

Take hawthorn. Herbalists and naturopathic doctors often tell their patients with angina to take hawthorn, an herb long used as a heart tonic, says Pamela Herring, N.D., a naturopathic physician at the Naturopathic Clinic of Concord in New Hampshire.

Hawthorn won't reverse atherosclerosis, a form of arteriosclerosis, but it may improve the overall functioning of the heart and make it more efficient, says Dr. Herring. Hawthorn also dilates coronary arteries.

Hawthorn, however, isn't one of those herbs that immediately makes you feel better when you pop it into your mouth. Its therapeutic effects take time to develop, usually over a period of weeks or months, says Dr. Herring.

Hawthorn comes in several forms: liquid, capsules, tea bags, and a concentrated extract that resembles a tarlike syrup. It's available in most health food stores and drugstores. If you have a cardiovascular condition, do not take hawthorn regularly for more than a few weeks without medical supervision. You may require lower doses of other medications, such as high blood pressure drugs. If you have low blood pressure caused by heart valve problems, do not use hawthorn without medical supervision. Be sure to follow the instructions on the product label.

Arthritis

Not all creatures get arthritis. Bats and sloths don't, for instance. They also spend most of their lives hanging upside down. Great for the joints, sure, but it's a mighty impractical lifestyle for the rest of us.

Yet short of living in this topsy-turvy fashion, arthritis may seem inescapable. After all, it is one of the nation's most common chronic health problems, affecting nearly 43 million Americans. One in every six people have some form of it, according to the Arthritis Foundation, based in Atlanta.

But even though it is prevalent, arthritis is *not* inevitable, and you don't have to turn your world upside down to beat it. In fact, by improving your diet, getting regular exercise, and using nutri-

tional supplements, you can dramatically diminish your risk of developing this painful joint disease, says Michael Loes, M.D., director of the Arizona Pain Institute and coauthor of *Arthritis: The Doctors' Cure*.

"You can be very elderly and not have a trace of arthritis," he says. "It's not necessarily related to aging."

And even if you have already developed arthritis, the same lifestyle changes that can prevent it can also help you corral it.

"To stop the fire of arthritis in the joints that is making life miserable, certain nutritional strategies are known to be not only helpful but in some cases curative, particularly if accompanied by exercise," Dr. Loes says.

WATER WORKS WONDERS ON MAN'S ARTHRITIC JOINTS

After he was diagnosed with arthritis in 1996, Roger Sizoo did exactly what his doctor ordered. Sort of. He took his pain medicine. But those stretches and flexibility exercises his doctor wanted him to do? Well, they got lost in the daily shuffle.

Within 6 months, Sizoo, a retired executive in southern California, couldn't bend over to pick up his morning paper. He had trouble even putting on his socks and tying his shoes.

"I was in real pain because I didn't have any flexibility in my joints at all," says Sizoo, who is in his late seventies. "I was in pretty tough shape." In fact, it got so bad that he told his doctor to go ahead and schedule hip-replacement surgery.

But then, with his daughter's help, Sizoo enrolled in an aquatic exercise program at a local YMCA. The 60-minute workouts three times a week, combined with daily flexibility exercises, worked wonders. Soon, the surgery was scrubbed, and the only painkiller he needed was an occasional aspirin.

"Life has taken on a new dimension. I sleep better. I feel better. I'm more flexible and mobile than I've been in years, and I don't feel any pain," he says. "You can take control of your arthritis pain. You don't want to roll over and feel sorry for yourself. You want to do something about it if you can."

HEAL THYSELF

Arthritis is hardly a new disease. Researchers have found evidence of it in dinosaurs. And it almost certainly racked our forebears—there are telltale signs of it etched in fossilized remains of humans dating back to the Ice Age. Yet up until a few decades ago, doctors knew relatively little about this ancient nemesis. Arthritis wasn't even fully described or named until the nineteenth century, and even then, doctors had few weapons to treat it.

"Our understanding of arthritis is dramatically better than it was 50 years ago. And the treatments are dramatically better as well," says Ted Fields, M.D., a rheumatologist at the Hospital for Special Surgery in New York City.

Doctors now know that arthritis, which literally translated from Greek means "fire in the joints," is not a single ailment. Instead, they have identified more than 100 different forms of disease that share a mutual trait: They all cause inflammation of the joints. The two most common among older Americans are the following:

▶ Osteoarthritis, the most prevalent form of the disease, afflicts 20.7 million Americans, mostly after age 45. Popularly known as a wear-and-tear disease, osteoarthritis affects the weight-bearing joints in the hips, knees, feet, and other parts of the body, and can attack the joints of the fingers and spine. It occurs when cartilage, the cushion between the bones, breaks down. Without this protective padding, bones rub against each other, resulting in pain, tenderness, swelling, and stiffness.

▶ Rheumatoid arthritis is a disease that occurs when the immune system, for some unknown reason, goes haywire and attacks the body's joints as if they were a foreign invader. As this attack progresses, a painful cycle of inflammation sets in, eroding cartilage and bone. Unlike osteoarthritis, rheumatoid arthritis seldom affects the lower spine, but it is common in the wrists, elbows, shoulders, knees, ankles, and feet. It is possible for someone to develop both osteoarthritis and rheumatoid arthritis.

Certainly, medications can help relieve these and other painful arthritic conditions. But they don't work in a vacuum. It will take some effort on your part as well.

"Older people often would rather just take medication than do exercise and other

RHEUMATOID ARTHRITIS VERSUS OSTEOARTHRITIS: WHAT'S THE DIFFERENCE?

The two most common types of arthritis—rheumatoid and osteoarthritis—are actually two different diseases with very divergent symptoms. Here's a quick look at some of the differences.

Rheumatoid Arthritis	Osteoarthritis
An autoimmune disease that often strikes in the prime of life (ages 25 to 50)	The age-related wear-and-tear-of-cartilage disease that usually occurs after age 40
May develop within weeks or months	Usually develops slowly over many years
Usually affects joints on both sides of the body (such as both knees)	Affects isolated joints, or joints on only one side of the body at first

self-help treatments. They want some sort of magical pixie dust that they can sprinkle over themselves to make their symptoms go away. For those of us who take care of older people, it is a constant struggle to get our patients to realize that self-help is extremely important in subduing arthritis pain," says Raymond Yung, M.D., a geriatric rheumatologist at the University of Michigan Health Sciences Center in Ann Arbor.

Here's a closer look at the most important things you can do for yourself to relieve arthritis pain.

Rheumatoid Arthritis	Osteoarthritis
Causes redness, warmth, and swelling of joints	Usually doesn't cause redness or warmth of joints
Affects many joints, usually small joints of the hands and feet, and may include the elbows, shoulders, knees, or ankles	Most commonly affects weight-bearing joints (such as the knees and hips)
Can affect the entire body, with general feelings of sickness and fatigue as well as weight loss and fever	Discomfort is usually related to the affected joints
Prolonged morning stiffness	Brief morning stiffness
Causes major fatigue	Rarely causes fatigue

EXERCISE: SQUEEZE OUT PAIN

Imagine a sponge sitting next to a kitchen sink. Day after day, as it sits there unused, it gets drier and drier until it finally crumbles. The same thing happens to your joints if you don't exercise them.

"If you don't exercise, your joints are only going to hurt worse," Dr. Fields says. "There's an old saying, 'Use it or lose it,' that is quite apt when it comes to arthritis. If you allow stiffness to win, if you give in to the pain and stop bending your joints, after a while you'll start developing scar

DRIVE ARTHRITIS OFF THE FAIRWAY

Arthritis shouldn't keep you off the links. In fact, if you enjoy the game, it can be a great way to improve your hand strength and keep your upper extremities—trunk, hips, and shoulders—mobile. The key is adaption. Your local pro shop or golf speciality store can help you keep up-to-date on the latest products designed to make golfing easier on arthritic joints. In addition, here are a few suggestions from the Arthritis Foundation that can make your day on the course as pain-free as possible.

▶ Use a lower-compression ball (a 90 instead of a 100, for instance) so there is more "give" to the ball when you hit it

▶ Use clubs with lightweight graphite shafts to help absorb shock better

▶ Use a perimeter-weighted head on the club, again, for better absorption

▶ Build up the grip size on your clubs with epoxy tape to help you hold them easier and to reduce stress and pain on your finger joints

▶ Try wearing wrist braces or gloves on both hands to stabilize your joints

▶ Use tees whenever you hit the ball—even on the practice range—to avoid striking the ground and jarring your joints

▶ Play from the 150-yard markers if you begin to get tired

▶ Listen to your body throughout the round—if you begin to tire, practice your chipping or putting, or play fewer holes

tissue that will make your movements even more difficult and painful."

In fact, exercise may not only stop pain, it can help reverse arthritis, says Dharma Singh Khalsa, M.D., a pain-management expert in Tucson, Arizona, and author of *The Pain Cure*. Among its many arthritis-reversing effects, exercise:

▶ Increases the flow of synovial fluid in and out of joints. Synovial fluid helps nourish and moisten cartilage and helps keep it from deteriorating.

▶ Strengthens bones. Exercise makes bones denser and helps pack them with minerals. This makes your bones far more resistant to arthritis.

▶ Strengthens muscles, tendons, and ligaments. Strong muscles and supporting tissue help counteract the stress and strain on your joints.

▶ Controls weight. Excessive weight aggravates arthritic joints.

▶ Increases bloodflow to your joints. Good blood circulation helps bring nutrients and oxygen into your joints and flushes out toxins and other waste that can aggravate arthritis.

In addition, exercise increases the production of three potent pain-fighting chemicals: endorphins, serotonin, and norepinephrine. When these natural pain relievers are released in your body, you'll not only feel less pain but you'll also be more capable of doing other things that are necessary to overcome your arthritis, Dr. Khalsa says.

The best anti-arthritis exercise program combines workouts that improve the range of motion, strength, and durability of your joints. A physical or occupational therapist—ask your doctor for a referral—can help design a specific exercise program to fit your needs. But later in this chapter, in "Exercises Just for Joints," on page 232, you'll find a few general exercises that can help you stay limber, strong, and arthritis-resistant.

DIET AND NUTRITIONAL SUPPLEMENTS: WHAT'S EATING YOU?

"Let food be thy medicine," Hippocrates wrote in the fifth century. And for centuries, that's exactly what our ancestors did, particularly for arthritis. Their remedies for joint pain included drinking vinegar and molasses or alfalfa tea or powdered rhubarb dissolved in whiskey. But mostly, they just ate well.

"A wholesome, natural diet has been the panacea for arthritis for ages," Dr. Loes says. "Our grandparents and great-grandparents may have had stiffness and

GET TO KNOW YOUR ARTHRITIS

Your joints feel stiff, sore, and swollen. But is it arthritis? And if it is, what kind is it and what can be done about it? It all depends on the diagnosis.

"Don't assume it's arthritis. It could be a joint infection or other problem," says Ted Fields, M.D., a rheumatologist at the Hospital for Special Surgery in New York City. "Even if it is arthritis, it's worthwhile getting a diagnosis because the treatments for many types of arthritis are very different. Rheumatoid arthritis, for example, is handled very differently from osteoarthritis. So it is well worth seeing your doctor if you develop joint pain."

Early detection and treatment of arthritis is important to prevent disability and deformity, says Raymond Yung, M.D., a geriatric rheumatologist at the University of Michigan Health Sciences Center in Ann Arbor.

"Many people self-diagnose their arthritis and don't get the appropriate therapy. Some people think, 'Oh well, I hurt a bit, so I'll decrease my daily activities.' And that's how their quality of life begins to deteriorate," Dr. Yung says. "So by the time

some wear and tear on their joints, but they usually avoided 'fire in the joints' because they were eating whole grains, nuts, and an ample supply of natural vitamins and minerals from the soil. The result was that more often than not, the more severe deformities and resultant disabilities were prevented. With the ad-

they do come in to see a doctor, it's kind of late in the ball game."

If you have pain, swelling, or stiffness in or around your joint for more than a few days, it's time to see your doctor, Dr. Yung says. Keep in mind that these symptoms can develop suddenly or over time. But only your doctor can tell if it is arthritis or other related problems.

When you see your doctor, be prepared to tell him:

- Where it hurts
- When it hurts
- When it first began to hurt
- How long it has hurt
- If you have noticed any swelling
- What daily tasks are difficult to do now
- If you have ever hurt the joint in an accident or overused it on the job or in a hobby
- If anyone in your family has had similar problems

All of this information will help your doctor make the proper diagnosis and plan the appropriate treatments, Dr. Yung says.

vent of processed food and the elimination of essential vitamins and minerals from our diets, we've seen a deterioration rather than an improvement in general joint health in America. Coupled with aging and lack of physical exercise, poor nutrition is having a crippling effect on our society."

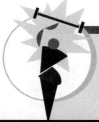

PUNCH OUT THE PAIN

Other natural-healing methods may be less invasive, but acupuncture has one mighty advantage: It's swift.

"It is one of the quickest-acting natural arthritis-pain relievers available," says Patrick LaRiccia, M.D., a physician and registered acupuncturist who works as director of the Acupuncture Pain Clinic at Presbyterian Medical Center of Philadelphia. "It's certainly a very powerful one because it is going to relieve a lot more joint pain than a TENS unit or a hot compress. If you had 100 patients with painful joints, I'd expect that the acupuncture may relieve at least 80 percent of them."

When acupuncture needles are inserted into the skin at the proper points, they reduce muscle spasms, inflammation,

Dietary changes won't cure your arthritis, but altering what you eat can reduce your painful symptoms by as much as 70 percent and lessen your need for anti-inflammatory medication, says James Scala, Ph.D., author of the *The New Arthritis Relief Diet*.

The key, say dietary advocates, is reducing consumption of foods such as dairy products, meats, fats, and sugars while increasing your intake of vegetables, beans, fiber, and vitamin and mineral supplements. Combined, these dietary changes can have a profound effect on your arthritis pain. In particular, these dietary changes suppress the production of free radicals, extremely unstable and destructive molecules that cause inflammation, pain, and pain associated with arthritis, he says. In addition, acupuncture helps increase the range of motion in stiff joints.

The needles likely stimulate the production of natural painkilling hormones called endorphins, and the anti-inflammatory hormone adrenalcorticotropin.

However it works, studies suggest that acupuncture does alleviate arthritis pain. In a pilot study, researchers at the University of Maryland in Adelphi found that 12 people who had osteoarthritis improved after acupuncture. And in another small study of 5 people, Dr. LaRiccia found evidence that acupuncture altered activity in portions of the brain that perceive pain.

"There is a clear physiological effect caused by acupuncture," he says. "It's not like people are just imagining it. It's not an imaginary technique. There is really something going on."

and joint damage, says Neal Barnard, M.D., president of the Physician's Committee for Responsible Medicine in Washington, D.C., and author of *Foods That Fight Pain.*

"We pay a terrible price for the foods we eat," he says. "Dietary changes can have more power than any prescription your doctor could ever write, because you're getting at the fundamental cause of your arthritis."

Now that you know about the importance of exercise, diet, and nutritional supplementation in the treatment of arthritis, here's how to put these and other natural remedies to work in conjunction with any medication your doctor has prescribed for you.

For Fast Relief

Press here. Acupressure, a treatment that involves applying pressure to the same points on the body that are used for acupuncture, can quickly squash arthritis pain, Dr. Khalsa says.

Although its effects are only temporary—lasting from 15 to 20 minutes—acupressure can help you get through painful moments when longer-lasting relief isn't readily available, he says. Acupressure triggers your brain to release endorphins, natural opiates that reduce your perception of pain.

To try it, apply pressure to the points that correspond to the joints that are hurting at the moment. Then hold that point until the pain dissipates, which should take from 3 to 5 minutes, Dr. Khalsa says. You need to press hard enough that your brain senses discomfort and releases endorphins. You can tell if you're pressing the right point because acupressure points are more sensitive than the areas around them.

▶ For arthritis of the wrist or hand, press at the top of the webbing between your thumb and index finger.

▶ For arthritis of the knee, press in the hollow beneath your kneecap.

▶ For arthritis of the shoulder, press on the inside of your elbow, on the same side as your thumb.

▶ For arthritis of the fingers and wrist, press on the hollow on the back of your wrist, behind your index finger.

For Lasting Relief

Chill the fire, warm the bones. Heat, cold, or a combination of the two can provide quick, temporary relief from arthritis pain, doctors say. Cold packs numb the sore area and reduce inflammation. Heat treatments stimulate circulation and relax muscles.

"In my experience, I'd say that 60 percent of my patients find that moist heat for 10 to 15 minutes is most helpful. But then there are 40 percent who say ice is better," Dr. Fields says. "I think you should use whatever works for you. No two people respond the same way to these things."

Although there is no ironclad rule, try this as a starting point, he suggests. Apply an ice pack wrapped in a thin towel for 10 minutes. Rest the area for 10 minutes. Then wrap the area with a moist, warm towel for 15 minutes. Repeat as needed.

Distract yourself. Over-the-counter liniments such as Bengay ointment or Icy Hot cream can temporarily distract your mind from your arthritis pain when used as directed, says Harry Shen, M.D., a rheumatologist at the Hospital for Joint Diseases in New York City.

AROUSE YOUR NATURAL DEFENSES

Kundalini yoga, a form of yoga that originated in India several thousand years ago, enhances your body's natural defenses, arouses your mental energy, and can help diminish pain signals from every joint in your body. At least once a day, practice the following exercise to help relieve arthritis pain. This exercise is particularly effective if it is done in conjunction with meditation.

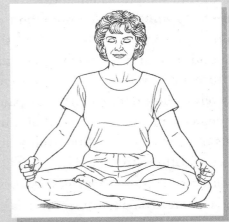

Sit in the pose shown, with your hands on your knees, your thumbs and forefingers touching, and your elbows straight. If it's too difficult for you to sit on the floor, you can do this sitting in a chair. Inhale through your nose until your abdomen is filled with air, then fill your lungs. Hold this breath for a moment, then exhale through your nose, emptying your lungs first, and then your abdomen. Near the end of your exhalation, pull your stomach in to force out as much air as possible. On each inhalation say, "Sat," and on each exhalation say, "Nam," a powerful mantra that literally means "to feel your true identity." Start with 5 minutes of practice. Then add 1 minute a day, to a maximum of 11 minutes.

"These liniments are basically counterirritants. It's like being at a cocktail party. How many people can you listen to at the same time? One, maybe two. The same principle applies to your body. If you create a sensation of warmth on the skin, your brain will be distracted from your painful joint," he says.

Beat the devil. Devil's claw, an anti-inflammatory herb, can slash pain caused by rheumatoid arthritis if taken regularly for several weeks, says Mark Stengler, N.D., a naturopathic physician in San Diego and author of *The Natural Physician*. He recommends taking two 500-milligram capsules three times a day. Devil's claw is available at most health food stores. Like other herbs, devil's claw is more effective if you take it at least an hour before eating. It's safe to take this until your symptoms subside.

Burst its bubble. A combination of the pineapple extract bromelain and the compound curcumin, which gives the spice turmeric its yellow color, helps to relieve swelling and dampen arthritis pain, Dr. Stengler says. Take 500 to 1,000 milligrams of bromelain and 500 milligrams of curcumin three times a day, at least 1 hour prior to eating, he suggests. These substances are available at most health food stores.

"Bromelain is the best natural anti-inflammatory substance available," he says. "And some experts compare the effects of curcumin to cortisone. It's a nice combination." It's safe to take this until your symptoms subside.

X hits the spot. If you have joint stiffness that lessens with heat, take two 6X pellets of the homeopathic remedy Rhus toxicodendron twice a day, Dr. Stengler says.

"Rhus tox is the number one homeopathic remedy for both osteoarthritis and rheumatoid arthritis," he says. "It can re-lieve most arthritis pain very quickly, sometimes within a day."

One of the following homeopathic remedies also may relieve your arthritis pain, Dr. Khalsa says. Like Rhus toxicodendron, these remedies are available at most health food stores. For best results, dissolve the tablets—in the dosage indicated—under your tongue every 15 minutes until the pain subsides.

▶ Cimifuga 30X is usually used for arthritis that flares up during cold weather or is worse in the morning.

▶ Bryonia 6X is good for people whose pain is aggravated by heat and soothed by cold.

▶ Ledum 6X relieves arthritis pain in your fingers, toes, and other small joints.

▶ Calcarea phosphorica 6X is a good remedy if your pain worsens when the weather changes.

Give a homeopathic rub. Traumeel tablets and cream contain a number of homeopathic substances, including chamomile, echinacea, belladonna, calendula, and arnica, that can ease arthritis pain, says Dr. Stengler. In some cases, Traumeel takes the sting out of painful joints in less than an hour.

If you have an arthritis flare-up, dissolve one tablet under your tongue every couple of hours until the pain begins to subside, Dr. Stengler suggests. As for the cream, rub that onto your painful joints as needed. Don't use it on broken skin. Traumeel cream and tablets are available at many drugstores and health food stores.

Get the red out. If possible, eliminate red meat from your diet, Dr. Scala urges. Beef and other red meats promote the production of an inflammatory substance called prostaglandin PGE-2 that aggravates arthritis pain. In fact, studies have shown that factors in red meat worsen symptoms in up to 20 percent of people who have arthritis.

Clip those wings. Poultry is a better choice than red meat because it contains fewer inflammatory substances. But you should limit your consumption of it to once or twice a week, Dr. Scala says.

Go fishing. Cold-water fish such as salmon, tuna, and halibut are loaded with eicosapentaenoic acid (EPA), a fat that helps fend off inflammation and, in turn, curbs arthritis pain, Dr. Scala says. He recommends consuming at least 3 grams of EPA daily. That's the equivalent of one 3½-ounce serving of tuna, flounder, or salmon. In fact, just eat salmon one meal a day and avoid meat and other animal products for the other two meals, and you will feel better without doing anything else, he says. If you don't like fish, try EPA supplements, which are available at most health food stores.

Skim the fat. Too much fat in your diet will spark the production of inflam-matory substances in your body, Dr. Scala says. Try to keep your fat intake below 25 percent of your total daily calories.

Figuring the percentage of fat in your meals can be tricky. So count grams instead because that's how fats are measured on nutrition labels. So if you eat 2,000 calories a day, for example, multiply 2,000 by 25 percent. That's 500 calories. Then, divide 500 by 9, the number of fat calories in 1 gram of fat. You get 56, the number of grams of fat you'll be allowed to eat in one day on this pain-relieving diet. Once you know that, you can read labels more critically and choose foods and cooking techniques that are less fattening, Dr. Scala says.

Turn off the triggers. Some foods such as dairy products, corn, meats, wheat, oats, rye, eggs, citrus fruits, potatoes, tomatoes, nuts, and coffee can trigger arthritis pain. So for 4 weeks, eliminate from your diet these and any other foods you suspect of aggravating your pain, Dr. Barnard suggests. If your symptoms improve or disappear during that month, chances are that one or more of the foods you eliminated was the culprit.

Every 2 days, reintroduce one of these foods back into your diet. If you develop a flare-up after eating a food, eliminate it again. Then, let your joints recover for a few days before reintroducing another food. Wait at least 2 weeks before trying a problem food a second time. Keep in mind

STORMY WEATHER, ACHING JOINTS?

olk wisdom has long contended that people with arthritis can predict the weather. Now, scientists are discovering that this notion isn't just a fairy tale.

"There is a bit of physiological reasoning to justify it. It's not just something people invented," says Robert N. Jamison, Ph.D., director of the pain-management program at Brigham and Women's Hospital in Boston and author of *Learning to Master Your Chronic Pain*.

In a four-city survey of 558 people who were in chronic pain, for instance, two-thirds of the respondents said weather changes affected their pain, and of those, a bit more than half said their pain was affected even before the weather noticeably shifted. In addition, those who had arthritis reported greater changes in their pain due to weather.

But curiously, the researchers also found that those living in a warm, dry climate actually reported greater sensitivity to weather changes than those who had to endure cold, damp conditions. This suggests that barometric pressure—rather

---

that more than one food may be causing problems for you.

"For some people, once they get away from their trigger foods, that's the end of the story," Dr. Barnard says.

Play it safe. Certain grains, fruits, and vegetables rarely contribute to arthritis pain, Dr. Barnard says. Try substituting some of the following foods for the ones you've eliminated from your diet.

than just cold or wet weather—is what actually ratchets up pain, says Dr. Jamison, who conducted the survey with his colleagues at Brigham and Women's Hospital.

Barometric pressure usually drops before the onset of inclement weather. And when air pressure outside your body falls, tendons, ligaments, and other tissues surrounding your joints adjust and expand. This, in turn, squeezes nerves that then send out pain signals to your brain, he speculates.

But if you don't like what the local weather is doing to your joints, moving may not be the answer.

That's because Dr. Jamison also found evidence that bodies adjust to a new climate fairly rapidly. So if you lived in Boston and went on a 2-week vacation in San Diego, for instance, you might notice that your aches and pain temporarily diminished. But if you moved to San Diego, within a few months subtle weather changes—even a modest temperature dip below 70°F—might trigger pains that would equal the ones you left behind in frigid New England.

If you sense painful weather changes coming on, pace yourself and adjust your schedule so that you'll have plenty of time to rest during the flare-up, Dr. Jamison suggests.

❱ Brown rice

❱ Dried fruits such as cherries, cranberries, pears, or prunes (but not citrus fruits, bananas, peaches, or tomatoes)

❱ Cooked green, yellow, and orange vegetables such as asparagus, broccoli, spinach, sweet potatoes, or squash

❱ Condiments: modest amounts of salt, maple syrup, and vanilla extract

▶ Water: plain water or carbonated forms such as Perrier are fine (other beverages, including herbal teas, can worsen your pain)

Dump the sugar bowl. Sugar sparks inflammatory reactions in your body and promotes pain in your joints, Dr. Scala says. Your best bet? Avoid sugar.

Feast on fiber. Dietary fiber, an indigestible substance in grains, beans, fruits, and vegetables, helps flush inflammatory toxins that aggravate arthritis pain out of the body, Dr. Scala says. Older people need 25 to 35 grams of fiber a day to ward off arthritis pain. Start your day with a bowl of bran flakes and a sliced banana, and you'll have 7 grams of fiber in your belly. Here are some other ways to add fiber to your diet.

▶ Eat whole fruits instead of drinking juice.

▶ Eat the skins of fruits and vegetables.

▶ Eat fruits with edible seeds, such as kiwifruits, figs, and blueberries.

▶ When preparing vegetables such as broccoli and asparagus, include more of the stems.

▶ Add beans, peas, and lentils to soups, stews, and sauces.

▶ Scrub vegetables instead of peeling them.

▶ Use pureed vegetables instead of cream to thicken soups.

▶ Add grated vegetables to casseroles and sauces.

Fill in the gaps. Most people who have arthritis don't eat well-balanced diets. And without the proper nutrients, they aren't able to fight off painful arthritis symptoms, Dr. Scala says. "Everything works better if all the nutrients are there. It's just that simple."

So take a multiple vitamin/mineral supplement every day, he suggests. For best results, your supplement should include 2,500 IU of vitamin A, 200 IU of vitamin D, 15 IU of vitamin E, 30 milligrams of vitamin C, 125 milligrams of calcium, 180 milligrams of phosphorus, and 50 milligrams of magnesium.

Get an oil change. GLA and ALA, two natural plant-based oils, have anti-inflammatory effects that can relieve arthritis pain, Dr. Barnard says. It can take several weeks for these oils to work and up to 6 months before you'll notice their full effect. Take each of the following every day with your evening meal.

▶ Borage, black currant, or evening primrose oil, containing 1.4 grams of GLA

▶ One tablespoon or four capsules of flaxseed oil

▶ 400 IU of vitamin E to prevent the other oils from oxidating

These supplements are available at most health food stores. It's safe to take these remedies until your symptoms subside.

Can it. Some older people find that commercial pectin products used to thicken homemade jams and jellies help relieve arthritis pain, says Sota Omoigui, M.D., medical director of the L.A. Pain Clinic in Hawthorne, California. These products contain ingredients that neutralize certain inflammatory compounds that cause some forms of arthritis.

Mix 2 teaspoons of pectin compound into 3 ounces of grape juice, then drink. Do this three times a day, he suggests. Cut back to 1 teaspoon of pectin in grape juice twice a day after your joints stop aching. Most people notice results within a month. Pectin products are available in the canning section of most grocery stores. It's safe to take this until your symptoms subside.

Take the bite out with bark. Pycnogenol, a pine bark extract, is a powerful herbal medicine that often can douse arthritis pain, Dr. Omoigui says. The extract is a natural antioxidant that blocks the formation of free radicals. Take 50 to 100 milligrams once a day. Pycnogenol is available at most health food stores. It's safe to take this until your pain diminishes.

Pass the (hot) pepper. Rub capsaicin creams such as Zostrix or Capsin into your sore joints four or five times a day, Dr.

Omoigui suggests. Capsaicin, an extract from spicy red peppers, is a natural analgesic. But be patient; it may take several days for these over-the-counter creams to soothe your arthritis pain.

Since capsaicin can cause discomfort if it is accidentally rubbed into the eyes, wash your hands carefully after use. In addition, test the cream on a small area of skin to make sure that it's okay for you to use, he suggests. If the cream seems to irritate your skin, don't use it. It's safe to use this remedy for as long as you need.

Slip in something more comfortable. Take 500 milligrams of glucosamine and 500 milligrams of chondroitin three times daily to curb joint pain, Dr. Khalsa suggests. Glucosamine, a sugar that is one of the body's natural building blocks, helps produce substances that keep cartilage in your joints slippery. Its partner, chondroitin sulfate, is a nutritional supplement that helps cartilage attract and hold lubricating fluids. Together, these "wonder" supplements have been shown to relieve joint pain without causing side effects. Be patient, he says, because it can take weeks for this combination to work. It's safe to take this combination until your symptoms subside.

Get help from Uncle SAM-e. In addition to glucosamine and chondroitin, take 600 to 1,200 milligrams of SAM-e, a form

(continued on page 237)

EXERCISES JUST FOR JOINTS

Stiff joints get stiffer if you don't move them. "Do your flexibility exercises," urges Harry Shen, M.D., a rheumatologist at the Hospital for Joint Diseases in New York City. "Without flexibility, your muscles will contract and you won't be able to move your joints fully."

Do 3 to 10 repetitions of each of these exercises at least twice a day, Dr. Shen suggests. Move slowly; do not bounce. Stop if you develop severe pain. Before beginning any exercise program, discuss it with your doctor.

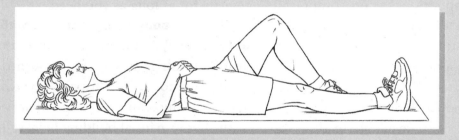

Knee and hip. Lie on your back with your left knee bent, your left foot flat on the floor, and your right leg as straight as possible.

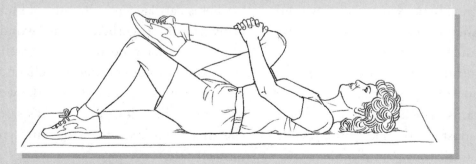

Bend the knee of your right leg. Use your hands to pull your knee to your chest.

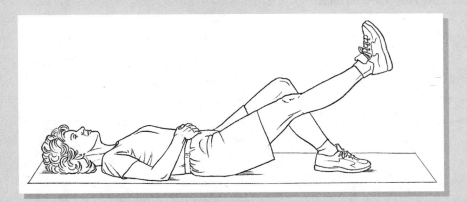

Push your right leg into the air and then lower it to the floor. Repeat with your left leg. If you feel pain in your knee, do not push your leg into the air. Just lower it to the floor.

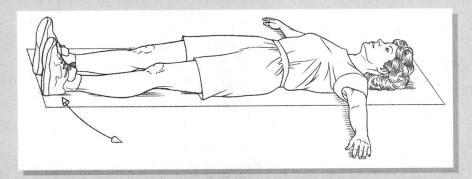

Hip. Lie on your back with your legs straight and about 6 inches apart. Point your toes up. Slide your left leg out to the side, then back. Try to keep your toes pointing up. Do not lift your leg. Repeat with your right leg. *Caution:* This exercise is not recommended for people who have had total hip replacements, who have lower-back problems, or who have osteoporosis.

(continued)

EXERCISES JUST FOR JOINTS—CONTINUED

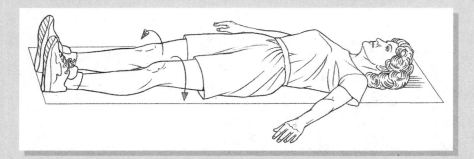

Hip and knee. Lie on your back with your legs straight and about 6 inches apart. Point your toes up.

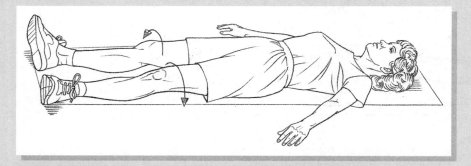

Roll your hips and knees in and out, keeping your knees straight and pointing your toes. To further strengthen your knees, while lying with both legs straight, attempt to push one knee down against the floor. Tighten the muscle on the front of your thigh. Hold this tightening for a slow count of five. Relax. Repeat with your other knee.

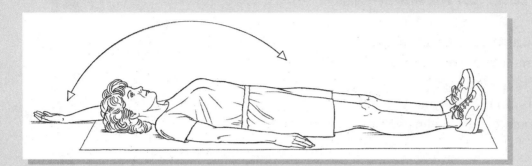

Shoulder. Lie on your back with your legs straight. Raise your left arm and then lower it, palm up, over your head and onto the floor, keeping your elbow straight. Keep your arm close to your ear. Return your arm slowly to your side by reversing this motion. Repeat with your right arm. (This exercise also can be done from a standing position.)

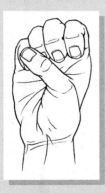

Fingers. Open your right hand, with your fingers straight and spread apart. Bend your top two joints of each finger, touching the top of your palm with your fingertips. Reach your thumb across your palm until it touches the second joint of your little finger. Stretch your thumb out and repeat. Repeat with your left hand.

(continued)

EXERCISES JUST FOR JOINTS—Continued

Chin and neck. Pull your chin back as if to make a double chin. Keep your head straight—don't tilt it down. Hold for 3 seconds. Then raise your neck straight up as if someone were pulling you by the hair.

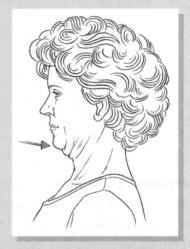

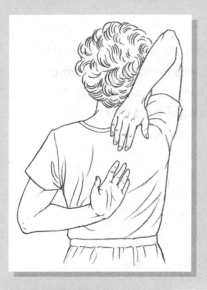

Back. Reach your right palm over your right shoulder to pat your back. Place the back of your left hand on your lower back. Slide your hands toward each other, trying to touch fingertips. (Note: Many people are not able to actually touch their fingertips together.) Alternate arms.

Ankle. While sitting, lift your toes as high as possible. Then return your toes to the floor and lift your heels as high as possible while keeping the balls of your feet on the floor.

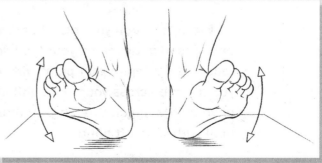

of the amino acid methionine, daily, Dr. Khalsa suggests. SAM-e stimulates the production of chondrocytes and proteoglycans, two essential substances needed to rebuild cartilage. In a study of 20,000 people with arthritis, according to Dr. Khalsa, about 80 percent of those who took SAM-e reported significant pain reductions. SAM-e is sold at health food stores.

Juggle. Pierre-Auguste Renoir, the famous impressionist painter, used to juggle balls for 10 minutes every morning to relieve his rheumatoid arthritis. And maybe you should too, says David Bilstrom, M.D., director of the physiatric medical acupuncture program at Christ Hospital and Medical Center in Oak Lawn, Illinois.

"Juggling is good exercise for the hands, elbows, and shoulders," he says. "Not only would that improve your flexibility, it would help you maintain fine muscle coordination." If you can't juggle, tossing and catching a bean bag or small, lightweight rubber ball in your hands for 5 minutes twice a day can help limber up your joints.

Knitting or playing a musical instrument such as a recorder in moderation also can limber up stiff fingers, Dr. Loes says.

Strike up the band. Vigorously conducting a recorded orchestra in the comfort of your home is great way to limber up your joints and get a terrific aerobic workout at the same time, says Kathleen Ferrell, P.T., a physical therapist and associate director of the Washington University Regional Arthritis Center in St. Louis.

"You don't need to go out. You don't need to change your clothes. You don't need special shoes. If you feel wobbly, you can do it sitting in a chair," she says.

Pick a 3- to 5-minute recording that you enjoy. It can be classical, swing, country, jazz. Use both of your arms to count out the beat. As you become more proficient, try conducting longer pieces. As you conduct, march in place to limber up your hips, knees, and ankles.

Make a splash. Aquatic exercises are kind to your joints, Dr. Bilstrom says. Because of its buoyancy, water enables you to flex your joints with less stress and discomfort. Simply walking in water for 20 minutes three times a week is a good exercise for the knees, hips, and lower back. And if you pump your arms as you water walk, you'll work out your upper-body joints as well. You can modify the intensity of your workout by walking in various depths of water. Start at 3 feet, then as you get stronger, gradually move up to chest height.

The Arthritis Foundation sponsors aquatic exercise programs in most communities nationwide. For more information, write to: The Arthritis Foundation, P.O. Box 7669, Atlanta, GA 30357-0669.

Step lively. Walking is the simplest, least expensive exercise you can do to keep your joints mobile and pain-free, Dr. Shen says. Start with a 3- to 5-minute walk around your neighborhood two or three times a day. Then add a minute to your walks every week until you're walking for 10 to 15 minutes two or three times a day.

Set your own pace, Dr. Bilstrom suggests. Remember, your goal isn't to win the Boston Marathon. You're just trying to keep your joints limber.

PAIN PREVENTERS

Kick off your heels. High heels can aggravate arthritis, says Andrew T. Weil, M.D., director of the program in integrative medicine at the University of Arizona College of Medicine in Tucson and author of *Spontaneous Healing* and *8 Weeks to Optimum Health*. In fact, high heels may be partly responsible for the fact that women are twice as likely to develop osteoarthritis of the knees, according to researchers at Harvard Medical School and Spaulding Hospital, both in Boston. The researchers recruited 20 healthy women who habitually wore heels at least 2 inches high. They asked these women to walk at a comfortable pace both barefoot and while wearing heels. Using video cameras and sensors, the researchers determined that walking on high heels increased the strain on the inner sides of the knees—the areas most prone to arthritic degeneration—by 23 percent.

At this point, no one knows how flat your shoes should be in order to avoid the risk of arthritis, but wearing flats is probably a whole lot safer than stressing your knees in heels, Dr. Weil says.

Knock off some pounds. If you're overweight, shedding a few pounds should be a high priority, Dr. Shen says. Because of body mechanics, every extra pound you carry around doubles the strain on the joints in your lower back and triples the pressure on your knees, hips, and ankles.

"You don't have to go crazy with weight loss to have an impact on your arthritis," Dr. Shen says. "Even if you lose 5 or 10 pounds, you'll probably notice that your joints aren't as sore. Every bit helps."

For starters, avoid keeping a large stash of finger foods like nuts, chips, and cookies in your house. Most people will eat more with their fingers than they do with a knife and fork, says Maria Simonson, Sc.D., Ph.D., director of the Health, Weight, and Stress Clinic at the Johns Hopkins Medical Institutions in Baltimore. If you must have these foods in your home, buy smaller packages and have only one open at a time.

Back Pain

No matter whether it occurs after a lifetime of pushing, pulling, and prodding or simply comes as a bolt out of the blue—golf legend Lee Trevino developed an excruciating case of it after he was struck by lightning during a tournament—back pain is one of life's most common and debilitating afflictions.

"Other than the common cold, back pain is the most frequent reason people go to see a physician or miss work," says Stephen Hochschuler, M.D., cofounder of the Texas Back Institute in Plano and author of *Treat Your Back without Surgery*. "We never know when it is going to strike. It can strike very suddenly. It can strike fear into you. One thing is certain: It's not a very pleasant experience."

By age 50, four out of every five Americans will have endured at least one serious backache. And by the time they reach age 70, arthritis of the spine, a major cause of back pain, is virtually epidemic, says Daniel Handel, M.D., president and medical director of the Forest Park Institute Center for Pain Management in Fort Worth, Texas.

"For most people, back pain is an inevitable part of living. We turn gray. We lose our hair. Our backs get worn. So you shouldn't be too surprised when you get it," Dr. Hochschuler says.

THIS OLD SPINE: A MARVEL OF EVOLUTION

Our prehistoric ancestors had it good. Scurrying across ancient plains and savannahs on all fours, they didn't put a lot of

TAME YOUR BACK SWING

Back problems are among the most common injuries that occur on the golf course. That's because when you start your swing, you shift your weight, and your spine essentially becomes a whip, says Russell Windsor, M.D., an orthopedic surgeon at the Hospital for Special Surgery in New York City. If the power that travels from the club through your legs and into the ball isn't uniformly distributed, you can end up with muscle spasms, or even a herniated disk in your lower back that can keep you sidelined for months.

Take a few refresher lessons to smooth out your swing, says Stephen Hochschuler, M.D., cofounder of the Texas Back Institute in Plano and author of *Treat Your Back without Surgery*. In particular, ask your golf pro to teach you the single-

strain on their backs. Then, somebody stood up and spoiled everything.

"Back pain is the price we pay for walking upright," Dr. Hochschuler says. "Instead of distributing our weight load evenly on four limbs, we're trying to do it on two. It changes the whole dynamic. Walking upright places more stresses and strains on the spine."

Standing, for instance, is 2 to 3 times more stressful on the back than lying down, Dr. Hochschuler says. Sitting places 4 times as much pressure on the spine as reclining. And lifting, particularly if you do it improperly, is up to 10 times more straining on the back than lying prone.

Fortunately, as we have evolved, the back has developed into a complex tower of bones, muscles, joints, and ligaments de-

axis swing, a technique that is much kinder to the back than conventional strokes.

A good stretch before you play also is important, Dr. Hochschuler says. The following stretches can help you limber up not only for golf but also for tennis and other racquet sports.

On the first tee, stand and raise one knee in your hands so that your thigh is about waist high. Gently cross your knee across your trunk until you feel a light tug. Hold for a count of 10, then repeat with your other leg. Do 5 to 10 repetitions of this stretch. Make sure to hold on to a wall, tree, or even a playing partner for balance.

Then, hold both ends of a golf club and put it behind your head, resting it on your shoulders. Gently rotate at the waist and turn from side to side, holding the stretch on each side for a slow count of five—one-Mississippi, two-Mississippi, and so on. These stretches will loosen up your back and prevent muscle strains.

signed to withstand these additional pressures. At its core is the spine—24 bony joints, called vertebrae, stacked upon one another like a child's building blocks. Each round, 1-inch-tall vertebra is made from the same stuff as seashell—calcium carbonate and calcium phosphate—and is just as strong and durable. Between the vertebrae are disks, jellylike shock absorbers that help cushion the movements of the spinal joints. Surrounding this tower are muscles and ligaments that act like guylines, keeping everything in place even under incredible strain, Dr. Hochschuler says.

"The back is a magnificent structure," he says. "It allows us to reach down to the ground and to reach up to the sky. It allows us to continue our daily lives. The problem we get into is when we move in unsupported ways—when we bend wrong, twist wrong, lift wrong—we set ourselves up for back injury."

GOT A BACKACHE? LET US COUNT THE WAYS

The joints, muscles, and disks in your back can withstand a lot of abuse, but there is a limit. And if you're not careful, a sudden stoop here or a jerk there can overtax muscles and leave you in agony. In fact, up to 80 percent of back pain is caused by muscle sprains and strains, Dr. Hochschuler says.

Facet joints, the bony projections that stick out from the vertebrae, are another common source of back pain. These joints secrete lubricant and act as hinges, allowing the vertebrae above and below them to bend, twist, and sway. But facet joints are fairly fragile, so an unexpected twist or turn can easily cause painful damage.

In other cases, particularly as you age, the following back problems can creep up gradually.

Disk degeneration. Around age 20, the blood supply to the disks ebbs. As a result, the disks slowly degenerate, becoming drier and flatter. Eventually, an outer wall surrounding one of the disks may bulge or rupture, allowing the jelly in the center of the disk to seep out and press on a nearby nerve. This process, known as herniation, also can cause leg pain.

Osteoarthritis of the spine. This disease, popularly known as wear-and-tear arthritis, causes degeneration of the joints and other bony structures in the back. Nearly a universal problem, some doctors consider it a natural consequence of aging.

"It's almost like opening and closing a door. Over time, the hinge of that door is going to get worn. Our backs get worn in much the same way. It's entirely normal," Dr. Hochschuler says.

Osteoporosis. A common problem with age, osteoporosis is a disease in which the bones lose calcium and become brittle and porous. Over time, the fronts of the vertebrae collapse, much like marshmallows squeezed between a pair of fingertips. Some studies suggest that up to half of all women over age 80 have evidence of spinal fractures attributable to osteoporosis, Dr. Hochschuler says.

Spinal stenosis. With age, the spinal canal narrows and can press on the nerves that pass through it. This condition, called spinal stenosis, causes backaches and numbness, weakness, and pain in the legs. The most common symptom of spinal stenosis is pain that worsens as you walk but subsides when you sit.

Some of these conditions, such as osteoarthritis, can be controlled with natural treatments and medication, but others, like spinal stenosis and disk degeneration, may require surgery, Dr. Hochschuler says.

Ironically, backaches are far more common in the lower back, where the vertebrae are larger and stronger, than in the upper back. That's because in addition to supporting the bulk of your upper body, your lower back bears the brunt of almost every movement you make, including sitting, standing, bending, and lifting, Dr. Hochschuler says.

Middle- and upper-back pain could be a warning sign of a heart attack, kidney infection, or other serious ailment and should be evaluated by a physician. In addition, see your doctor if you develop severe or shooting back pains, get numbness or tingling in your back, or have back pain that is accompanied by fever, difficulty walking, loss of bladder or bowel control, or blood in your urine or stool.

TAKE BACK YOUR LIFE

Although it may seem as if you're up against an intractable foe that will torment you forever, keep in mind that most acute back pain goes away on its own within 2 to 3 weeks. During that time, it's not uncommon for doctors to recommend painkilling drugs such as aspirin and ibuprofen. But there are also plenty of nondrug steps that you can take to hasten back pain's departure and lessen its frequency and severity as you age.

For Fast Relief

Learn your ABCs. Aside from drugs, immediate relief boils down to four fundamental steps that Dr. Hochschuler calls the basics of back pain.

1. Stop what you're doing. "It's hard to believe, but some golfers will hurt their backs on the second hole yet continue to play until putting out on the last green. That's simply not smart," he says. "If you think you've hurt your back, you are much better off stopping immediately, no matter what you're doing."
2. Lie down in a comfortable position. Often, lying on your back with pillows under your knees or lying on your side with pillows between your legs will help ease your pain during the first 12 to 24 hours, he says.

FIRST-AID STRETCHES

These simple stretching exercises are terrific remedies for most backaches, according to Stephen Hochschuler, M.D., cofounder of the Texas Back Institute in Plano and author of *Treat Your Back without Surgery*. Hold each stretch for 10 seconds, then relax. Do 5 to 10 repetitions once an hour when your back hurts.

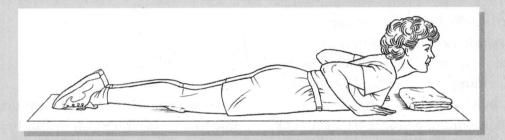

Pain-relieving back extension. Lie on your stomach on the floor or a bed with your toes pointed, your palms on the ground under your shoulders, and your forehead resting on a rolled-up towel. Using the muscles in your upper back, slowly lift your upper body slightly, straightening your arms a bit and raising your head to look straight ahead. Don't push up with your arms. Keep your hips in contact with the floor and avoid tightening the muscles in your lower back.

3. Get up and go. Even though rest is important, too much of it—even during the first 24 hours—can weaken back muscles and worsen your pain. So at least once an hour while you're awake, get up and do something physical. Even a mild stretch will help.

If your pain worsens while you are stretching, stop. But try again an hour or two later. The more you stretch, the better your back will feel, Dr. Hochschuler says.

4. Ice, then heat. Ice is good treatment for the first 48 hours after back pain sets in

Alternative pain-relieving back extension. If you have difficulty lying down, try this alternative. Stand facing a wall with your feet shoulder-width apart and your toes a couple of inches away from the wall. Then, place your hands, fingers down, on the tops of your buttocks. Using your hands to support your lower back, arch your spine, pushing your hips forward so that they touch the wall.

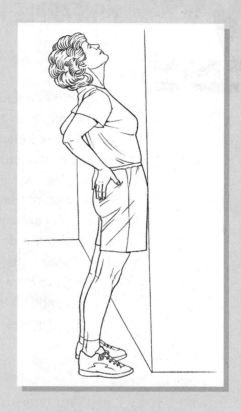

because it helps numb the area and prevent swelling, Dr. Hochschuler says. You can simply wrap a bag of frozen vegetables in a towel and place it over the sore spot. Ice can be used about once an hour, but don't apply it for more than 15 minutes at a time—excessive cold can injure your skin. After 48 hours, you can place a warm, well-wrung towel on your sore back for 10 to 15 minutes two or three times a day. Once the pain subsides a bit, try doing a few stretches to keep your back limber after you remove the heat.

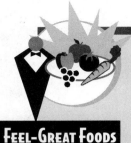

FEEL-GREAT FOODS

PINEAPPLE KO's BACK PAIN

Pineapple is a good source of bromelain and papain, two enzymes that help flush toxins out of your body and relieve painful back inflammation, says David Molony, O.M.D., a licensed acupuncturist, a doctor of oriental medicine in Catasauqua, Pennsylvania, and executive director of the American Association of Oriental Medicine. He recommends eating half a pineapple daily until your back pain subsides. Be sure to eat as close to the core as possible, because it is a rich source of bromelain. Many people tend to discard the core because it is tough to chew, but try running it through a food processor first and eating it like applesauce or spooning it over cereal or fruit, he suggests.

For Lasting Relief

Although the fast-relief plan suggested by Dr. Hochschuler can take the sizzle out of back pain, it's often just a starting point.

Years ago, the best remedy for a backache was thought to be 2 weeks of bed rest. No longer. Doctors have discovered that extended rest actually aggravates back pain because it weakens muscles and stiffens joints in the spine. So as soon as possible after your backache develops, preferably within 48 hours, start exercising, Dr. Hochschuler urges. Thirty minutes of brisk walking followed by simple muscle stretches is a good place to start. You can always increase your exercise from this point, but make sure to consult with your physician before beginning any exercise program.

"Exercise is the mainstay of a healthy back. It's not just back exercises. Your whole body has to be in shape," he says. "Everything in your body is interrelated. It's like a kinetic chain. If one part of the chain doesn't work, the rest doesn't work. So if your legs aren't strong and in good shape, for example, then you're carrying more of a load on your back."

Exercise also triggers the release of morphinelike substances that can diminish your backache and slash your need for ibuprofen and other painkilling medication, he says.

"You must actively participate in the rehabilitation of your spine," Dr. Hochschuler says. "That means improving your aerobic conditioning, flexibility, and strength. They're all important." Here are some exercises and other remedies that can shatter your pain and hasten recovery.

Fold and hold. Yoga is an excellent way to strengthen your back, balance nerve function, promote flexibility, and neutralize stress, says Andrew T. Weil, M.D., director of the program in integrative medicine at the University of Arizona College of Medicine in Tucson and author of *Spontaneous Healing* and *8 Weeks to Optimum Health*.

In particular, a simple tabletop technique can relieve painful muscle tightness and stiffness in your lower back, says Judith Lasater, P.T., Ph.D., a physical therapist in San Francisco and author of *Relax and Renew*.

Stand in front of a large, uncluttered table with your feet parallel and hip-width apart. Gently bend forward from your waist and rest your upper body on the table. Keep your legs straight and your feet on the floor. Your upper body and legs should be at a 90-degree angle. (If you're not at 90 degrees, stack one or more single-folded blankets on the table, then resume the position.) Stretch your arms out in front of you, bend your elbows, and rest your forehead on your forearms.

Breathe slowly and easily. Slightly bend your knees and let the weight of your legs drop toward the floor. Allow your back and neck to lengthen on each exhalation. Do this for 2 minutes as needed to relieve back pain, Dr. Lasater suggests. To prevent further aggravation to your back, keep your knees bent and use your arms to help lift yourself into a standing position after you finish this exercise.

Let love conquer all. Many older people with back pain avoid having sex because they fear it will aggravate their condition. But in reality, just the opposite is

(continued on page 251)

BACK STRETCHES

Stretching improves back flexibility and is a good starting point for any exercise program, says Stephen Hochschuler, M.D., cofounder of the Texas Back Institute in Plano and author of *Treat Your Back without Surgery*. For long-lasting relief, do these stretches two or three times a day.

Caution: Never jerk or bounce abruptly during your stretches. Instead, move slowly and steadily until you feel a gentle tension in your muscles. Then hold that position for 10 to 30 seconds. If you feel pain while exercising, stop.

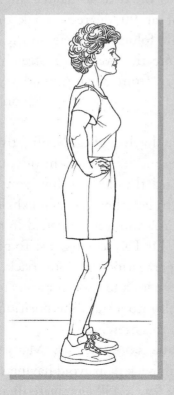

Partial squat. Stand with your feet shoulder-width apart, your knees slightly bent, your toes facing forward, and your hands on your hips.

With your weight balanced on the balls of your feet, slowly drop your buttocks toward the ground while keeping your back straight and upright. Keep your heels on the ground and don't let your knees go beyond your toes. Hold for 10 seconds. Do 5 to 10 repetitions.

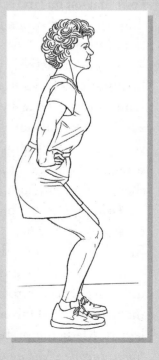

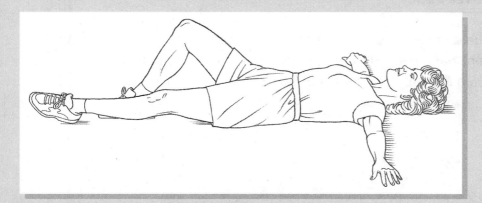

Back-pain-relieving lumbar rotation. Lie flat on your back on the floor or a bed with your legs straight and your arms out to your sides. Bend your right knee at a 90-degree angle and place your right foot flat on the floor or bed.

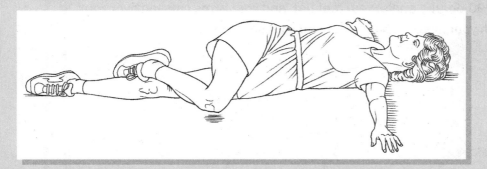

Slowly cross your right leg over your body so that your bent knee points toward the left side of your body. Bring your knee as close to the floor as possible. Try to keep your shoulders flat against the floor or bed. Hold for 10 seconds, then return to the starting position and repeat with your left knee. Do 5 to 10 repetitions. Then, raise both knees, keeping your feet flat on the floor or bed, and slowly lower both knees to one side. Hold for 10 seconds, then repeat on the other side of your body. Again, do 5 to 10 repetitions.

BUILD A BETTER BACK

Inadequate muscular support of the spine is one of the primary causes of persistent back pain. Here is a basic exercise that can help support back muscles and subdue your ache. Do this exercise at least once a day.

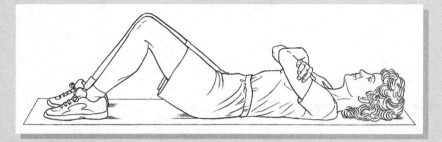

Diagonal curl. Lie flat on your back on the floor or a bed with your knees bent at a 90-degree angle, your feet flat, and your arms crossed over your chest with your fingers pointing toward your shoulders.

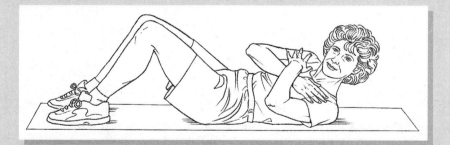

Do a partial situp, lifting your right shoulder off the floor, while pointing your right elbow at your left hip. Don't strain or pull on your neck—keep your head in line with your shoulders. Repeat on your left side. Do 20 repetitions. This exercise strengthens your abdominal muscles, which support your back muscles and protect them from future strain.

true. Sexual intimacy, Dr. Hochschuler says, triggers the release of natural morphinelike substances in the body that temporarily mask pain signals to the brain. So much so, in fact, that you might not feel the symptoms of your backache for hours afterward. So don't be afraid of a little romantic distraction.

"There is no reason why you can't have sex," he says. "You just need to remember that the person with the back pain should be on the bottom."

Rub it out. Massage is a terrific additional treatment for back pain, but don't count on it to relieve all of your discomfort. "Massage does help. It promotes blood circulation into the painful area, and most patients find it very comforting," Dr. Hochschuler says. "You don't want to rely exclusively on it—you have to continue to stretch, strengthen, and exercise your back."

For a simple self-massage, put a couple of tennis or racquet balls into a sock and tie off the open end. Sit down in a chair so that the sock is under the small of your back with one ball on each side of your spine, Dr. Handel suggests. Take a deep breath. As you exhale, let your body relax into the balls, and roll from side to side to get the full massage effect. You can do this for 5 to 10 minutes, as needed, to relieve your back pain.

"If you stretch, do some exercise, apply some heat, and then do this self-massage or get a massage, that's wonderful therapy," Dr. Handel says.

Get away from it all. Take time out of your day to relax, especially on those days when you feel overwhelmed and stressed out, Dr. Hochschuler says. Relaxation techniques such as guided imagery help loosen up tense back muscles and trigger the release of endorphins and other natural painkillers that can quell backaches.

Allow yourself a full 30 minutes to relax. Permit nothing to intrude on this time; otherwise, you may sabotage the process. Slowly close your eyes and take several deep breaths. Concentrate on how your chest rises and falls with each inhalation and exhalation. Imagine that with each breath you are releasing more and more tension from your body. If your mind begins to wander, refocus your attention on your breathing.

When you feel at ease, imagine yourself in a pleasurable, relaxing setting such as a beautiful meadow on an early spring morning. Allow your imagination to take hold. Imagine breathing in the cool, crisp air; notice the dew on the grass at your feet. Try to put yourself in that scene. See yourself bending down and marveling at the splendid color of blooming shrubs and flowers. Continue on with the scene,

(continued on page 254)

POOL EXERCISES

Water's buoyancy enables you to exercise your back with less stress and discomfort. Here are two pool exercises that can ease back pain. To prevent slips and falls, wear pool shoes or aqua socks (most sporting goods stores carry them). Initially, you may need to use buoyant devices, like a kickboard, or hold on to the side of the pool to keep your balance.

Water stretch. In chest-deep water, stand up straight a few inches away from the side of the pool with your back pressed against the side. Interlace your fingers under your right knee. Draw your right knee toward your chest.

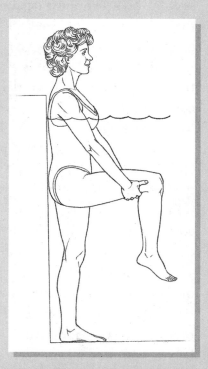

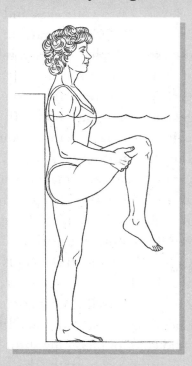

Pulling up with your hands, draw your right leg closer to your chest. Maintain your back position. Hold for 5 to 10 seconds. Do 10 repetitions. Then, repeat with your left leg. Leaning against the pool wall may help with balance.

Trunk stabilization. Stand in chest-deep water with your feet shoulder-width apart and your right foot slightly ahead and to the side. Bend forward from your hips while keeping your back straight. Cross your hands and forearms in front of your upper thighs with your palms facing your body, and make fists with your hands.

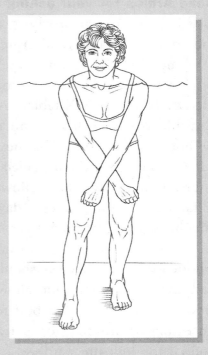

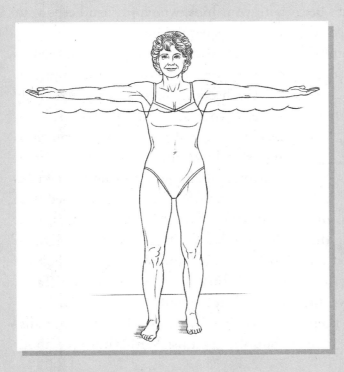

Stand straight up as you open your hands and twist your forearms out, pushing your arms up and out sideways until they're above the water level, with your thumbs pointing up. Time the movement of your arms and trunk so that each completes its movement at the same time. Repeat the exercise 10 to 15 times a day.

adding smells, noises, and other sensations that help you unwind.

Take Arnica for your aching back. Arnica is a good homeopathic remedy, found in most health food stores and even some drugstores, for acute back spasms, bruises, and other trauma, Dr. Weil says. Take four 30X tablets as soon as possible after the injury, and repeat every hour until bedtime. The next day, cut down your doses to four tablets every 2 hours. In the days that follow, take four tablets just four times a day. You may continue this treatment for 4 to 5 days.

Homeopathic remedies should be placed under the tongue and allowed to dissolve, Dr. Weil says. For best results, avoid eating or drinking for at least 15 minutes before and afterward.

PAIN PREVENTERS

Once you have recovered from a sore back, it's important to continue doing the stretches and exercises recommended on the previous pages to prevent another injury or a relapse, Dr. Hochschuler says. In addition, here are a few more ways to keep your back in tip-top shape.

Sleep sunny-side up. Lying on your stomach while snoozing can hyperextend your back and put pressure on your pelvic joints. Worse, if you prop up your head with pillows and turn to the side, you're stressing your neck and upper-back muscles.

To give your spine a rest, sleep flat on your back with a pillow under your knees, Dr. Handel says. This position relieves pressure on your spine and restores a natural curve to your back. Or, you can sleep on your side with your knees slightly bent and a pillow propped between your knees. That keeps your shoulders better aligned with your hips, which in turn keeps your spine in its natural line.

Arise wise. Rolling out of bed is easier on your back than bolting upright, Dr. Hochschuler says. When you're ready to begin your day, roll onto your side toward the edge of the bed, with your hips and shoulders moving together. Avoid twisting. Then, gently bring your knees up until your feet dangle off the bed. Use your hands and elbows to push up against the edge of the bed. Use the weight of your legs as a counterbalance to help hoist yourself into an upright position. From there, simply stand up.

To sit down in a chair without discomfort, try this: With your feet about shoulder-width apart, touch the backs of your knees to the chair. While holding the armrests firmly, exhale as you lower yourself to a sitting position at the edge of the chair, then scoot back, Dr. Hochschuler suggests. To get up again, use the armrests to scoot yourself to the edge of the chair. Inhale, then use your legs to get into a standing position.

Go straight. Keep your back straight, Dr. Hochschuler urges. Slouching takes your back out of its natural arch, which in turn puts more pressure on your spine. The simplest way to keep your back straight—no matter if you are sitting or standing—is to imagine that you have a skyhook attached to you that is pulling your chest upward.

"If you do that, you develop the normal curvature in the back and tighten your back muscles," he says. "That's the proper stance, and it definitely makes a difference."

Use props. Prolonged standing can damage the facet joints. If you must stand for long stretches, prop one foot up on a small stool, phone book, railing, curb, stoop, or other platform, Dr. Hochschuler says. If you're doing dishes, for instance, open the cabinet below the sink and prop your foot on the ledge. Every few minutes, alternate feet to ease the pressure on your spine.

Be sure to stretch every 30 minutes while standing, he says. Bend over and touch your toes with your knees slightly bent. (If you can't reach your toes, reach as far down toward your ankles as you comfortably can.) It will help loosen up your back muscles, joints, and ligaments.

Stake out a good seat. To minimize back strain when you're seated, pick a chair that has armrests; they'll help decrease the load on your back and shoulders. The height of the chair should let your feet rest comfortably on the floor, allowing for better lumbar support, Dr. Handel says. Position the chair so that you'll be directly facing the activity you're watching or participating in. That way, you'll be less likely to twist and turn awkwardly, he says.

Sit so that your buttocks are aimed at the point where the seat and the backrest meet, Dr. Handel says. If you're sitting in a straight-back chair, wedge a rolled-up towel or a back-support pillow between the small of your back and the chair. It will help you maintain the natural arch of your back as you sit.

Keep your knees slightly higher than your hips, Dr. Hochschuler suggests. It will help keep your back aligned and straight.

If you're working on a project, sit as close to the activity as possible so that you

LET YOUR MATTRESS MELT BACK PAIN

Traditionally, a firm mattress is the best choice for a bad back. But "firm" is a subjective sensation, and there are many orthopedic mattresses available these days that are very good for the back.

So visit a few bedding stores and try out the mattresses in the showroom. When you think you've found one that suits you, find out if that mattress is used in any hotels or motels in your area, suggests Stephen Hochschuler, M.D., cofounder of the Texas Back Institute in Plano and author of *Treat Your Back without Surgery*. The salesclerk may know, but you also may need to make a few phone inquiries. If it is used in a local hotel, check in and spend the night there. If you sleep well and your pain diminishes, you've found the right mattress.

It may seem like an expensive solution, but considering

don't have to lean or reach for things. Leaning and reaching put additional weight and strain on your back, Dr. Hochschuler says.

Lift like an elevator. When lifting, imagine that your back is an elevator that can only go up or down, Dr. Handel says. So when you want to pick up a trash can, grocery bag, golf bag, or other object, bend at the knees and slowly lower your back down in a straight line. Then when you lift, push up with your legs—let them do the work—while your back gently rises straight up.

Before lifting, spread your feet to shoulder width and squat down as close as possible to the object. Give it a test tug to make sure you can lift it easily, Dr. Hochschuler suggests. (If it's too heavy,

that you're buying something you'll spend 8 hours a day on, it's worth spending a little time and some extra money to evaluate it properly.

You also might want to investigate high-tech bedding products, such as temperature-sensitive foam mattresses and pillows, which can help you sleep better as well as relieve back pain and prevent it from recurring, Dr. Hochschuler says. Also known as visco-elastic or memory foam, temperature-sensitive foam was originally developed by NASA to help relieve g-forces on astronauts.

The material, which senses weight and temperature, compresses like a marshmallow when you lie on it and conforms to the shape of your body. As you sleep, the mattress relieves pressure on your hips, shoulders, spine, and other joints. Once you arise, the foam returns to its natural shape. Temperature-sensitive foam products are available at speciality stores such as Brookstone and Relax the Back.

get some help or ask someone else to lift the object for you.) Bring the object up to about knee height, then continue lifting with your legs. Remember, keep the object as close to your body as possible at all times; it will lessen the strain on your back.

If you're retrieving a box or other object from a car, put one knee on the seat in front of you, pull the box toward you, then lift, Dr. Hochschuler recommends. If you're hauling luggage out of the trunk, put one foot on the bumper, then reach in and pull the bag out. Using these techniques will help keep your back straight as you lift.

Hug, don't lug. A visit with your grandchildren will be far less than grand if you strain your back while lifting them, says David Flemming, M.D., a pain-management specialist at American Whole Health in Chicago. To prevent that, squat down to their level and let them hug you, or sit in a chair and let them crawl up into your lap. If you must lift a child, be sure to use all the proper lifting techniques: Squat down, keep your back straight, keep the child close to your body, and lift with your legs. Also, be sure to test the load—your grandchild may have put on a few pounds since you last picked him up.

Push, don't pull. Pushing is easier on your back than pulling, Dr. Hochschuler says. When you push, most of the weight is propelled by your leg muscles. But when you pull, your back does most of the work, and that can lead to strained muscles or even herniated disks.

Brace yourself. Braces and corsets can help prevent back pain, but they need to be used in conjunction with exercise and stretching, Dr. Hochschuler says.

"Back supports are good to a point," he says. "They shouldn't be used at the expense of strengthening exercises for the back. If you're wearing one to avoid exercising or to avoid lifting properly, that's not good. If you're wearing one to remind yourself to lift properly and to be careful when you exercise, then that's fine."

Get hip. Two simple hip exercises can actually help keep your lower back in shape and pain-free, says Patrick B. Massey, M.D., Ph.D., a pain-management specialist and president and director of the ALT-MED back-pain program and the Alternative/Complementary Medicine Referral Service at Alexian Brothers Medical Center in Elk Grove, Illinois.

Hip circles stimulate bloodflow to your lower back and pelvis, reducing your risk of inflammation and muscle spasms. With your feet about shoulder-width apart and your hands on your lower back, move your hips in a circular motion, Dr. Massey says. Keep the circles small—your hips should look like a washing machine on the gentle cycle. Start by doing 20 hip circles four to eight times a day. From this starting point, your aim is to *increase* the number of hip circles you do consecutively and *decrease* the number of times a day you do the exercises.

Next, hold on to the wall or a doorway for support and stand with your right leg elevated on a thick phone book, Dr. Massey says. Slowly swing your left leg back and forth 10 times. Swing your leg only as far as it feels comfortable. Remember, you're not a chorus-line dancer and you do not have to kick your leg as high as the ceiling. If you feel pain, reduce your swing. Switch legs and repeat. Many of the muscles in your lower back attach around the hip joint. So when you do these leg swings, you're not only strengthening your hip but also gently stretching the muscles in your lower back. As a result, your lower back will be less susceptible to muscle spasms.

Steer clear of road hazards. Like a shock absorber, your spine sops up every bump, thump, and whump of the roadway. So before you hit the highway, it's important to take precautions that will make your trip less grueling on your back.

Sit with your back and buttocks completely up against the rear of the seat, Dr. Handel says. Adjust the lumbar support—if you have one—in the seat; or place a rolled-up towel in the small of your back. Make sure that your left foot rests comfortably on the floorboard.

"What you don't want is to have that foot dangling in space so that all of the pressure is on your lower back and buttocks to support you," Dr. Handel says.

When possible, stop once an hour in a rest area, get out of the car, stretch, and adjust the seat into a slightly different position before getting back behind the wheel.

It will help keep your back from getting stiff and sore.

When you arrive at your destination, take a few minutes to walk around and relax before getting your luggage out of the trunk. It will stretch out your back muscles so that they'll be more resistant to injury when you do this chore, Dr. Hochschuler says.

Use your turn signal. When getting out of a car, lift and swing both legs out of the door before standing, Dr. Handel urges. By rotating on your rear, instead of twisting your pelvis, you'll lessen the strain on your back. If there is a handrail built into the door, use it to support yourself as you rise. It will help lessen the strain on your back even more.

When you're getting into a vehicle, reverse the process. Sit down so that you are facing the opened door, then swing your legs into the car.

Soar without soreness. If you're traveling by air, use luggage with wheels or use a cart to haul the bulk of your luggage so that you don't have to do so much heavy lifting, Dr. Hochschuler says. Once you've checked your luggage, divide your carry-on items into two bags, weighing no more than 5 to 10 pounds each. Carry one bag in each hand to evenly distribute the weight of the load. If you must use an overhead bin, ask a flight attendant to help lift your bags. If your back hurts—even just slightly—check all of your luggage.

As soon as you board the aircraft, ask a flight attendant for two pillows, Dr. Hochschuler suggests. Put one pillow in the small of your back to support your lumbar region. Place the other one on your knees. Then put your book or other reading material on top of that pillow. That way, you won't lean over as much as you're reading. As soon as possible after takeoff, recline your seat back and prop your feet up on any baggage stowed under the seat in front of you. Get up and walk about the cabin for a few minutes every hour or so.

Shuffle your footwear. Worn-out shoes are terrible shock absorbers that allow the force of every step you take to rattle up your legs, jostle your knees, and aggravate your back, Dr. Handel says. So if your shoes are worn, get a new pair or at least replace the insoles. Better yet, have at least two pairs of well-maintained, comfortable shoes so that you can wear a different pair on alternating days. It will save wear and tear on your shoes and your spine.

Avoid wearing shoes with heels that are more than 1 inch high, Dr. Handel warns. High heels are the worst shoes for your back because they exaggerate the natural curve in your lower spine and can trigger back pain.

Uproot your wallet. Take your wallet out of your back pocket when you sit down, Dr. Handel suggests. If you don't, you'll be sitting lopsided on your wallet. That, in turn, causes your spine to twist ever so slightly and increases your risk of a painful back injury. If you need another good reason to remove your wallet before sitting, consider this: Your billfold will press on your sciatic nerve and could trigger sciatica—a burning, tingling pain in your legs and buttocks.

Shun shoulder bags. Big purses with sling-on shoulder straps put a tremendous amount of unnecessary pressure on your spine, Dr. Handel says. A hand purse that you can tuck under your arm or a fanny pack are better ideas. If you insist on using a shoulder bag, keep your load to a minimum—no more than 2 to 3 pounds—and switch the bag between shoulders frequently.

Snuff the puffs. Smoking reduces bloodflow to disks in your back and makes them more susceptible to injury, says Sota Omoigui, M.D., medical director of the L.A. Pain Clinic in Hawthorne, California. So if you smoke, quit.

Take a load off. For every 10 pounds

you lose, you eliminate 200 pounds of stress on your spine and other joints, Dr. Omoigui says. If you're overweight, the pain-relieving exercises in this chapter will help you burn calories. But to really shed unwanted pounds, you'll also need to modify your diet. Small changes in your eating habits can add up to a big difference in your waistline and go a long way toward relieving back pain. If you want to lose ½ to 1 pound a week, you have to shave only 150 calories a day from your menu. That's the equivalent of a slice of cheese pizza or five gingersnaps.

To get started, plan your meals first thing in the morning. Jot down when you're going to eat, where you're going to eat, and what you're going to eat, and try to stick to it. Eat six smaller meals instead of three large ones. Use smaller plates—it will remind you to take smaller portions. Serve yourself directly from the stove and immediately put leftovers away. All of these strategies will discourage overeating.

Bursitis and Tendinitis

At age 50, Lolita T. Shirley wanted to add an exercise to her fitness routine. So she began walking on her hands.

Several years later, the Idaho native—a grandmother in her sixties and a longtime gymnastics teacher—demonstrated her flexibility for a national audience on the *Late Show with David Letterman*. Standing with her feet on a pair of chairs spread shoulder-width apart, she bent over backward and plucked a handkerchief off the floor with her teeth, without touching the floor.

"When I can move like that, I feel younger," she says.

Many of us, though, didn't have that sort of limberness when we were younger. And as we age, our joints become more prone to feeling the pain of tendinitis and bursitis, which can flare up throughout the body but have a particular fondness for the shoulders.

ANATOMY OF THE PROBLEM

Tough cords called tendons anchor our muscles to our bones near the joints. Also, about 150 sacs of fluid called bursae are scattered throughout our joints to allow muscles, tendons, and skin to slide smoothly over our bones.

Though the bursae don't change as we age, many older peoples' tendons become stiff and inflexible, much like dried-out rubber bands, says Wade Lillegard, M.D., codirector of sports medicine at Saint Mary's/Duluth Clinic in Duluth, Minnesota. When you overuse a muscle in an activity—like when you rake a yard full of leaves or hammer too many nails into a carpentry project—you can make tiny cracks in a tendon, leading to a painful case of tendinitis.

Excessive leaf raking can cause bursitis in your shoulder as well, either from too much friction rubbing directly on the bursa or from inflammation spreading to it from a nearby irritated tendon, he says. Either condition will make the area around your joint flare in pain when you move it, then quiet down when you rest it, though bursitis often has a more constant achy quality.

You should get medical attention if a joint suddenly becomes hot and painful and you can't think of a recent exertion to blame. Though it's rare, a bursa may have become infected by bacteria through a cut in your skin, Dr. Lillegard says.

Over-the-counter medications like ibuprofen can help reduce inflammation and pain, but drugs are just one way to solve the problem. Many people can heal their tendinitis and bursitis on their own if they follow some basic tips for resting the aching part and quieting the inflammation. But if a week or so of self-care hasn't made your joint feel any better, see your doctor.

pineapple that works as an anti-inflammatory, advises Luke Bucci, Ph.D., vice president of research at Weider Nutrition International in Salt Lake City and author of *Healing Arthritis the Natural Way*.

With bromelain, "you can expect some noticeable reductions in pain and swelling and all those other signs of inflammation overnight. Then, you can expect to heal the situation sooner than usual," he says.

Take 250 to 750 milligrams of bromelain on an empty stomach three times a day until your symptoms subside. Find a kind with 1,800 to 2,000 gelatin-digesting units or milk-clotting units, which is how its potency is measured.

Because its potency degrades quickly on the shelf, you may need to try several brands to find one that works well for you. Bromelain can be found in health food stores and nutritional supplement catalogs.

For Fast Relief

Take a tropical treatment. Try capsules or tablets containing bromelain, which is a type of enzyme derived from

For Lasting Relief

Cool it. "Ice can be magic if applied right," particularly if you're treating a hurt tendon or bursa near the surface of the skin, like in your elbow, Dr. Lillegard says.

BURSITIS-PAIN BANISHERS

Regular stretching is an important way to decrease your chances of developing bursitis and tendinitis or send them away after they strike, many health-care professionals say.

Try these stretches for prevention and flare-ups, suggests Wade Lillegard, M.D., codirector of sports medicine at Saint Mary's/Duluth Clinic in Duluth, Minnesota. Do 10 repetitions of each stretch, but as you begin a stretch, don't reach as far as you can. Slow progression is key.

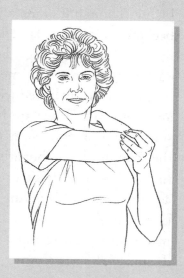

Shoulder stretch. Hold your right arm across your chest at shoulder level, with your palm facing back behind you. Grasp your right elbow with your left hand, then press the crook of your elbow into your chest. Repeat with your left arm.

Fill a foam or paper cup with water and freeze it. Then, peel away the top edge until you have a smooth surface of ice sticking out. Rub the ice onto the painful area for about 5 minutes four times a day. It may hurt for the first minute, he warns, but then the area will grow numb. Make sure to keep the ice moving over your skin.

Give it a break. "Simply put whatever you've hurt in a resting position," advises

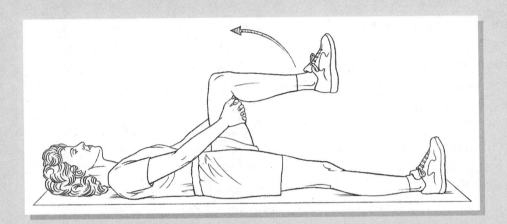

Hamstring stretch. Lie on your back on the floor. Raise your left leg, bending your knee and keeping your left thigh perpendicular to the floor. Clasp your hands behind your left knee. Try to straighten out your left knee until the back of your left thigh feels tight. Repeat with your right leg.

Mark Taranta, P.T., a physical therapist in Philadelphia. "Don't work through the pain—rest that thing for a few days." Later, when you can move the affected body part through its full range of motion without pain, you can gradually start using it again.

Curb pain with curcumin. Another natural anti-inflammatory that Dr. Bucci recommends is curcumin, which, like

GET STRONGER

A strengthening routine will help keep your joints free from tendinitis and bursitis pain, says Leonard Kamen, D.O., a physiatrist with Moss Rehabilitation Hospital in Philadelphia. "The principle I use for the strengthening and endurance building is that you need to work toward your own level of exertion, but not exhaustion."

For an individual strengthening program, you may want to consult a physical therapist. But try the shoulder-flexion exercise shown here. Sit in a sturdy, armless chair with your back straight and your feet flat on the floor and shoulder-width apart. Hold 1- to 4-pound hand weights down at your sides, with your palms facing inward. Don't lock your elbows. Lift your arms in front of you until they're parallel with the ground, keeping them out straight. At the same time, rotate your arms so that your palms are facing up when your arms are lifted. Increase the repetitions, or number of times you lift, until you feel as though you're exerting yourself, Dr. Kamen says. As you increase the repetitions and gain confidence that you are not hurting yourself, slightly increase the resistance or weight levels by 1 to 2 pounds and start the cycle of building up repetitions once again.

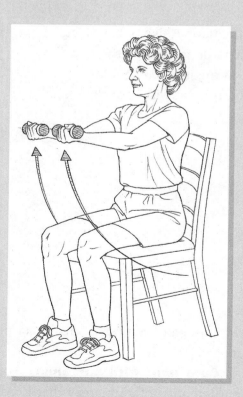

bromelain, can be found in health food stores and nutritional supplement catalogs. Take 200 to 400 milligrams of curcumin three times a day, between meals, until your pain goes away.

Sleep carefully. If tendinitis or bursitis has made your shoulder its target, sleep in a position with your arms near your body, Taranta advises. People who sleep on their stomachs or backs often bend their arms over their heads, which aggravates their shoulders and makes them heal more slowly.

PAIN PREVENTERS

Limber up. Though a diverse number of stretches work your many body parts, here are some overall tips on stretching correctly.

First, give your body a chance to warm up before you stretch; don't do it first thing in the morning, advises Elton Strauss, M.D., chief of orthopedic trauma and reconstructive surgery at Mount Sinai Hospital in New York City. Take a hot shower to loosen yourself up, walk around to work your arm and leg muscles, and *then* start stretching.

As you stretch an area, extend yourself gradually and slowly and hold the position, rather than bouncing around, Dr. Strauss says.

As for how hard to push yourself, "stretch the area to your own individual tolerance," recommends Leonard Kamen, D.O., a physiatrist with Moss Rehabilitation Hospital in Philadelphia. "Stretch until you feel like you're exerting yourself, but not to the point that it's so painful that you can't go ahead and repeat it."

A physical therapist or yoga instructor may be able to help you develop a stretching routine suited to your needs.

Know your limits. Because tendinitis and bursitis are often brought on by a sudden burst of unaccustomed exercise, keep a realistic view of what you can physically accomplish, recommends Catherine Amendolara, P.T., a physical therapist at Mount Sinai Hospital in New York City.

"If you've been inactive, don't expect that you're going to go out and do something you did 10 years ago without paying the consequences," she says.

Take bite-size chunks of chores. Similarly, you shouldn't do the same strenuous activity for a long period of time. If, say, you're going to rake leaves, break the chore up into short periods instead of an hour at a time, Amendolara suggests.

Or divide your time between different activities, Taranta says. "Mix your gardening in with some other activity in which you aren't stooped over, but rather you're reaching or you are in an upright position."

Cancer Pain

Toward the end of the Oscar-nominated film *Hoosiers,* the coach of a 1950s Indiana high school basketball team leads his players into an empty gym where they will play for the state championship later that evening. Looking around, the players, who are from a small rural town, are clearly intimidated by the cavernous coliseum that dwarfs their tiny home court.

Then, the coach pulls out a measuring tape and asks the boys to check the height of the baskets. They're both 10 feet. Regulation height—just like at home. It's still the same game, the coach says, no matter where you play. In that instant, the awesome challenge of playing in that huge gymnasium dwindles. That night, the team wins the game.

Like the formidable surroundings these players faced, cancer pain is certainly intimidating. Just the mere thought of it can send a shiver down your spine. In a 1993 survey of 1,000 Americans, cancer pain was rated the worst pain imaginable, topping a stabbing or gunshot wound, childbirth, arthritis, and other painful maladies.

But if you could objectively measure it against those other discomforts, you might be in for a surprise: Cancer pain really isn't different from any other serious pain you've ever encountered. To be sure, you may be involved in the battle of your life. And the emotional upheavals of this struggle can make your pain and suffering seem overwhelming. But the bottom line is that if you can keep cancer pain in perspective—if you realize that it responds to treatment just like any other pain—odds are that you can keep it under control and continue living as fulfilling a life as possible.

"Mentally, we've been trained to think of cancer pain as something that is above and beyond all other types of pain," says Karen Syrjala, Ph.D., a psychologist at Fred Hutchinson Cancer Research Center in Seattle and author of *Relieving Cancer Pain*. "But at its fundamental level, it really isn't. Ultimately, cancer pain is just a pain like any other."

PAIN IN PERSPECTIVE

Virtually every older American has experienced or knows of someone who has experienced the pain and emotional suffering that often accompanies cancer. In fact, more than half of all cancers occur among people 65 and older. Of those older Americans who do develop cancer, at least 70 percent experience pain at some point during their disease—usually caused by a tumor pressing on bones, nerves, or organs, says Fred N. Davis, M.D., an anesthesiologist and cofounder of Michigan Pain Consultants, based in Grand Rapids. But what most older Americans don't realize is how much of that pain can be corralled. According to at least one survey, for instance, only 1 in 10 Americans believe that all or al-

most all cancer pain can be relieved. That perception, doctors say, is a myth.

"We're in a very different place in terms of treating cancer pain than we were even just a few years ago. There have been tremendous advances," Dr. Syrjala says. "We're demonstrating that people can truly be comfortable despite having cancer."

Many drugs are available to relieve cancer pain, and your doctor will likely prescribe one or more of them to help keep you pain-free. For best results, it's important to take these medications exactly as directed by your physician, Dr. Davis says. But painkilling drugs are only a starting point.

"There are some very potent complementary approaches that have made substantial differences in not only pain but also quality of life and length of life in cancer patients," Dr. Davis says. Here are a few ways you can help yourself cope with cancer pain in conjunction with medical treatment. Be sure to discuss these remedies with your doctor first.

For Fast Relief

Try a little tenderness. Gently rubbing a sore spot with menthol creams, lotions, liniments, or gels such as Bengay or

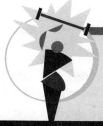

Take the Jab Out of Cancer Pain

Acupuncture, an ancient Chinese healing technique that involves the insertion of very thin needles into specific parts of the body, can dramatically diminish cancer pain and subdue many of the disagreeable side effects associated with treating the disease, says David Bilstrom, M.D., director of the physiatric medical acupuncture program at Christ Hospital and Medical Center in Oak Lawn, Illinois.

In one large study of 183 people with cancer, researchers found that acupuncture was particularly effective for dampening pain involving veins or arteries, muscle spasms, and bone cancer. The technique also excels at clamping down on nausea, vomiting, fatigue, and other adverse effects of cancer treatment that can intensify your pain and suffering, he says.

Depending on the type of cancer, a single acupuncture treatment may be able to take the edge off your pain for several days. Ask your oncologist for a referral to an acupuncturist in your area, Dr. Bilstrom suggests.

Heet can help relieve cancer pain for several hours, says Pamela Haylock, R.N., past president of the Oncology Nursing Society and coauthor of *Cancer Doesn't Have to Hurt*. As these over-the-counter products are rubbed onto the skin, they produce warmth and other pleasurable sensations that numb your discomfort.

Follow label directions carefully, Haylock says. If you have been advised not to take aspirin, check with your doctor or nurse before using menthol rubs, since some of these products contain a similar ingredient. Do not use a heating pad over an area coated with menthol; it can cause a burn. Do not use menthol on open wounds or areas treated with radiation.

For Lasting Relief

Soak in some heat. Warm baths, showers, and other types of moist heat can help tame muscle spasms and flush painful toxins out of cancerous organs and tissues, says Richard Patt, M.D., president of the Patt Center for Cancer Pain and Wellness in Houston and coauthor of *You Don't Have to Suffer*. You can soak in the tub as needed to relieve your pain.

For a drip-dry alternative, consider specific kinds of heating pads called hydrocollators, which create their own moisture, Haylock says. Hydrocollators are available at many drugstores and medical supply stores, or ask your pharmacist to order one.

Apply the heating pad to the sore spot for no more than 10 minutes every 1 to 2 hours, Haylock says. Keep the heat at a medium setting or below, and place a soft towel or cloth between the pad and your skin to prevent burns. Keep in mind that some people find that heat doesn't relieve their cancer pain and in some instances actually heightens their discomfort. If this happens to you, try applying cold instead, she says.

Visit ice land. Cold compresses can quickly relieve nerve pain, muscle spasms, and other types of discomfort caused by cancer, Haylock says. Plastic-sealed gel packs, available at many drugstores, are one of the most convenient ways to apply cold. They are less cumbersome and messy than ice cubes and can easily be held in place with an elastic band. You also can make your own inexpensive cold packs, she says. Mix 1/3 cup of rubbing alcohol with 2/3 cup of water in a sealable plastic bag. Put the bag in the freezer until the mixture forms a slush. Like the commercial packs, this homemade pack can be used over and over again.

Ice or cold packs can be applied to a painful area for up to 10 minutes every 1 to 2 hours, as needed. If you begin shivering or the treatment causes pain, remove the cold pack immediately, Haylock says.

Be sure to wrap the cold pack in a soft cloth or towel to prevent skin damage. Notify your doctor or nurse if your skin becomes irritated. Never apply cold to any area that has been treated with radiation therapy, Haylock warns. Radiation causes nerve and skin damage that can be aggravated by cold.

Snag three-in-one relief. St. John's wort, an herbal remedy, can spark a three-pronged assault on your cancer pain, says Sota Omoigui, M.D., medical director of the L.A. Pain Clinic in Hawthorne, California. First, it has analgesic properties that dampen pain in general. Second, it helps fend off depression, an emotion that can lower your pain threshold and intensify your discomfort. Third, it specifically helps soothe nerves damaged by cancer. He suggests taking 200 to 300 milligrams of St. John's wort two or three times daily to fight the pain. It's safe to take this until your pain diminishes.

Sow some seeds. Grape seed extract is a potent alternative cancer-pain reliever, Dr. Omoigui says, based on his experience. Cancer increases the production of free radicals, unstable molecules that damage cells and other tissues in your body and, in turn, intensify your pain. The extract, which is available at most health food stores, can block the formation of these pain-producing molecules. He suggests taking 50 to 100 milligrams daily while you are battling cancer.

Go tropical. Bromelain, an enzyme extracted from pineapple, is a natural anti-inflammatory substance that can relieve cancer pain, Dr. Omoigui says. He recommends taking 250 milligrams of the enzyme four times a day while you have cancer. Bromelain is available at most health food stores.

Tackle it gingerly. Gingerroot tea is an ancient Chinese home remedy that can help relieve cancer pain and the nausea that often accompanies the disease and its treatment, Dr. Omoigui says. Some people in his practice who use this remedy report that the tea slashes pain by 50 percent or more.

Ginger is a natural pain blocker and anti-inflammatory compound, he says. For best result, use fresh gingerroot, which is usually available at most grocery stores. Chop the root into several large pieces and pulverize it in a food processor. Then, put about a handful of the pulverized root into a mixing bowl filled with 2 cups of water. Microwave for 2 to 3 minutes. Allow the mixture to steep overnight in your refrigerator. Then strain through a coffee filter. In an 8-ounce cup, pour hot water over ¼ cup of the concentrated tea. (You can store the remaining tea concentrate in a covered container in your refrigerator for up to a week.) Ginger has a bitter flavor, so add honey to taste, Dr. Omoigui suggests. Drink up to three cups a day while you have cancer pain.

If you don't have a food processor or a microwave, or you simply want to make one quick cup of the tea, cut off two or three penny-size slices of the root. Remove the skin if you prefer, dice the ginger, and add to a pot of simmering hot water for 2 minutes. Pour into an 8-ounce cup, add honey to taste, and drink, he suggests.

Pop out of gear. In just a couple of minutes, relaxation techniques such as autogenic training can help relieve anxiety, muscle tension, and other signs of stress that aggravate cancer pain, Dr. Patt says.

In a darkened or dimly lit room, sit in a comfortable chair, then shut your eyes, Dr. Patt suggests. Take a deep breath in through your nose, letting your abdomen expand. Hold the air in for a count of five, then slowly exhale through your mouth. Repeat three or four times. This will help enhance the effects of the autogenics. When you feel comfort, begin thinking about your body. Focus on a body part, such as your hands, and slowly begin repeating your thoughts aloud in four or five different ways. So, for instance, you might say:

"My hands are heavy and warm, very heavy and warm.

"My hands are getting even heavier and warmer.

"My hands are sinking . . . sinking down to the floor."

Repeat these statements as you focus on each body part, substituting legs, neck, feet, back, arms, head, and so on as you go, Dr. Patt says. As you practice this relaxation technique, try to visualize warm sunshine, a warm fire, or another image that conjures sensations of warmth and pleasure. When you complete the sequence, take a few more deep breaths. As you exhale, repeat to yourself three times, "When I open my eyes, I will remain relaxed and refreshed."

Then, open your eyes and take a moment to move your hands, arms, legs, and feet around a bit. Notice how much better you feel and how much the pain has diminished. Use this technique whenever you feel your cancer pain surging, Dr. Patt suggests.

Get away from it all. Any imagery that consumes your attention and revolves around an activity that you adore can be a stupendous painkiller, Dr. Syrjala says.

Your brain is constantly interpreting and responding to pain signals produced by the cancer, she says. But if you can occupy your brain with an image, the pain

(continued on page 276)

IMAGERY HELPED HER CRUMPLE CANCER PAIN

In the far southeastern reaches of the Show Me State, Missourian Carmen Love has seen far too much cancer. So much cancer, in fact, that she knew how to deal with the pain and emotional stress of the disease long before she was diagnosed with it in 1990.

"Breast cancer is very dominant in my family. My sister died of it, my grandmother had it, my mother had it, my first cousin, my aunt. . . . So in lots of ways, I'd gotten myself prepared for it," says Love, a retired Dexter, Missouri, schoolteacher in her late fifties.

When her sister Bonita's cancer spread to her liver and bones, for instance, Love spent months by her side, helping her overcome the pain. A cornerstone of their approach involved mental imagery, which Love had learned from the book *Getting Well Again* by O. Carl Simonton, M.D.

"Mainly, you imagine yourself in a relaxing place. You're supposed to think of the place where you remember feeling the most at peace," Love says. For her image, Bonita traveled back in time to a memorable camping trip near an isolated stream in the Ozarks.

"(She recalled) how she floated on an air mattress all afternoon," Love says. "The sun was shining down, there were trees all around, and she said that was the most peaceful moment that she'd ever remembered having."

Once, the sisters stayed awake all night blocking out Bonita's pain with this image. When the sun rose the next morning, Love recalls with a laugh that her sister quipped, "We made it, but I'm waterlogged from being on that air mattress all night long."

Five years later, when the time came for her to deal with her own cancer, Love created an image in her mind of the rocking chair on her front porch, where she enjoys the peacefulness of the surrounding countryside.

Though her treatment included a modified mastectomy and 9 months of chemotherapy, she says the experience was uncomfortable rather than painful, which she credits almost totally to the imagery-forming techniques.

Since 1991, Love has remained cancer-free. She now works with a support group that she started in her small town and frequently lends an ear to others dealing with the disease. They often use laughter and conversation as a way to draw their fears and pain out into the open, and most also use spiritual faith to calm their worries.

"When you're mentally in a turmoil, you're not going to be able to handle physical pain," she says.

will seem less severe. The key is finding the right imaginary activity.

"Traditionally, when you do guided imagery, you're supposed to imagine waves gently lapping up on a beach, snow falling, or some other relaxing scene. But those kinds of passive images aren't always the best for cancer pain because they may not be engaging enough to counteract the pain messages that your brain is receiving from your body," Dr. Syrjala says. "The goal of imagery is to get yourself away from the pain for a while. And to do that, you really need to create an active scene in your mind."

So whenever you feel pain creeping up, create an image in your mind of an activity you enjoy. Use all of your senses to explore the scene. You might imagine yourself going on a camping trip. Picture yourself hiking through a meadow. What color are the flowers? How does the grass feel as it brushes up against your legs? How is the footing? Is it muddy and slippery or is it dry and rocky? What types of birds do you see? How does the air smell?

Feel the warmth of the sun; take in all of the sounds. Who is traveling with you? Your children? Your spouse? Your best friend? Have an imaginary conversation with these people about what is going on around you. Hear the snap of the camp-fire. What is behind you? Make the scene a complete 360-degree experience, Dr. Syrjala says. The more elaborate the image, the more active the scene, the more senses you involve, the more your brain will shove pain aside. As the scene evolves, you'll be able to spend more time there. Strive to create an image that you can picture for 5 to 10 minutes at a time, she suggests.

If you're not fond of the wilderness, you can create more cosmopolitan scenes. One woman with cancer, for instance, simply enjoyed imagining herself sitting on her stoop hearing the sounds of the city—people yelling, kids playing, the cars going by, Dr. Syrjala recalls.

"That gave her a real sense of home, a sense of familiarity that felt good to her," she says. "It also was a scene filled with tons of action that helped her control her pain."

Name that tune. In his memoir, *A Whole New Life*, novelist Reynolds Price recalls that when he had cancer, he listened to music as if it were "life-or-death food." And with good reason. Music can help decrease muscle tension, anxiety, nausea, vomiting, and pain associated with cancer and its treatment, Haylock says. All you need is a CD or cassette player and a pair of headphones.

You might be surprised by what you

find calming. During his battle with cancer of the spine, for instance, Price couldn't bear vocal music, particularly the comic operas of Mozart and Rossini, even though these works had helped lift his spirits in the past. Instead, he found baroque compositions by Bach, Handel, and Vivaldi more to his liking.

"I'd lie alone, as still as I could manage, with both eyes shut, and concentrate on letting the actual visible line of harmony enter my mind—coiling as baroque lines do, luxuriantly but in strict logic—till that line reached the core of my spine," Price wrote. "Its lucid conclusion in benign order seemed to help me crowd out the idiot killer encysted in me."

So experiment a bit. Spend about 20 minutes a day listening to different types of music such as classical, country, rock, jazz, blues, or folk. Once you discover the right mix of tunes, record a 20- to 30-minute tape that you can listen to as needed to cope with your pain, Haylock suggests.

Dental Pain

Buddha survives. Well, one of his teeth does, at least. And nothing—not cremation, not the ravages of time—has been able to eradicate it. Even now, more than 2,400 years after his death, disciples still regard Buddha's tooth as one of the world's most holy relics.

A miracle? Hardly. Of all the parts of your body, your teeth are the most indestructible. Capable of enduring for more than 30 lifetimes, teeth tend to be so reliable that they are often taken for granted. Yet when teeth or gums hurt, they can quickly torment even the most stoic among us.

"Tooth pain is one of the worst afflictions known to man," says James R. Hladik, D.D.S., chairperson of the department of dentistry at the Carl T. Hayden Veterans Affairs Medical Center in Phoenix. "At the very least, it is enough of a pain to drive some people to try extreme measures."

Over the centuries, people have embraced dozens of wacky (and useless) remedies for their aching teeth such as placing cooked earthworms in the opposite ear from the ache, squashing a ladybug onto the tooth, and holding fresh cow dung on the side of the face where the tooth is aching.

These days, of course, dentistry is much more sophisticated and truly less torturous, but your teeth—or the lack of them—can still be a major cause of pain as you age. Tooth sensitivity, toothaches, and denture soreness all can trigger intense discomfort for older Americans, Dr. Hladik says. Here's a look at these three pain makers and what you can do to relieve them.

TAKE THE SIZZLE OUT OF TOOTH SENSITIVITY

Ranging from a distracting irritant to a full-blown ache, tooth sensitivity affects an estimated one in four American adults over age 18. But age does have some advantages. Tooth sensitivity actually may dip as people get older, says Stephen K. Shuman, D.D.S., director of the Oral Health Services for Older Adults program at the University of Minnesota in Minneapolis. To understand why, it's important to know a bit about your teeth.

Beneath the outer surface of your tooth's enamel is a hard substance called dentin, which protects the pulp chamber, the heart of the tooth that is filled with blood vessels and nerves. As a tooth ages, the dentin thickens, the pulp chamber shrinks, and it becomes harder for nerves to detect painful sensations like hot coffee or cold air on the tooth's surface.

"We certainly do see some people in their early sixties who develop tooth sensitivity. But as a general rule, teeth get less sensitive with age. In fact, so much so that we often are able to do minor restoration work on older people without local anesthetic," Dr. Shuman says.

If you do develop tooth sensitivity, more than likely your gums have receded, exposing dentin along the root surface of the tooth, just below the enamel. Tooth sensitivity, whether it is persistent or just occasional, should be discussed with your dentist, Dr. Shuman says. It's important that the dentist rule out other causes of sensitivity such as tooth decay. Without proper treatment, tooth sensitivity can transform brushing and flossing into a painful ordeal and, in turn, lead to neglect of your teeth.

Here are a few things that you can do to take the sting out of sensitive teeth.

For Fast Relief

Slip on some oil. If you suspect that your sensitivity is caused by a tooth abrasion or by gums that have receded to the point that the root surface of the tooth is exposed, try coating the sensitive spot with warm olive oil, recommends Richard D. Fischer, D.D.S., a dentist in Annandale, Virginia, and past president of the International Academy of Oral Medicine and Toxicology.

First, place a piece of gauze or cotton onto the tooth to dry it and keep it saliva-free. Meanwhile, heat a few drops of olive oil in a small bowl by sitting it in a larger bowl of hot water. Take a cotton swab, dip it in the oil, and gently wave it in the air two or three times or blow on it to cool the oil a bit. Remove the gauze from your mouth and dab the warm oil on your dry tooth and gums. Allow the oil to dry for a couple of minutes, then apply a second coat.

This simple treatment can effectively eliminate tooth sensitivity for up to 6 months. "The oil acts just like a sealant. It's a great home remedy that works about 90 percent of the time," he says.

For Lasting Relief

Sneak in supplements. Nutritional supplements can diminish the sensitivity of your teeth, says Dr. Fischer, based on his experience. He suggests taking 600 to 800 milligrams of calcium and 300 to 400 milligrams of magnesium a day. Without adequate amounts of these two nutrients, your teeth will have some sensitivity, particularly to hot or cold. If nutritional deficiencies are causing your tooth-sensitivity problems, these supplements will relieve the problem within 7 to 10 days.

Take the bite out of your toothpaste. Specialized toothpastes such as Sensodyne or Thermodent can help take the sting out of brushing, Dr. Shuman says. These toothpastes contain protective ingredients such as potassium nitrate that within 2 to 3 weeks will begin blocking the painful sensations being sent to your tooth's nerves.

Remember that whiter isn't always brighter. Avoid using toothpastes that promise to whiten or brighten your teeth. Some of these products are so abrasive that they can actually erode enamel and heighten the sensitivity of your teeth, Dr. Shuman says.

Brush off hard bristles. Always use a soft-bristled toothbrush, Dr. Shuman says. Hard bristles cause tooth abrasion and tears in the gums that aggravate tooth sensitivity. Even if you use soft bristles, be sure to dampen them in warm water for 5 to 10 seconds before putting the brush in your mouth. Doing that will help soften the bristles even more.

"Sometimes, abrasions appear at the spot where the person starts his brushing routine," he says. "That's a sign that the bristles still aren't soft enough."

Any brush designated as "soft" on the label should be okay, Dr. Shuman says. In addition, be sure to look for brushes with bristles that are end-rounded and polished. These brushes will lower your risk of tooth abrasion and sensitivity. If you're unsure, ask your dentist or hygienist for specific brand recommendations.

Ditch the ancient brushes. An old brush with worn bristles will not remove plaque well. This, in turn, can contribute to tooth sensitivity if plaque accumulates at the gum line and causes the gums to recede, Dr. Shuman says. He recommends replacing your toothbrush every 2 to 3 months.

TAME YOUR TOOTHACHE

Like tooth sensitivity, toothaches are generally less common among older Americans, Dr. Shuman says. In fact, only about 1 in 10 Americans will develop a toothache after age 55. Toothaches and tooth sensitivity may be less common as we age for the same reason: Thickening dentin makes it harder for nerves in the tooth to register pain.

But if you do develop a toothache, it's important—particularly if you are over age 60—to seek immediate dental care, Dr. Fischer says. Although a toothache is usually just an early sign of a cavity, it can be caused by inflammation of the gums, an abscess (an infection that develops in the tooth root or between the tooth and gum), a cracked tooth, or a dislodged filling. A toothache also can be sign of a sinus infection or, in rare instances, angina or even a heart attack.

"Any time you have a toothache, your body is sending you a signal. The only way to figure out what that signal really means is to see your dentist for a complete evaluation," says Andrea Helene Brockman, D.D.S., a dentist in Philadelphia and a board member of the Holistic Dental Association.

The following remedies can help soothe your tooth pain while you're waiting for an appointment.

For Fast Relief

Floss. Sometimes, a toothache is caused by something as simple as popcorn, poppy seeds, or other food particles trapped between your teeth. These food particles actually irritate your gums, but the pain can radiate into the surrounding teeth, Dr. Brockman says. So try rinsing your mouth with warm water to loosen any food particles. Then, floss or use a water-irrigating device to clean between your teeth. But even if this technique relieves your pain, you should still consult a dentist to make sure that other, more complex dental problems aren't contributing to your toothache, she says.

HOLY MOLARS! PRAYER EASES DENTAL PAIN

faced with a stark choice between her teeth and her faith, Apollonia made a memorable sacrifice.

A young convert to Christianity during a time when it was outlawed in the Roman Empire, Apollonia was jailed for her beliefs because they were contrary to Roman law. She was imprisoned, and each day the Romans would demand that she renounce her religion. Each day that she didn't, they extracted one of her teeth for punishment. Finally, in agony, Apollonia concocted a ruse. Promising to recant, she asked for a bonfire to be made to pray for their gods. Accepting her promise, she was released from her cell and taken to the bonfire. But instead of repudiating her God, she threw herself into the bonfire and was engulfed by the flames.

"Because of this martyrdom, she was regarded as a saint and a legend; and for centuries afterward in Christian societies, whenever someone suffered from a toothache, they would pray to her to relieve their pain," says Milton B. Asbell,

For Lasting Relief

Chomp on cloves. Grab a couple of cloves from your spice rack and place them between your aching tooth and your cheek,

Dr. Fischer suggests. First, let the hard, seedlike cloves soak in your mouth's saliva for several minutes to soften them up. Then, gently chew on them—like you would on gum—so that the soothing oils within the cloves are released into the area around

D.D.S., historian at the University of Pennsylvania School of Dental Medicine in Philadelphia. "They prayed because it was the most reasonable thing they could do. The vast majority of people in the Middle Ages didn't have access to dental care."

But even today, in this era of state-of-the-art dentistry, we can still learn a thing or two from those devout peasants, says Michael F. Roberts, D.D.S., executive director of the Christian Dental Society.

"Turning to God when you are challenged with an ordeal does help ease pain a great deal," Dr. Roberts says. "Oftentimes, I will bow my head and pray with my patients, asking God to bring His peace, comfort, and strength to bear and help us all go through a dental procedure without difficulty and discomfort. Many times, my patients have told me that these prayers have helped them tremendously."

So the next time you have toothache or other dental problem, try repeating a simple prayer, such as "God, grant me peace and serenity," until the pain subsides. It may be one of the best methods you can use for quelling dental discomfort, Dr. Roberts says.

the aching tooth. Swish the mixture between your aching tooth and your cheek. Leave it in place for about 30 minutes, or until the pain subsides, and then spit it out. Continue this treatment as needed until you can see a dentist, he suggests.

Try the oil alternative. Essential oils made from cloves, peppermint, or eucalyptus also can do wonders for an aching tooth. Simply dip a cotton swab in one of these oils and dab the solution onto your sore gums and teeth as needed, Dr.

Brockman recommends. These oils are soothing antibacterial agents that quickly penetrate into the tooth and the surrounding gum tissue. Essential oils are available at many drugstores and health food stores.

Concoct a paste. Mix 1 tablespoon of baking soda, 1 teaspoon of sea salt, and 3 or 4 drops of hydrogen peroxide into a soothing paste, Dr. Brockman suggests. The salt will help reduce inflammation, while the baking soda and peroxide will kill off harmful bacteria that might be aggravating your toothache. You can either dab the paste directly onto the offending tooth or brush with it as needed.

Crack a leaf. Aloe vera gel is another great way to get instant toothache relief, Dr. Brockman says. Derived from the aloe vera plant, the gel has long been used as a natural painkiller.

If you have the plant, break open a leaf, extract the gel, and dab a fingertip-size dollop onto your sore tooth and gums with a cotton swab, as needed. You also can purchase aloe vera preparations at most drugstores. Use these products as directed, she says.

Soothe with a salt rinse. Rinsing your mouth with warm salt water can help reduce gum swelling, disinfect abscesses, and relieve tooth pain, Dr. Fischer says.

Mix 1 teaspoon of salt into an 8-ounce glass of warm water and use as needed for discomfort, he suggests. Swish each mouthful for 10 to 30 seconds, focusing the salt water on the painful area as much as possible. Spit it out, then repeat until the glass is empty.

If you have high blood pressure and are on a sodium-restricted diet, use Epsom salts instead of table salt, Dr. Fischer suggests. Epsom salts are made with magnesium and, unlike table salt, shouldn't adversely affect your blood pressure.

Freeze it. Wrap an ice pack in a towel and apply it to the outside of your mouth for 15 to 20 minutes every hour until your pain subsides, Dr. Hladik suggests. The ice will reduce swelling and calm agitated nerve endings in your aching tooth.

Load up on minerals. Take 500 milligrams of calcium and 200 to 300 milligrams of magnesium at the first sign of toothache, Dr. Fischer suggests. Increasing your intake of calcium and magnesium can help soothe nerves and temporarily ease tooth pain, he says.

Breathe deep. Relaxation techniques such as deep breathing can distract your attention from your pain and relieve muscle tension in your mouth and jaw that may be aggravating your tooth pain, Dr. Brockman says. To try it, slowly breathe in through your nose for a count of eight.

Hold your breath for a slow count of four, then slowly breathe out for a count of eight. As you do this, focus all of your attention on the sensation of the air rushing in and out of your lungs. If your mind starts to wander, refocus your attention on your breath. After three or four breaths, you'll probably notice your pain starting to diminish. Do this deep-breathing exercise as needed to control your tooth pain, she suggests.

Dim the lights. Your imagination is a powerful healer that can help you dampen tooth pain, Dr. Fischer says.

To try it, imagine that the pain in your tooth is a red light attached to a dimmer switch. First, turn up the intensity of the light—make it bright red. Then, slowly start dimming the red until the light is completely out. As you do this, your tooth will feel less and less painful. Do this imagery for 1 to 2 minutes, as needed, says Deena Margetis, a certified clinical hypnotherapist specializing in dental care in Annandale, Virginia. If you prefer, you also can imagine that as the aching red light dims, it is replaced by a cool blue that soothes your painful tooth.

"Using the dimmer switch to control the pain is an extremely powerful imagery technique that I have found to be very effective with many of my patients," Margetis says.

Sip a soothing tea. Herbal teas made with chamomile often can quell mild toothache pain, Dr. Brockman says. You can buy these teas premade in the tea section at your health food store. Prepare them as directed and use them as needed.

X it out. Belladonna, Magnesia phosphorica, and other homeopathic remedies may help relieve your toothache, Dr. Fischer says.

If cold weather or foods worsen your tooth pain and light pressure on your jaw makes it feel better, reach for a 30X dose of Magnesia phosphorica every 30 to 60 minutes, as needed. If you have a throbbing toothache that develops suddenly, try a 30X dose of Belladonna every 30 to 60 minutes until the pain begins to ebb. If you develop a toothache after a fall or a blow to the mouth, try a 30X dose of Arnica every 30 minutes, as needed, Dr. Fischer suggests. Homeopathic remedies are available over the counter at many health food stores.

SILENCE SORE DENTURES

Like the eight-track tape, the slide rule, and the 3-cent stamp, full dentures are rapidly becoming relics of the past. Thanks to better oral hygiene, more older Americans are keeping their teeth throughout their lives. In 1960, for instance, nearly half of all Americans 65 and older were toothless. By the early 1990s, only about one in three seniors were wearing full dentures.

Even if you do have full or partial dentures, more than likely they're far more comfortable than those available back when Alan Shepard first zoomed into space or Roger Maris cracked his 61st home run.

"In the old days, after 2 or 3 years, the plastic teeth on the dentures would literally wear down to nubs," says Flora Parsa Stay, D.D.S., author of *The Complete Book of Dental Remedies*. "But now, the technology has improved, so we have more choices on how to make better-fitting, longer-lasting dentures that cause fewer problems and less pain."

But even the best pair of dentures won't necessarily fit well forever. That's because as time goes by, your gums and the bone supporting them continue to change shape. So a pair of dentures that fit perfectly 5 years ago may not conform to your gums as well now. The result is sore, painful gums—a clear signal that you may need new dentures.

If you are getting dentures for the first time or having an old pair replaced, expect some discomfort, particularly in the first few days after you get a new set, Dr. Hladik says.

"It's going to take awhile for you to get comfortable with them," he cautions. "For the first 2 or 3 weeks, you might have some discomfort and difficulty chewing. But you really shouldn't be in too much pain. It should be more of a discomfort. If you're really in pain, you probably should go back and see your dentist for an adjustment."

Here are a few suggestions that can help you minimize your discomfort while you are adapting to your new pair of dentures.

For Fast Relief

Seek an herbal solution. Dab a bit of aloe vera gel or eucalyptus oil on a cotton swab and apply it directly to your gums where the dentures are causing pain, Dr. Stay says. These products, which are available at most health food stores, soothe and heal sore gums. You can use the gel or oil as needed, but for best results, avoid eating for at least 1 hour after applying these products.

For Lasting Relief

Stick with what is comfortable. When you first get your dentures, continue eating what you have been eating until you get accustomed to them.

"The worst thing a dentist can hear is a patient who says, 'Boy, the first thing I'm going to do after I get my dentures, doc, is go out and eat a steak.' That's just not wise, even if you've worn dentures in the past. Maybe you can do it in 3 weeks or a month, but not that first night," Dr. Hladik says. Remember, your mouth needs time to adjust to having two pieces of plastic inside it. So continue eating what you were eating before you got your dentures until you feel comfortable and confident that you can chew your food well, he recommends.

Give your gums the night off. Don't leave your dentures in too long, especially when they are new; otherwise, your gums will rebel. So take your dentures out for at least 6 hours a day, either while you're sleeping or when you're at home doing household chores, advises Jeffrey Astroth, D.D.S., chief of dentistry at the University of Colorado Center on Aging in Denver. If your gums do get sore, call your dentist to make sure that you don't need an adjustment. If you can't get an appointment right away, take your dentures out and set them aside, except for when you're eating, until you see your dentist, he recommends.

Make them sparkle. Without regular cleaning, adhesives can build up on your dentures and become a breeding ground for bacteria, fungi, and other germs that can cause irritating infections in your mouth, Dr. Shuman says. Plus, old adhesives can alter your bite and make your dentures fit less snugly. The net result is sore gums.

So get in the habit of taking your dentures out of your mouth before bed, brushing them thoroughly with a denture cleanser, then placing them in a glass of water overnight, he suggests. Whenever you use a new denture cleanser, read and follow the directions carefully.

"If these cleansers aren't used correctly, they can cause gum irritations, particularly if they aren't rinsed off the dentures thoroughly," he says. "Sometimes, people will use bleach in the water to brighten their dentures up, and that can cause major irritations as well. So don't do it."

Avoid using regular toothpastes, because they are too abrasive for most dentures, Dr. Shuman says. These pastes can damage your dentures to the point that they don't function properly, which will cause—that's right—sore gums.

Rely on Arnica. A 6X dose of Arnica, a homeopathic remedy, taken three times a day can help subdue denture pain, Dr. Fischer says. Arnica is available at many health food stores.

Handy isn't always dandy. Never attempt to adjust or repair your dentures on your own, Dr. Shuman warns. The handyman approach can cause irreparable damage to your dentures, harm your health, complicate your treatment, and ultimately boost the cost of your dental care.

So avoid over-the-counter denture products such as home reliners. Improperly repaired or relined dentures simply irritate your gums and cause mouth sores. In extreme cases, dentures damaged in this way can traumatize the underlying tissue and actually accelerate the shrinkage of bone under your gums, he says, causing the dentures to be looser and function poorly. So leave any necessary adjustments or repairs to your dentist, he urges.

Foot Pain

In 1948, Earl V. Shaffer became the first person to hike from one end of the Appalachian Trail to the other in one trip, a feat that carried him across more than 2,000 miles of mountains, meadows, and streams between Georgia and Maine.

Fifty years later, to celebrate the golden anniversary of his hike, the Pennsylvania man marched his 79-year-old feet—often sockless in a pair of boots—step by wearying step along the entire trail yet again.

When he finished the 5-month trek, he shared his euphoria with reporters. "I'm mighty, mighty, mighty glad it's over," he said. "If I had to go another week, I would fall on my face."

Even if you've never hoofed across 14 states at a time, the normal wear and tear you've put on your feet during your lifetime can give them plenty of reason to ache, too.

But that doesn't mean that you should accept foot pain as a consequence of aging, says Arthur E. Helfand, D.P.M., professor of community health and aging and chairperson of the department of community health, aging, and health policy at the Temple University School of Podiatric Medicine in Philadelphia. After all, he says, the two factors that most determine how active we'll be as we get older are the keenness of our minds and our ability to keep walking.

Though you don't have to accept foot pain, nature will probably try to send you some anyway. Your feet are susceptible to a host of problems, in part because of their complexity and the function they serve.

DIABETES FOOTNOTE

If you have diabetes, take extra care of your feet, paying close attention to any changes they show. Because the disease can slow down the blood circulation to your feet, injuries there may heal much more slowly than normal—and you may not feel any pain at all on account of a loss of nerve function. Thus, a tiny cut, bruise, or blister on the foot can become infected without your knowing it, creating a serious health threat.

The following are suggestions from the National Institute of Diabetes and Digestive and Kidney Diseases and Arthur E. Helfand, D.P.M., professor of community health and aging and chairperson of the department of community health, aging, and health policy at the Temple University School of Podiatric Medicine in Philadelphia.

Keep your eyes on your feet. Set a time each day to carefully inspect your feet for cuts, sores, red spots, swelling, and infected toenails. If you have trouble bending down, use a mirror to look at your feet or have a loved one or friend do it.

If an injury isn't healing after a day, call your doctor.

Keep them clean. Wash your feet in warm water every day, but don't soak them. Be sure to first test the water with a body part that has feeling, such as your elbow, to make sure that it's not too hot.

Dry your feet well, including between your toes. Dust between your toes with talcum powder to keep the area dry.

Keep them supple. Rub skin lotion or cream onto the tops and soles of your feet to keep them soft and smooth. Dr. Helfand suggests that you do this after your daily bath as a way to keep more moisture in your feet. He cautions, however, against applying anything greasy to your feet, which could lead to a bathroom fall.

Keep your nails straight and orderly. File your nails straight across with an emery board, making sure that the corners of your nails aren't taken down next to the skin, Dr. Helfand says. Be careful using clippers, as there's a higher risk of jabbing or cutting yourself and exposing your feet to infection. Filing your nails straight across will keep them from growing into the tender skin next to them, which can lead to an infection.

Cover those feet. Wear shoes and socks or nylons whenever you're walking around, either inside or out, to protect your feet from objects on the ground. Also, check the insides of your shoes for foreign objects before you put them on.

Go with the flow. Avoid tight socks or garters around your legs that restrict the blood circulation to your feet. Also, instead of crossing your legs, put your feet up on a stool or chair when you're sitting down.

Trouble Underfoot

Each foot is an assembly of 26 bones, 33 joints, 19 muscles and tendons, and more than 100 ligaments. Each day, the weight that your feet must carry step-by-step can add up to several hundred tons.

Over the years, problems in your feet that may have been minor in your youth, such as the misaligned bones found in bunions and hammertoes, can grow more serious, says Jeffrey Cohen, D.P.M., chief of podiatric surgery at Englewood Hospital and Medical Center in New Jersey.

Improper choices in the shoes you wear can lead to foot pain as well as to conditions ranging from dry skin to reduced circulation to arthritis.

Then there's diabetes, a disease that often gets special mention in discussions of foot problems since it can impair arteries and nerves to the feet, making them especially prone to harm.

Despite the potential for problems, many people tend to be cavalier about maintaining their feet—perhaps because these body parts are usually hidden out of sight under shoes and socks, agree Dr. Helfand and Dr. Cohen.

If you have foot pain that doesn't get better after a few days, you should see a podiatrist or your primary doctor to find out what's wrong, Dr. Helfand urges. Until then, stay well-acquainted with these southernmost reaches of your body so that you can maintain their health and stamp out painful problems soon after they begin.

For Fast Relief

Use the RICE remedy. Though there are many different things that can cause foot pain, an overall pain reliever that you may try is RICE, which stands for rest, ice, compression, and elevation, says Robert Mendicino, D.P.M., medical director of the Foot and Ankle Institute of Western Pennsylvania in Pittsburgh.

Wrap a hand towel over your foot to protect it, then place a bag of ice or frozen vegetables on the site of your pain. Wrap an elastic bandage over the bag to keep it in place and provide compression. Then, lie down and elevate your aching foot on a pillow so that it's above your heart.

The ice will help reduce pain and inflammation in your foot, and the elevation and compression will reduce swelling. Dr. Mendicino recommends that you do this for about 20 minutes out of every waking ½ hour for 24 to 72 hours.

Note: This treatment not generally recommended for people with diabetes, Dr. Mendicino says.

For Lasting Relief

Get those doggies moving. A common cause of foot pain is arthritis, and exercise is a great way to keep its pain in check, says Frank Spinosa, D.P.M., associate professor of radiology at New York College of Podiatric Medicine in New York City and president of the New York Podiatric Medical Association.

"It can be likened to a rusty hinge on a door. If you keep the door moving and oiled, it will have less tendency to stiffen up and not work," he says. "You don't want to overdo it, but seniors need to move."

This advice is echoed by Dr. Cohen. He recommends at least 30 minutes of exercise three times a week. The type you choose depends in part on your abilities, but he recommends walking as the best form. If stiffness is bothering you, try swimming or walking in a swimming pool.

Stretch it out. One source of foot pain is the tough band of tissue called the plantar fascia that runs across the arch of your foot from the base of your toes to your heel. If this tissue becomes inflamed, you might feel a sharp pain in your heel when you take your first few steps after getting out of bed or up out of a chair.

For relief, place your palms against a wall, stand a few steps away with your feet flat on the floor, and gently lean forward against the wall, Dr. Spinosa says. Hold this stretch for about 30 seconds, relax, and repeat. Continue this for about 10 minutes to stretch out the plantar fascia and Achilles tendon. Another way to help relieve these pangs is to roll your foot over a tennis ball until it feels better.

Give them a work over. A massage can help relieve pain and swelling by moving around fluids that may have settled into your feet, Dr. Spinosa says.

Dr. Helfand recommends the following technique: Use your fingertips to knead the ball of your foot, pressing along your sole until you reach your heel. Then gently push each toe back and forth to relax the muscles there.

PAIN PREVENTERS

Leave the operations to the doctors. Resist the urge to practice do-it-yourself surgery on a thickened callus or corn on the skin of your feet, Dr. Helfand says.

You may lack the eyesight and coordination—not to mention the knowledge—required to safely treat your own feet. He also advises against burning off thick skin with over-the-counter liquids containing salicylic acid.

Give Your Feet a Happy Home

Just as our feet steadily change shape as we get older, the type of shoes we put them in needs to evolve, too. Ill-fitting footwear can add a lot of ache to the feet inside them.

As we age, our arches flatten out and our feet grow longer, says Jeffrey E. Johnson, M.D., associate professor in the department of orthopaedic surgery at Washington University School of Medicine and chief of foot and ankle service at Barnes Jewish Hospital, both in St. Louis. Despite these and other changes, however, people often keep wearing their old shoes that no longer fit or replace them with *new* ones that don't fit either, he says. These wrong shoes can cause bones in the feet to bend painfully out of shape into bunions and hammertoes or make these conditions worse.

He offers the following advice on finding the right shoe to put around your foot.

"These things should be professionally taken care of. If you had chest pain, you wouldn't take care of it yourself," Dr. Helfand says.

Put your feet in padded cells. Wear shoes with enough cushioning to compensate for the loss of your foot's natural padding. In one of life's little ironies, the layers of fat that act as shock absorbers in your feet tend to shrink up as you get older and the rest of your body needs more protection from the force of walking, says Jef-

Shop late in the day. Throughout the day, blood circulating in your body tends to settle in your feet, making them swell as much as 5 percent larger than normal. Look for shoes in the afternoon or later so that they'll fit when your feet are at their largest.

Don't settle for conformity. In many regular shoe stores, shoes grow in size proportionally—so if you need a shoe that's a little wider, you'll probably have to buy one that's a little longer. Plus, these stores may carry only the popular sizes, which may not be the right choice for you. You may need to shop at a specialty shoe store that carries footwear in the size you need if yours is unusual.

Don't feel like a heel. If you must wear high-heeled shoes, do so for only a short time, for a specific event. A shoe with a 3-inch heel will put seven times more stress on the front of your foot than will a shoe with a 1-inch heel.

Prevent break-ins. You shouldn't have to break in your shoes to make them feel comfortable—they should feel good when you wear them out of the store.

frey E. Johnson, M.D., associate professor in the department of orthopaedic surgery at Washington University School of Medicine and chief of the foot and ankle service at Barnes Jewish Hospital, both in St. Louis.

He recommends that you buy shoes with removable insoles so that you can switch the insoles with soft, insertable cushions more to your own liking. These cushions are available at many variety stores and shoe stores that carry products for people with special footwear needs.

Gas

The Goodyear blimp floats peacefully above the landscape, even though it's swollen with at least 202,700 cubic feet of helium—more than enough gas to fill a party balloon for every man, woman, and child in North Dakota.

But while gas in a blimp's belly makes it light and graceful, a feeling of gassiness in your abdomen is more likely to cause pain, discomfort, and bloating.

It's normal for your digestive system to hold less than ½ pint of gas at any given time. It's also normal—though not always encouraged—to expel up to 1½ quarts of gas during the course of 14 or so, ahem, releases each day.

This gas gets into your system in two ways. You swallow the air surrounding you throughout the day as you eat and drink. Also, bacteria found naturally in your intestines produce gases as they ferment undigested foods you've eaten.

A little bit of gas goes a long way in making you feel uncomfortable. Research has shown that when you feel "gassy," you may have just a normal amount of wind inside you. The discomfort you feel may be on account of other conditions that either make you sensitive to normal amounts of gas or mimic its feeling.

As you age, you're more likely to develop tiny pouches in the lining of your intestine, called diverticula, that make you more sensitive to distress in that area, says Patrick Okolo, M.D., a gastroenterologist and assistant professor at the Pennsylvania State University College of Medicine in Hershey.

People complain of gas, bloating, and constipation as they age. The reasons for this are unclear since their intestines appear to work without a significant change when compared to those of younger subjects, he says.

And in a study of 170 postmenopausal women in California, close to half of them reported flatulence or a sense that their bowels were functioning differently, so it's possible that menopause may somehow affect digestion.

The next time you feel as if internal pressure is puffing you up like a blimp, try some of these tips to help you deflate.

For Fast Relief

Shake it out. Simple exercise like walking promotes the rhythmic motion of food through your digestive tract. For this reason, sustained aerobic activity should improve your constipation and sensation of gassiness, Dr. Okolo says.

He also suggests 15 to 20 minutes of walking, jogging, swimming, or other aerobic activities two or three times a week. But simply moving around more in your day-to-day life can ease your digestion, too. For example, park farther away at the mall so that you'll have to walk a bit more, or take the stairs instead of the elevator.

For Lasting Relief

Feel finer with fennel seeds. This spice, found on supermarket shelves and sometimes served in Indian restaurants, may help ease your digestive pain. Chew ½ teaspoon of fennel seeds at the end of a meal or when you feel gassy, suggests Andrew T. Weil, M.D., director of the program in integrative medicine at the University of Arizona College of Medicine in Tucson and author of *Spontaneous Healing* and *8 Weeks to Optimum Health*.

Make yourself minty. Peppermint tea can be effective in fighting gas pain, suggests David Edelberg, M.D., founder of the American Whole Health Center in Chicago. Drink the tea when you feel digestive discomfort; or try peppermint tincture, following the label directions for its use. People with heartburn, however, should avoid peppermint since it can worsen that condition.

PAIN PREVENTERS

Choose your fiber wisely. Fiber is your friend, but it is one of those friends that can get you into trouble if you let it.

Use Caution with Charcoal

You might see activated charcoal promoted as a remedy to soak up gas and take it out of your body, but it may be ineffective and can even cause you harm. A recent study by the Minneapolis Veterans Affairs Medical Centers found that activated charcoal didn't significantly reduce either production of gas or symptoms from it.

But what charcoal might do is interfere with the absorption of many of the vital medications you take, says J. Patrick Waring, M.D., associate professor of medicine at Emory University School of Medicine in Atlanta. Talk to your doctor before taking products that contain charcoal.

An ample amount of fiber in your food helps keep digesting material moving through your system. Soluble fiber, however, the kind found in beans and fruits, contains chemicals that aren't absorbed in your small intestine. When it gets to your large intestine, friendly bacteria there break the fiber down, forming gas. Beans, broccoli, cabbage, and onions are infamous gas producers.

Insoluble fiber, such as wheat bran, isn't changed much during digestion and doesn't cause as much gas.

You should eat 25 to 35 grams of fiber from a variety of sources each day, which would be at minimum the equivalent of a raw apple with skin, 1 cup of raisin bran cereal, 1 cup of cooked black beans, and a baked potato.

If you need more fiber in your diet, increase it gradually, or "the gas is going to come on," says Anne Dubner, R.D., a registered dietitian and nutrition consultant in Houston and a spokesperson for the American Dietetic Association. Bring the extra fiber into your meals slowly over several months, she recommends. For example, bolster your meals with ½ cup of raw vegetables here and a salad there, with a bran cereal for breakfast.

You should observe which types of fiber-rich foods give you gas, Dr. Okolo says. To help you keep track, make a food diary, taking note of what you eat and how you feel afterward.

Drink up. Fiber needs plenty of fluid to help it move through your digestive system, so don't forget to drink enough water, at least eight 8-ounce glasses per day, Dr. Okolo says.

Knock the wind out of beans. Beans are famously flatulent, but a little planning can stifle the gas-making potential of these so-called musical fruits.

"Beans are really the most gas-producing foods of all time," Dubner says. To cut down on the gas they make, she recommends that you soak the beans for a few hours before you cook them, changing the water several times. Then, cook them in fresh water.

This approach leaches out some of the compounds from the beans that are difficult to digest, says Pat Baird, R.D., a regis-

tered dietitian, nutrition consultant, and author of *Be Good to Your Gut*.

What works for fresh beans won't work for the canned variety. About all you can do is eat smaller quantities and gradually build up a tolerance, Baird says. You also may want to eat beans in combination with other foods, such as rice and pasta, to reduce the gaseous effect.

You can also put a food additive called Beano on your beans. This additive contains an enzyme that helps some people digest beans with less gas, Baird says. Beano, which is also intended for broccoli, onions, and other gas-causing foods, is widely available at supermarkets and drugstores. Follow the label for dosage amounts.

Trim your milk mustache. If milk or other dairy products give you gas and abdominal pain, you may have trouble digesting the natural sugar in them called lactose. As we get older, our bodies produce less of the enzyme needed to digest lactose. If that's the case with you, try a reduced-lactose milk, or even try soy milk, which is available at many supermarkets. In addition, before you eat or drink dairy products, you can take a supplement such as Lactaid that contains this necessary enzyme, lactase, Dr. Okolo says.

Breathe it, don't swallow it. You can reduce the amount of gas in your digestive tract simply by swallowing less air. For example, avoid water fountains and drinking liquids through a straw, says J. Patrick Waring, M.D., associate professor of medicine at Emory University School of Medicine in Atlanta.

You can also limit misdirected air by cutting out smoking, gum, and hard candy.

Examine those ingredients. If you do choose to eat or chew sugar-free candy or gum, check to see if it contains the sweetener sorbitol, as this chemical can promote gas production, Dr. Waring says.

Keep your belch to yourself. Forcing yourself to burp may seem like a dandy way to release air, but you should avoid it. Often, people push down a gulp of air to trigger a belch, but wind up taking in more than they release, Dr. Okolo says.

Avoid the bubbly. Minimize carbonated beverages, including sodas and beer, since their tiny bubbles can carry gas into your gut, Dubner says.

Headache

Of all the everyday aches and pains that flare up in our bodies, headaches seem to have a special way of bringing out the creative storyteller in each of us:

"Each hair on my head feels like a raw nerve."

"I feel like little men with hammers are working on the inside of my head."

"I feel like I have bricks lying on my eyeballs."

Artwork depicting headache pain is just as colorful. One collection of such works on the Internet shows people whose heads are under attack from drills, knives, jackhammers, and grinning demons.

Most of us have the chance to come up with metaphors for our own headaches at some point. It should come as no surprise to you that about 9 out of 10 people have had at least one headache in the past year, and about 45 million Americans get them repeatedly.

As the stories of personal torment imply, *headache* is one word that covers many types of pains from many potential causes.

Tension headaches tend to bring a dull, nagging discomfort that feels like a vise tightening around the head and neck, often following times of stress.

Migraine headaches have earned an especially fearsome reputation. Though they often create considerable pain on one side of the head—their name comes from the Greek *hemicrania*, or "half of the head"—the pain is only one element of the ailment. People in the grip of a migraine may see sparkling lights in their vision before the headache hits, then feel dizziness, nausea, and confusion during the course of the attack, which can last from hours to several days.

Rebound headaches are a case of too much of a good thing. They occur, ironically, if you use pain medications too often, especially if you're also drinking too much caffeine.

Cluster headaches are rare, and good thing, too. They're considered to be the absolutely most painful type of headache—a short-lived but severe stabbing pain around one eye that can totally incapacitate the sufferer. Cluster headaches often attack chronic smokers, especially after they drink alcohol.

HEADING OFF HEAD PAIN

As we age, all these headaches tend to hit less often, even migraines. But, especially after the age of 55 or so, a headache may signal a serious health problem, particularly if it gives you a type of pain you've never felt before.

You should get medical help right away if you're hit by a "thunderclap" headache, which is sudden and feels like "the headache of your life," says Carol Foster, M.D., director of the Valley Neurological Headache and Research Center in Phoenix. Such a sudden headache could be a warning of an impending problem such as a stroke or cerebral hemorrhage.

You should also see a doctor if your headache occurs along with numbness in an arm, dizziness, loss of speech, or a stiff neck and fever. And, since long-running yet mild headaches also can have serious causes, you should get help if your headache has been nagging you so long that you find yourself regularly putting a bottle of aspirin on your shopping list.

Fortunately, headaches are seldom caused by an ominous development like a stroke or tumor and are more likely to be just another run-of-the-mill pain. And science has produced a small pharmacy's worth of medications—both prescription and over-the-counter—to help silence these sorts of throbs.

But sometimes, those common painkillers aren't much help or are off-limits because of other medications you're taking. In that case, you can also take charge of your own headache relief with some simple do-it-yourself remedies, or better yet, avoid them with commonsense planning.

For Fast Relief

Get away from it all. If you feel the early twinges of a headache settling in for

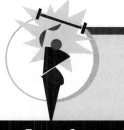

EXTRA-STRENGTH PAIN RELIEF

BANISH THAT BRAIN BUSTER WITH BIOFEEDBACK

You can teach yourself to squelch tension headaches and migraine headaches with the help of biofeedback, says Kenneth Lofland, Ph.D., director of the headache program at the Pain and Rehabilitation Clinic of Chicago.

If your headaches grow out of your tense shoulder and neck muscles, a biofeedback therapist may stick painless electrodes onto the area and connect them to a computer. The computer will show you a picture or play a sound that changes as you gradually loosen your muscles. As you learn how it feels to take control of your relaxation, you'll start to be able to do it without the machine.

To treat migraines, the setup is similar, but this time you change the image or sound on the computer by making your fingertips grow warmer, which is measured by a sensor on your finger. As you warm your fingers, you divert blood to the edges of your body, leaving less of it to throb away in your brain and aggravate the pain of your migraine, Dr. Lofland says.

Typically, you should need only 6 to 12 biofeedback sessions before you're able to control your headaches without special equipment.

a visit, find a dark, quiet, relaxing place to rest for a while.

"I often say that headache is like a forest fire—it's important to catch it early," says Marc Husid, M.D., a neurologist with the Headache and Neurology Center in Birmingham, Alabama. "In the people I deal with, they might be at work and things are stressful and they start to get a little headachy. Then they just ignore it, and the headache gets worse." If this sounds like you, learn to stop yourself from pressing on despite the head pain. Recognize the pain when it's mild and stop what you're doing. Try to find a restful place where you can close your eyes and relax for a while. If the weather is nice, find a shady, quiet area, such as a park, where you can go for a walk or sit on a bench, he says. Give yourself a few minutes of rest in a comfortable, quiet place. Often, that's all that's needed to end a headache.

For Lasting Relief

Try an herbal "aspirin." Salicin is one of the active ingredients in regular over-the-counter aspirin, and it's found in abundance in the herbal remedy willow bark. You can buy it as a powder or tincture in health food stores, and you can use it for migraine and other types of headaches. Unless you're allergic to aspirin, it is worth a try, says Ellen Kamhi, R.N., Ph.D., of Oyster Bay, New York, a professional member of the American Herbalists Guild and host of the nationally syndicated radio show *Natural Alternatives*. Follow the instructions on the label. If you can't take regular aspirin, you should avoid willow bark as well.

Turn your body loose. Tension headaches—the most common type—often arise during times of stress as your neck and shoulder muscles grow tight.

Kenneth Lofland, Ph.D., director of the headache program at the Pain and Rehabilitation Clinic of Chicago, remembers a city bus driver who would succumb to tension headaches each autumn. They'd first start at 3:00 P.M.—about the time unruly school kids would board his bus—then gradually begin earlier and earlier in the afternoon as he dreaded their arrival.

"What we found was that he was clutching his steering wheel tightly with two fists. His shoulders were raised up, squeezing his shoulder muscles, and he was causing enough muscle tension to create his own headache," he says. Once the frazzled driver learned to relax, his headaches faded away.

You should keep tabs on stress building

up in your body, so you can know when to reduce it, says Justin Nash, Ph.D., a psychologist with the headache-management program at Miriam Hospital in Providence, Rhode Island. "Spend a moment at different times during the day to develop an awareness of where your muscle tension is, then use a simple breathing strategy to relieve some of that tension," he says.

Breathe deeply so you draw the air down to your diaphragm and the breathing pushes out your belly, as opposed to taking shallow breaths that just make your chest rise and fall. Concentrate all your awareness inward on the simple act of breathing in and out. "Once you focus on that, then relaxation will naturally occur," Dr. Nash says.

You can also try a form of relaxation in which you concentrate on repeating calming phrases over and over. For example, silently repeat to yourself, "My arms and hands feel warm, heavy, and relaxed" and "I feel calm, I feel at peace, and I feel at ease."

Put the squeeze on pain. Many headaches really begin in your neck and shoulders due to muscle tension, so when you start to get head pain, a little self-massage of your neck and shoulders can help the muscles relax and stop a headache.

When you massage this area, you increase blood circulation to the muscles, relaxing them and reducing tension pain, says Patricia Benjamin, Ph.D., dean of the Chicago School of Massage Therapy and coauthor of *Tappan's Handbook of Healing Massage Techniques*.

Grasp the back of your neck with one hand, with your elbow pointing upward. Gently but firmly squeeze the sides of your neck and release, as if you're kneading dough. While massaging your neck, you can also use your thumb to rub and press into the muscles alongside your spine. You shouldn't do any of these so hard that it hurts.

With the same kneading motion, gently massage your trapezius muscles, which run from the base of your neck out to the tops of your shoulders (they're the thick muscles above your collarbones). Finally, with your fingertips, make small circles moving the skin over your temples and above your ears.

Try these massages for 3 to 5 minutes at a time, Dr. Benjamin suggests.

Use a cold/hot combo. Press an ice pack wrapped in a thin towel against your head wherever it's hurting, suggests Debra Elliott, M.D., clinical associate professor of neurology and codirector of the Tulane Headache Center in New Orleans. The coldness slows down the pain messages traveling along the nerves and constricts the flow of blood in the area.

You can also place a warm compress on the back of your shoulders and neck at the same time to help relax the muscles there. Both the cold and warm compresses

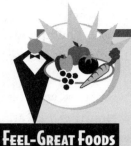

DAGWOOD THERAPY

Sometimes, when a patient calls Carol Foster, M.D., director of the Valley Neurological Headache and Research Center in Phoenix, she recommends that the patient eat something for the pain.

But not just any food will do. Here's what she suggests: Start with two pieces of whole-wheat toast since it contains an ingredient called tryptophan that your brain uses to boost its own levels of a natural pain-fighting chemical called serotonin. Toss on some fresh turkey and a slice of American cheese, which adds even more tryptophan. You've assembled not just a turkey sandwich but also a meal that fights headache.

should be used only if they improve the discomfort and only as long as they are comfortable—about 5 minutes at a time over a period of an hour, she adds.

PAIN PREVENTERS

Have fewer migraines with feverfew. Some studies have shown that people can cut down their numbers of migraines when they take the herb feverfew, a plant related to the chrysanthemum.

Considering that many prescription migraine drugs have a hit-or-miss chance of working for you, feverfew is at least worth a try to see if it will help. She suggests taking a brand that will provide you with a daily dose of 250 milligrams and making sure that the label says it contains at least 0.2 percent parthenolide, the active chemical. Follow the label for specific dosage information. Try it for 3 months before deciding if it is helping your headaches, Dr. Elliott says. It's widely available at health food stores.

Decaffeinate yourself. Caffeine isn't just another ingredient in coffee, tea, and sodas, it's a drug that affects the chemicals coursing through your brain, Dr. Foster says. After you consume caffeine, it triggers a chain of events in your brain that causes an important chemical called serotonin to dwindle.

"Serotonin is your calm chemical. As you get older, you produce less of it," she says. "If you're 60 years old or older, you don't have any serotonin to be wasting on a cup of coffee." In addition to this effect, if you've consumed caffeinated beverages regularly for years and then skip your morning coffee or other regular caffeine jolts, you can get a withdrawal headache.

As a result, you should keep your caffeine intake under 100 milligrams a day, which is about one cup of coffee or two cans of soda, says Dr. Foster. If you're drinking more than that, taper it off gradually over several weeks to avoid withdrawal headaches.

Get the message about MSG. As you get older, you may be allowing yourself the indulgence of prepackaged or frozen meals, which are certainly easier and more convenient to prepare than making a meal from scratch. But that convenience comes at a price—these foods may be giving you a headache.

That's because prepared foods often contain MSG, or monosodium glutamate, an ingredient that enhances flavors but may also enhance headaches, says Dr. Foster. She thinks that MSG plays a big part in the headaches that assault America each year, and the chemical makes many other headache experts' lists of potential causes too.

One way to cut down on MSG is to try to eat more fresh produce, dairy, and lean meats and to cut down on the instant sauces and just-add-water foods. If you miss the convenience of prepared foods, at least try to look for foods that contain no MSG (it'll say so on the label).

Shake a leg. Exercise is a great way to dampen the pain of many ailments, including headaches, Dr. Foster says.

Dr. Husid agrees, recommending that you walk at least 30 minutes four times a week.

If walking isn't comfortable, find a swimming pool that offers water aerobics classes, Dr. Foster suggests.

Ease 'em with magnesium. Some studies have shown that you may make yourself less of a target for migraine attacks if you take regular magnesium supplements.

The recommended amount is 400 to 500 milligrams a day, Dr. Elliott suggests. People with heart or kidney problems should check with their doctors before taking supplemental magnesium. It may cause diarrhea in some people.

Make a beeline to riboflavin. Another supplement that may cut down on migraine frequency is riboflavin. In one study conducted at the University of Liège in Belgium, a majority of the patients who took 400 milligrams of the vitamin each morning cut the number of days they had migraines by at least half. Since this is a large dose of riboflavin, however, you should discuss this dose with your doctor before trying it, Dr. Elliott suggests.

Take the hurt out of HRT. Menopausal women taking hormone-replacement therapy, or HRT, should follow some extra precautions with these treatments since they may trigger migraines, says Ninan Mathew, M.D., director of the Houston Headache Clinic in Texas.

Take the hormones in as steady and uniform an amount as possible, he says. Skin patches that consistently deliver the hormones are ideal. But if you take tablets, take them in small, evenly spaced doses.

Know when to say no to painkillers. Over-the-counter painkillers pose a frustrating dilemma: While they can ease a headache when used sparingly, taking too many of them can *give* you one.

To avoid such rebound headaches, don't take nonprescription headache pills more than 2 days a week. If you're using them more than that, it's time to see your doctor, Dr. Husid says.

Steer clear of this sweetener. Another chemical Dr. Foster urges patients to avoid is the artificial sweetener aspartame.

Avoid pulling your food triggers. Certain foods such as chocolate, cheese, and citrus fruits are thought to trigger migraines and other headaches. They may affect some people and not others, or they may kick off a migraine only when you're stressed out or fatigued.

While the list that Dr. Foster provides her patients includes dozens of foods, here are some of the main ones to watch. Trim these from your diet to see if your migraines decrease.

- Aged, cured, or processed meats
- Red wine
- Peas
- Kidney, fava, and lima beans
- Chickpeas
- Aged cheeses
- Doughnuts
- Sourdough breads
- Yeast extracts
- Onions
- Olives
- Pickles
- Sauerkraut

❱ Avocados
❱ Nuts
❱ Sunflower seeds
❱ Soy products

Feed your head. One way to provoke a headache is to miss a meal, Dr. Husid says. Your blood sugar drops, your internal chemistry goes askew, and before you know it, you have drills, jackhammers, or other metaphors of your choice pounding at your head.

If you don't like eating three substantial meals a day, eat five smaller ones, he suggests.

Get out of the sack to avoid attack. "Oversleeping is a big trigger of migraine," Dr. Husid says. Too much sleep throws off the body's internal clock and may be a factor in why many people get migraines on Saturday. Lack of sleep may cause trouble as well. So do your best to go to bed and wake up at the same time every day.

Become a journalist. Keep a headache diary, which may help you and your physician learn what time of day you tend to have your attacks and what may cause them, Dr. Lofland says.

The American Council for Headache Education also recommends that you keep a headache diary, each day noting the amount of headache pain you feel, from no pain to severe; what steps you took to relieve it; and what may have triggered it, such as food, stress, or sleep problems.

Water down your headaches. Dehydration can put a throb in your head, so be sure to drink at least six to eight 8-ounce glasses of water a day, so long as you don't have a kidney or heart condition that limits your fluid intake, Dr. Foster says.

Heartburn

A pack of no-nonsense reporters fiercely questioned President Clinton's press secretary one summer afternoon. Scandal and matters of state had to wait until later—the newshounds wanted to go immediately for Clinton's throat. More precisely, his esophagus.

The spokesperson had revealed that Clinton was feeling a pain that unites him with millions of his fellow Americans, both young and old. News flash: The president had chronic heartburn.

"The thing about heartburn is that it's common in everybody. There are just more reasons for older people to develop heartburn," explains Gary Salzman, M.D., a geriatrician and director of the geriatric fellowship program at Good Samaritan Regional Medical Center in Phoenix.

The signs of a heartburn flare-up, such as a burning sensation in your chest and a bitter taste and a rush of saliva in your mouth, are triggered when digestive juices from your stomach venture out where they don't belong.

A valve at the bottom of your esophagus normally keeps these harsh digestive juices, including acids and enzymes, out of your esophagus. When you eat or drink, the valve opens like a gate to let the food or beverage pour into your stomach, then it closes. When contents from your stomach slip up through that valve, called the lower esophageal sphincter, they may irritate your esophagus enough to trigger a case of heartburn. Even though heartburn doesn't actually involve your heart, it understandably can be confused with a heart attack since it does cause a pain in your chest.

As a general rule of thumb, heartburn will usually occur after you eat, while a heart attack is more likely to follow exertion, explains Charles Gerson, M.D., associate clinical professor of medicine and attending physician in the division of gastroenterology at Mount Sinai School of Medicine of the City University of New York in New York City. But you should seek medical treatment if your painful condition lasts longer than 30 minutes and includes pain running down your left arm, pain accompanied by a rapid heartbeat, shortness of breath, heaviness in your chest, or sweating, he says. See your doctor if food gets stuck on the way down your esophagus or if the heartburn is chronic.

As you age, you can be more prone to feeling the effects of heartburn because your esophagus becomes less effective at pushing acid back down before it does damage and because you also may produce less saliva to help wash away acid, Dr. Salzman says.

Regardless of how old you are, though, you can douse heartburn's fire or even prevent the blaze from starting with a few simple remedies and lifestyle changes.

For Fast Relief

Lick heartburn with licorice. As a natural way to douse heartburn, try eating some licorice, recommends Bill Caradonna, R.Ph., N.D., a registered pharmacist and naturopathic physician with the Queen Anne Naturopathic Center in Seattle. The sort of licorice used for heartburn relief is called deglycyrrhizinated licorice, which means a chemical that can raise blood pressure has been removed. Also known as DGL, this remedy is found in health food stores as chewable lozenges. DGL helps soothe your esophagus when taken during heartburn flare-ups and is also used as a long-term therapy, he says.

Dr. Caradonna recommends taking one or two lozenges before each meal until symptoms resolve. (Underlying causes, such as low amounts of stomach acid, must be corrected for a more permanent solution.)

For Lasting Relief

Sit up straight. When you start feeling the heartburn, you may want to

GIRD YOURSELF AGAINST GERD

Americans are showing an exuberance for treating their heartburn (which may actually be gastroesophageal reflux disease (GERD) instead) with tablets and spoonfuls of antacid, sometimes for years, without ever making a trip to the doctor's office. This approach has some medical professionals concerned.

That's because heartburn is one of your body's ways of letting you know that your stomach and esophagus aren't working in sync. Quelling the heartburn pain without examining the underlying problem is akin to pulling the low-oil warning light out of your car's dashboard instead of adding more oil, says Bill Caradonna, R.Ph., N.D., a registered pharmacist and naturopathic physician with the Queen Anne Naturopathic Center in Seattle.

This underlying problem, in which stomach fluids repeatedly leak into your esophagus and irritate it, can also cause such symptoms as coughing, hoarseness, and asthma. And if your esophagus is irritated for long enough, it can form

reach for an over-the-counter antacid. That's fine. Just sit upright when you take it, advises Lawrence Kim, M.D., a gastroenterologist at South Denver Gastroenterology in Colorado. When you sit up, you reduce the pressure of your stomach's contents against that crucial valve, so they'll be less likely to trespass into the esophagus.

Go the extra mile with chamomile. You can also lessen heartburn pain with a cup of chamomile tea, which has anti-in-

scarred constrictions or grow abnormal cells in an effort to protect itself, which is a serious condition called Barrett's esophagus. This condition can in rare cases proceed to cancer and, therefore, must be closely monitored if present.

Doctors from the Oklahoma Foundation for Digestive Research at the University of Oklahoma Health Sciences Center in Oklahoma City conducted a study on the long-term use of antacids. They concluded that lifestyle changes and over-the-counter remedies, including antacids and acid blockers such as Pepcid AC and Zantac 75, are safe to treat occasional heartburn. Long-term heartburn, though, calls for more help.

"If you're taking these medications chronically for more than a 2- to 3-week period, you should see a doctor," says Fred Sutton, M.D., associate professor of medicine in the division of gastroenterology at Baylor College of Medicine in Houston.

Don't wait it out if you also develop nausea, vomiting, weight loss, black stool, or trouble swallowing, which are all signs of more serious digestive problems, adds Lawrence Kim, M.D., a gastroenterologist at South Denver Gastroenterology in Colorado. See your doctor as soon as possible.

flammatory properties, suggests Susanna Reid, N.D., Ph.D., a naturopathic physician with the Center of Natural Medicine in Darien, Connecticut. Anywhere from one to four cups should do the trick, according to Dr. Reid.

PAIN PREVENTERS

Keep troublemakers off your table. Doctors say that the following foods can compound heartburn trouble, either because they weaken the esophageal sphincter

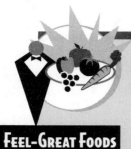

CHEWING OUT HEARTBURN

When you want to extinguish heartburn, gum in your mouth can work like a water hose in the hands of a firefighter.

The gum can stimulate your mouth to produce more saliva, which contains bicarbonate, an ingredient that helps neutralize acid. As the saliva runs down your throat, it can also wash acid back into your stomach.

Just be sure to avoid spearmint- and peppermint-flavored gum, which may worsen your heartburn, advises Fred Sutton, M.D., associate professor of medicine in the division of gastroenterology at Baylor College of Medicine in Houston.

that keeps acid in your stomach or because they just irritate your esophagus: fatty foods, spicy foods, citrus juices, tomato products, onions, chocolate, coffee, hot tea, colas, and alcohol. Try to minimize their use.

Avoid the burn by not lighting up. Smoking has the same effect on your lower esophageal sphincter as Delilah had on Samson when she gave him a haircut: It weakens it, says Dr. Kim. So to help keep that barrier strong, avoid smoking.

Here's a hint: Don't eat mints. Peppermint and spearmint can also make things worse by weakening the sphincter, says Fred Sutton, M.D., associate professor of medicine in the division of gastroenterology at Baylor College of Medicine in Houston. So curb that urge next time you're tempted to dip into the bowl of mints next to the cash register at the restaurant.

Make a detour between the table and the bed. Stay upright for 2 to 3 hours after you eat, Dr. Kim advises, and certainly don't eat a large meal right before bedtime. This advice may be easier to give than to heed. Sometimes, that contented feeling after a nice meal practically demands a good snooze.

If you have a dog, take it out for a walk after dinner, advises Jan I. Maby, D.O., medical director of the Cobble Hill Health Center in Brooklyn, New York. You could also schedule a simple chore to be done after the meal—one that keeps you upright to aid digestion, such as watering your plants or washing dishes. If you've just eaten out at a restaurant, walk around nearby and do a little window-shopping.

Also, if you eat early enough in the evening, the remaining daylight will make outdoor activities more inviting.

Keep your chin up. When you do hit the bed, another way to keep acid out of your esophagus is to prop up your upper body while sleeping, according to Dr. Maby. One traditional piece of advice has been to raise the head of the bed a few inches with blocks, boards, or other lifts. A simpler variation on this remedy is to buy a foam-shaped wedge that elevates your upper body when you lie on it. These can be found for about $30 in some medical supply and department store catalogs.

Give yourself some space. Avoid wearing snug clothing around your midsection, including tight belts, corsets, and girdles, Dr. Sutton says. These put more pressure on your belly and, therefore, your lower esophageal sphincter.

Don't eat and run. The body likes to digest food in a resting state, Dr. Caradonna states, and not in the tense, hurried mood that we find ourselves in more often than we'd like. "Relax and enjoy your meal," he says. "People need to chew their food well. There's a reason why we have a mouth and teeth—so when food hits the stomach, the stomach has less work to do."

Check your choppers. If you're having trouble chewing your food because of ill-fitting or missing dentures, get them fixed or eat softer foods, Dr. Maby says.

Examine your medicine cabinet. A large number of medications can increase your chances of heartburn, Dr. Sutton advises. These include some asthma medications and sedatives, nonsteroidal anti-inflammatory drugs like ibuprofen, and cardiac and high blood pressure medicines like calcium channel blockers. If you or your physician are sleuthing around for potential causes of your fiery condition, always consider your medications as potential contributors, he says.

Hip Pain

You don't have to take hip pain in stride.

"Hip pain isn't something you should necessarily chalk up to aging, nor should you presume you have to live with it the rest of your life," says Patrick B. Massey, M.D., Ph.D., a pain-management specialist and president and director of the ALT-MED back-pain program and the Alternative/Complementary Medicine Referral Service at Alexian Brothers Medical Center in Elk Grove, Illinois. "It doesn't have to be debilitating. In most cases, it isn't serious and is reversible."

Even though the joint itself is located deep within the body and is protected by the large muscles of the upper leg, doctors say that the hip is one of the body's most vulnerable joints and a common source of pain and suffering. In fact, about one in three people who have hip problems report a great deal of discomfort, according to the National Center for Health Statistics.

"The hip is the one joint in the body that really absorbs most of the shock as we move. It literally is the major hinge we use to bend, lift, and twist. Even sitting can put a tremendous amount of stress on the hips," Dr. Massey says.

Among older Americans, hip pain is often caused by hip fractures, bursitis, arthritis, gout, and osteoporosis. In addition to being in the hip, the pain sometimes can be felt in the groin, outer thigh, and down the leg to the knee. And, in some cases, hip pain is a sign of trouble elsewhere in the body.

"I have seen older patients come to me with hip pain, convinced they have arthritis. Yet when we look into it, we discover they have prostate problems, a bladder or kidney problem, or another underlying condition that is causing pain to spread into the hip," says Keith O. Javery, D.O., an anesthesiologist at Michigan Pain Consultants, based in Grand Rapids.

So consult with your doctor to make sure there isn't an underlying medical problem that could be the real cause of your pain, Dr. Javery says. Once you've done that and have a diagnosis, here are some things you can do to subdue hip pain.

For Fast Relief

Dab on a cream. Rub an over-the-counter capsaicin cream such as Zostrix or Capzasin-P onto your painful hip, as needed, suggests John Catanzaro, N.D., a naturopathic physician specializing in pain management and director of the Health and Wellness Institute in Seattle. Capsaicin, an extract from spicy red peppers, is a natural analgesic that usually soothes aches in about 10 minutes.

Since some people are sensitive to the compound, test a tiny amount of the cream on a small area of skin to make sure that it's okay for you to use. If the cream

seems to irritate your skin, don't use it. And be sure to wash your hands once you've applied the cream. Pepper cream may work wonders on the hip, but it could cause more discomfort if you accidentally rub it on any sensitive area such as your eye.

For Lasting Relief

Use a combination to lock out pain. Traumeel ointment or tablets, available at many drugstores and health food stores, contain a number of homeopathic substances, including chamomile, echinacea, belladonna, calendula, and arnica, that are known to ease pain, Dr. Catanzaro says.

"Traumeel works well. Many people who use it report pain relief within an hour of using it," he says. If you are having a lot of acute pain, he recommends that you dissolve one tablet under your tongue every couple of hours until the pain begins to subside. As for the ointment, rub that on your painful hip as needed. Use the ointment every day during periods of acute pain.

Let ice melt swelling. Cold is your best choice for relieving painful inflammatory conditions of the hip such as bursitis or rheumatoid arthritis, Dr. Javery says. Although heat will initially feel good

(continued on page 320)

HIP HELPERS

Stretching exercises that improve the flexibility of muscles surrounding your hip can often relieve pain, says Sherry Brourman, P.T., a physical therapist in Los Angeles and author of *Walk Yourself Well*. This is especially true after you've warmed the joint up with heat.

Side-to-side stretch. Stand with your feet a little more than hip-width apart. Then, gently sway from side to side, shifting your body weight from hip to hip. Do this for about a minute five times a day. It will help stretch and strengthen the muscles around both hips. Once you get used to this movement, you can try making small circles with your hips.

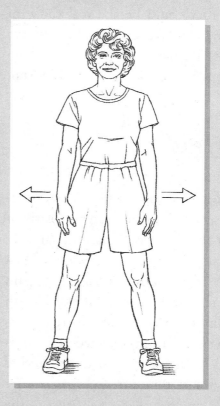

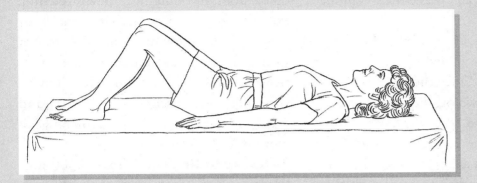

Lower-back, hamstring, and buttocks stretch. Lie on your back on the floor or a bed and bend your knees so that your feet rest flat on the floor or bed. For comfort, you also can prop up your head with a couple of pillows, if necessary.

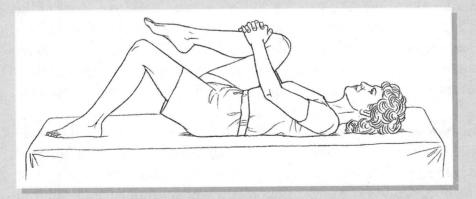

Clasp your hands around your right knee and slowly bring it up toward your shoulder. Hold for a count of five, then slowly put your knee back down. Then repeat with your left knee. Do this five times with each knee.

if you have one of these conditions, warming swollen tissue will draw more blood to the area and make the inflammation even worse.

Preparation is the key, he says. Fill 6-ounce disposable paper cups with water and freeze them. Once they're frozen, tear the first inch or two off the top of a cup so that the ice is exposed but you can still use the bottom of the cup as a handle. Then when you feel an ache, rub the cup of ice over your hip in a brisk, circular motion. This ice massage will help the cold reach the deepest layers of muscle and tissue surrounding your hip. Do this for 5 minutes three times a day.

Feel the heat. If you have osteoarthritis, a condition that causes degeneration of the hip, apply heat instead of ice, Dr. Javery says. Heat will improve mobility of the hip and boost bloodflow of vital nutrients into the joint that can help heal it and reduce pain.

Place a warm, well-wrung towel on your sore hip for 20 minutes two or three times a day. Avoid using a heating pad, Dr. Javery warns. "The hottest towel is going to cool off rather quickly, and it won't burn the skin like a heating pad might. Heating pads? I tell my patients to throw them away. They're just too dangerous."

Stand up for yourself. In most cases, inactivity will only worsen your pain, not relieve it, Dr. Javery says. Walking to the post office, swinging your hips on the dance floor, or doing just a few stretching exercises are all better activities than just sitting there allowing your hips to get weaker. Try to do at least 20 minutes of activity daily, such as gardening. It will make your hips less susceptible to aches and pains and help you maintain a full range of motion in the joints.

Get back to basics. Take 1,500 milligrams of glucosamine and 1,200 milligrams of chondroitin daily to curb pain, says Luke Bucci, Ph.D., vice president of research at Weider Nutrition International in Salt Lake City and author of *Healing Arthritis the Natural Way.*

Glucosamine, a sugar that is one of the body's natural building blocks, and chondroitin sulfate, a nutritional supplement, have been shown to relieve hip and other joint pain without causing side effects, Dr. Javery says.

Be patient, because it can take weeks for this combination to work. "With non-steroidal anti-inflammatory drugs such as ibuprofen, you get immediate relief, but you gradually need more and more of it to have the same effect," Dr. Bucci says. "With glucosamine and chondroitin, the relief sets in slowly, but it gradually gets better and better until about one in four people are actually pain-free."

Lighten up. If you are overweight, shedding a few pounds will help reduce strain on your hips and may alleviate your pain, says James N. Dillard, M.D., D.C., a pain-management expert and instructor at the Columbia University College of Physicians and Surgeons in New York City. Each pound you lose will take 2 to 3 pounds of pressure off your hips and surrounding muscles.

Slip in some supplements. Vitamin and mineral supplements strengthen your nervous system, help your body maintain and rebuild cartilage and tendons, and help reduce pain in your hips and other joints, researchers say. Here's what they suggest.

▶ Vitamin A: Take 5,000 IU a day. It helps build cartilage and tendons, Dr. Catanzaro says.

▶ Vitamin B_6: Try 50 milligrams a day. B_6 helps control pain, Dr. Catanzaro says.

▶ Vitamin C: Take 2,000 milligrams twice a day for a total of 4,000 milligrams of vitamin C daily, Dr. Bucci suggests. If taking this much gives you diarrhea, reduce the dosage.

▶ Vitamin E: Try 400 IU daily. Scientists in Germany and Israel have found that regular doses of vitamin E can cut the need for pain-relieving medication by 50 percent in just 2 weeks, Dr. Bucci says. He speculates that the vitamin helps regulate the production of anti-inflammatory prostaglandins, some of the body's natural painkillers.

▶ Niacin: Take 500 milligrams a day, Dr. Catanzaro suggests. Niacin promotes blood circulation to the hip. Doses above 35 milligrams must be taken under medical supervision.

Eliminate nightshade foods. Eating tomatoes, potatoes, eggplants, peppers, and other nightshade foods can actually trigger painful inflammation in your hips and other joints, Dr. Catanzaro says.

"Many older people who eliminate these foods from their diets notice that their joint pain ebbs significantly. If a person is suffering a 10 on the pain scale, once you eliminate these foods, it goes down to a 6 very quickly." High-fat foods can also provoke inflammation, he notes.

Dump the toxins. Detoxifying teas made with dandelion root, milk thistle extract, echinacea, red clover, and sarsaparilla root help cleanse your body of toxins that aggravate hip pain, Dr. Catanzaro says. At least two companies, Celestial Seasonings and Traditional Medicinals, make commercial versions of these teas. Drink two to three 6-ounce cups of the hot tea daily. It's best to ingest the teas on an empty stomach, so

(continued on page 324)

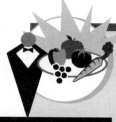

Flax Conquers Aches and Pains

It was a staple of the ancient world long before the Egyptians built the pyramids. And now, researchers are discovering that flax, a diminutive sesame seed look-alike, may be one of nature's best pain relievers, particularly for hip and other joint discomfort.

"Flax is the wonder nondrug," says Keith O. Javery, D.O., an anesthesiologist at Michigan Pain Consultants, based in Grand Rapids. "It's what I immediately recommend for anyone who has degenerative arthritis of the hip and other joints."

Flaxseed is a tremendous source of alpha-linolenic acid, which has a proven ability to seep into painful joints like the hips, soothe them, and improve mobility.

"In a sense, taking flax oil is like giving your joints a lube job," Dr. Javery says. "I prescribe it frequently. It's over-the-counter, you can get it in any health food store, and it's cheap. A 32-ounce bottle will last you months."

He recommends taking 1 to 2 tablespoons of flaxseed oil no more than twice a day or eating ½ cup of ground flaxseed once a day. You should begin noticing significant pain relief within 3 to 4 weeks, Dr. Javery says. If you use flaxseed, freshly grind it in a coffee grinder—a blender won't do the job. Grind only as much as you need for one day. The ground seed can be sprinkled on cereals, used as a topping on desserts, and used in making muffins and other baked goods. As for the oil, it can be mixed with apple juice, orange juice, or another cold juice or beverage. But avoid heating it. When it is subjected to sustained heat, flaxseed oil oxidizes and should not be consumed. Flaxseed oil should be stored in the refrigerator. To get you started using flaxseed as a hip fixer, here is a tasty recipe.

FLAXSEED MUFFINS

This recipe delivers 25 grams of flaxseed per muffin, which should give your hips plenty of help. Although this muffin is higher in fat than what is usually recommended, nearly half the fat is alpha-linolenic acid—the plant version of omega-3 fatty acid, which is sorely missing in most diets. It's worth finding room for this muffin in your daily low-fat plan.

⅓–½	cup light molasses	1¼	cups flour
¾	cup fat-free milk	3	cups ground flaxseed
2	tablespoons canola oil	1	tablespoon baking powder
½	cup egg substitute		

Preheat oven to 350°F. Coat a 12-cup muffin pan with no-stick spray.

In a medium bowl, stir together the molasses, milk, oil, and egg substitute.

In a large bowl, whisk together the flour, flaxseed, and baking powder. Stir into the molasses mixture until just blended.

Pour into the prepared muffin pan. Bake for 18 minutes, or until a toothpick inserted in the center of one muffin comes out clean. Can be frozen for use as needed.

Makes 12 muffins.

Per muffin: 196 calories, 12.4 g fat, 8 g fiber, 110 mg sodium, 25 g flaxseed

avoid eating for at least an hour before or after drinking it.

Lean on a friend. Don't think of a cane or walker as an impediment you should avoid. It can be your best friend if it eases your hip pain and helps you stay independent, Dr. Javery says.

If you need a cane or walker for stability, be sure it is the right size. An ill-fitting device will increase your hip pain, not relieve it. Ask your doctor to refer you to a medical supply store where you can be properly measured and outfitted with an appropriate cane or walker. Also, be sure to ask your doctor for a referral to an occupational therapist who can help you learn how to use the device correctly in your everyday life.

"If you're going to use a cane or walker, you need to learn to use it in a way that will prevent pain, not aggravate it," Dr. Javery says. "So I highly recommend at least one visit with an occupational therapist to work out the kinks. It's an hour visit that is well worth the cost."

Let the cane bear the load. If you do use a cane, hold it in the hand opposite your painful hip, Dr. Dillard says. Move your cane forward at the same time you take a stride on your aching hip, so that you are distributing weight onto the cane and away from your bad hip as you take a stride on the opposite foot.

PAIN PREVENTERS

If you don't have hip pain—or you feel only the occasional twinge—you can still take steps to prevent it from disrupting your retirement years, says Dr. Massey.

"Preventing a hip problem is always better than trying to find a cure, because it takes a lot less effort," he says. "If you develop hip pain, you're not going to be walking as much. If you have hip pain, you're not going to be using that joint as much. If you're not using your hip, then you're not using your knee or ankle either, and those joints will start to degenerate and become painful. So whatever you can do to prevent hip pain, do it." Here are a few ways to keep your hip in tip-top shape.

Take the trip out of falls. Falls are one of the top preventable causes of hip pain and disability, Dr. Massey says. Make sure that you have secure rugs, good lighting throughout your home, sturdy handrails on stairways, nonskid strips and grab bars in the bathtubs, and slip-resistant carpeting on the bathroom floor.

Stroll away from trouble. Walking is a weight-bearing activity that can help strengthen your hips in several ways, Dr. Massey says. Walking helps your body absorb calcium, a mineral that helps keep your hip joints strong and pain-free. A good stroll increases bloodflow to your hips and helps you maintain range of motion in the joints. It also improves your balance and reflexes, making you less likely to fall and injure a hip. Try brisk walking 20 minutes a day, 7 days a week, he suggests. Aim for a pace that boosts your heart rate, causing you to break a mild sweat yet still allowing you to carry on a conversation.

Go feet first. When getting out of a car, lift and swing both legs out of the door before standing, suggests Dr. Javery. By rotating on your rear—instead of twisting your pelvis—you'll lessen the strain on your back and hips. "If you put one leg out so that you're only halfway out of the car, you're putting a lot of unnecessary torque on the back, hips, and knees," he says.

Similarly, when you're doing household chores like dishwashing, avoid twisting your lower back and hips as you dry and stack your dishes, Dr. Javery adds. Instead, pivot on your feet so that your whole body is facing the direction in which you are working. "Some patients will tell me, 'Doing that makes me look like a robot.'

And I'll tell them, 'That's exactly what it should look like,'" he says.

Cork the bottle. Drinking alcohol will thin your bones and, in large amounts, will hinder the formation of new bone. This can eventually weaken your hips and contribute to the onset of pain, Dr. Massey says.

Snub the smokes. Smoking increases your risk of hip pain and fracture by speeding up the rate at which your body burns up estrogen, the hormone that helps prevent rapid bone loss. In addition, lighting up can slow the healing of your hip and surrounding muscles, Dr. Massey says.

Say yes to yucca. Take 500 milligrams of yucca root capsules four times a day to prevent hip pain, suggests Dr. Catanzaro. Yucca, a medicinal herb, does a couple of things that stop pain before it starts. It helps you maintain strong cartilage, plus it strengthens connective tissue surrounding the joint. Yucca is available at most health food stores.

Knee Pain

It was a small bump—nothing more than a thump, really. And after the initial pain of banging his knee while getting into a car subsided, Vice President Richard Nixon, the 1960 Republican nominee for president, shrugged off the seemingly minor injury. But within weeks, his aching knee would do much to unhinge his first presidential bid.

At first, Nixon simply applied hot compresses to his knee and waited for the injury to heal itself. But 12 days later, he developed intense pain in the knee and was hospitalized for treatment of a severe infection in the joint. He recovered but had lost 2 valuable weeks on campaign trail. Then, incredibly, in late September, Nixon cracked the same knee again—this time getting out of a car just hours before his first televised debate with his Democratic rival U.S. Senator John F. Kennedy. Standing on his painful knee throughout much of the crucial debate, Nixon looked pale, pasty, and wan. "After the program ended," Nixon wrote in his memoirs, "callers, including my mother, wanted to know if anything was wrong, because I did not look well."

It was a bad omen. And 6 weeks later, Kennedy narrowly defeated Nixon in one of the nation's closest presidential elections.

Certainly, painful knees seldom change history, but they do change lives every day.

"If your knees are free of pain, it really gives you license to be active. And activity will help your heart work better, help keep your brain in tip-top condition, and improve your overall quality of life as you age. But if your knees are painful, it limits your life in many ways that are bound to have detrimental effects," says Jordan Metzl, M.D., a sports-medicine specialist at the Hospital for Special Surgery in New York City.

ANATOMY OF A KNEE JOINT

More than just a simple hinge, the knee is a stout pillar of muscles, bones, ligaments, and cartilage that endures an extraordinary pounding every day. When you walk down a staircase, for instance, your knees support a force that is equivalent to 4½ times your body weight. Jump, and your knees absorb a vertical impact that is equal to 7 times your body weight.

"The knee is the strongest joint in the body," Dr. Metzl says. "It has a very remarkable design that is meant to stand up to a lot."

Three bones—the femur (thighbone), the tibia (shinbone), and the patella (kneecap)—form the knee, the largest and most complex joint in your body. The ends of these three bones are covered with cartilage called articular cartilage and are interspaced with meniscus cartilage. A tough, elastic material that helps absorb shock and prevents the bones from rubbing against each other, cartilage allows your knees to bend and swivel. This mechanism is bound together by a snarl of ligaments, tendons, and muscles, including the quadriceps, the strongest group of muscles in your body, which are attached to the kneecap.

Yet as sturdy as it seems, the knee is actually one of the most vulnerable joints in the body, particularly among people older than 60. In fact, more than 600,000 seniors seek medical care for knee problems each year, according to the National Center for Health Statistics.

Your knee is particularly susceptible to injury because, unlike your hip, it isn't well-protected by muscle or fat, Dr. Metzl says. Bursitis, tendinitis, infections, cysts, and chondromalacia—a softening of the cartilage on the back of your kneecap—also can trigger immobilizing knee pain.

But by far, the most common cause of knee pain is osteoarthritis, a degenerative joint disease that affects more than 20 million Americans, most of them over age 45. As osteoarthritis progresses, the cartilage that protects the bony structures in your knee wears down, allowing bones in the joint to literally gnash against each other, causing pain and loss of mobility.

"A one-time knee pain usually isn't a problem. But if it is ongoing, it should be checked out," Dr. Metzl says. "The earlier you find out what is causing your knee pain, the more that can be done to correct the problem and prevent it from getting worse." So see your doctor if:

▶ Your knee pain or stiffness lingers for more than a week.

▶ Your pain is severe or unexplained.

▶ Your knee is hot, red, swollen, or painful.

▶ You feel pain radiating down your leg.

▶ You have recently injured the joint, particularly with a sharp blow.

▶ Your knee swells following activity.

Often, knee pain can be relieved without surgery, Dr. Metzl says. In fact, once you are diagnosed, your doctor may suggest some of the following simple, non-invasive strategies. Here's how to get a head start.

For Fast Relief

Trample trouble with Traumeel. Traumeel tablets and cream, available at many drugstores and health food stores, contain a number of homeopathic substances, including chamomile, echinacea, belladonna, calendula, and arnica, that are known to ease knee pain, says John Catanzaro, N.D., a naturopathic physician specializing in pain management and director of the Health and Wellness Institute in Seattle. In some cases, Traumeel snuffs out pain in less than an hour.

If you have acute knee pain, dissolve one tablet under your tongue every couple of hours until the pain begins to subside, he suggests. As for the cream, rub that on your painful knee as needed. Don't use it on broken skin.

For Lasting Relief

Follow the master plan. Rest, ice, compression, and elevation are four of the best initial treatments for knee pain, Dr. Metzl says. So for the first 24 to 48 hours after the pain develops, stay off your feet as much as possible, prop your leg up on a pillow or two, wrap your knee snugly—but not too tightly—with an elastic bandage, and apply cold packs to the sore joint for 15 minutes every hour.

For icing, a bag of frozen peas wrapped in a thin towel is probably your best bet since you can easily mold the bag so that it conforms to the shape of your knee, he says. In addition, if you feel tingling or numbness or see discoloration in your foot, loosen the elastic bandage because it is probably wrapped too tightly.

Flex your muscles. Plunge into exercise, particularly any routines that stretch and strengthen the muscles, tendons, and ligaments surrounding your knee, Dr. Metzl says.

The sooner you get started, the better. If you rest your knee for more than 48 hours, the muscles and other tissues that stabilize the joint and help keep it flexible will begin to weaken and atrophy. That, in turn, will aggravate your pain.

Weak quadriceps, for instance, can make it harder for you to control how hard your feet hit the ground as you walk and can increase the strain on your knee and hasten the breakdown of cartilage within the joint.

But simple exercises that promote flexibility and strength will dampen your pain and help fend off further discomfort, Dr. Metzl says. In fact, preliminary data suggest that when 30 people with osteoarthritis of the knee followed an at-home strength-training program, they averaged a 37 percent reduction in pain and an 82 percent increase in strength of the affected leg. After 4 months, they were more active and confident, with fewer limps and hobbles, according to researchers at Tufts University in Boston, who conducted this study.

Dive in. Swimming, water walking, and other pool activities are terrific exercises if you have aching knees, Dr. Metzl says. You should try water exercises even before you try land exercises. Because of its buoyancy, water enables you to flex the joint with less stress and discomfort.

Forward, march! Just taking a walk for 30 minutes or longer three or four times a week can relieve knee pain, says Walter Ettinger, M.D., executive vice president of Virtua Health in Marlton, New Jersey.

In an 18-month study of 439 people age 60 and older with knee problems, those who walked three times a week reported a 12 percent reduction in knee pain as well as increased mobility when negotiating stairways and getting in and out of vehicles.

Walking probably dampens knee pain in several ways, says Dr. Ettinger, who conducted this study at Wake Forest University School of Medicine in Winston-Salem, North Carolina. It helps strengthen the muscles surrounding the knee, stabilizes the joint, and makes it less susceptible to pain. It also may increase the production of pain-blocking substances called endorphins. Finally, as walkers noticed improvement, they developed an I-can-do-it attitude that lessened their perception of pain.

If you have severe knee pain, consult your doctor before starting a walking program. Before and after you walk, do the stretches suggested in "Knee Routine I" on page 330. You may feel some soreness and pain as your body gets used to being active. But if you stick with it, you'll have less pain over time, Dr. Ettinger says.

(continued on page 334)

KNEE ROUTINE I

The stronger the muscles around your knees, the better your chances of preserving your knee performance into your eighties and nineties. Use a sturdy, straight-back chair to do 10 to 15 repetitions of each of these exercises twice a day.

Knee extension. Wrap an ankle weight around each ankle. Sit with your thighs supported. Slowly extend your right leg until it is straight, but not locked. Hold for a count of eight. Slowly lower it. (If this is uncomfortable, start with your foot on a low stool.) Repeat with your left leg.

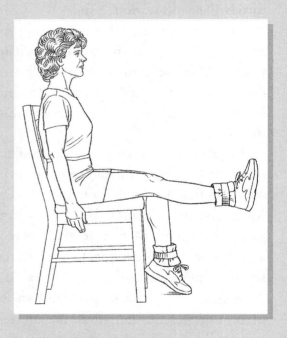

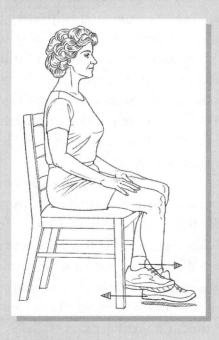

Resisted knee flexion. Sit and cross your legs above your ankles. Your legs can be almost straight, or you can bend your knees as much as you like. Try several positions. Push forward with your back leg and backward with your front leg. Exert pressure evenly so that your legs do not move. Hold for 10 seconds.

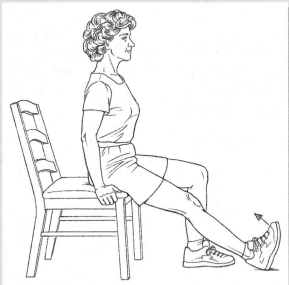

Thigh firmer. Sit on the edge of the chair with your right leg extended and the heel resting on the floor. Tighten the muscle that runs across the front of your knee by flexing your toes and foot. Hold for 5 seconds. If your leg is sore the next day, don't do this exercise. Repeat with your left leg.

Quads stretch. Stand on your right foot to the left of a chair. Hold on to the chair with your right hand for balance. With your left hand, draw your left foot as close to your buttocks as you can. Keep your knees relatively close together. Press your left knee forward without actually letting it move more than a few inches in front of your right knee. Hold this position for 20 to 30 seconds on each side, then repeat.

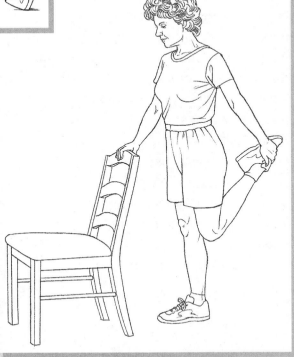

KNEE ROUTINE II (IN THE WATER)

These three pool exercises can ease knee pain. To prevent slips and falls, be sure to wear pool shoes or aqua socks when doing this workout. Initially, you may need to use buoyant devices or hold on to the side of the pool to maintain your balance when doing these exercises.

Knee flexion in water. In chest-deep water, stand facing the side of the pool. Hold on to the pool ledge with your left hand to support yourself. With your right hand, gently pull your left ankle toward your buttocks, as shown. This will produce a stretching sensation at the front of your left thigh. Be sure to keep your back straight. Hold for 5 to 10 seconds, then lower your leg. Do 5 to 10 repetitions with each leg.

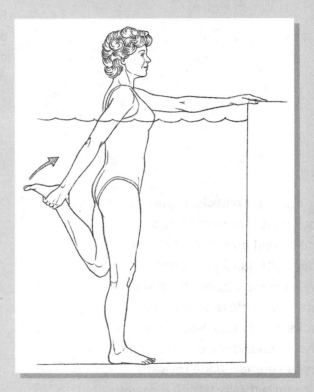

Knee extension in water. In chest-deep water, stand with your back against the side of the pool. Raise your right leg and link both hands under your knee. Keep your back straight and gently extend your right knee until it is straight but not locked. Hold for 5 to 10 seconds, then relax. Do 10 to 15 repetitions with each leg.

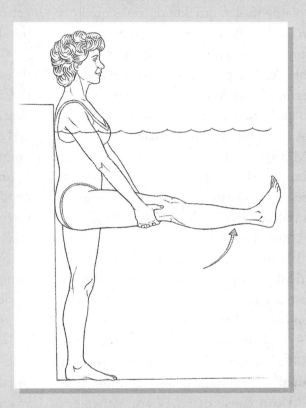

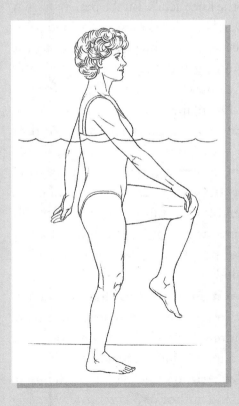

High-knee water walking. In chest-deep water, walk across the pool with high knees and exaggerated arm swinging, as shown. Do this for 2 to 5 minutes, and gradually increase your endurance so that you can do it for 10 to 15 minutes three times a week. Remember to keep your back straight.

Give it a (M)ighty (SM)ack. Methyl-sulfonylmethane (MSM), a nutritional supplement, can quickly douse acute knee pain and with regular use may dampen chronic joint pain as well, says Stanley Jacob, M.D., professor of surgery at the Oregon Health Sciences University in Portland and coauthor of *The Miracle of MSM*.

A component of dimethyl sulfoxide (DMSO), a pain medication used worldwide, MSM is an analgesic that also reduces inflammation and muscle spasms. But unlike DMSO, MSM is available over the counter at drugstores and most health food stores and has fewer side effects. In particular, MSM doesn't produce the distinctive fishlike taste in the mouth that often plagues DMSO users, Dr. Jacob says.

A typical dose of MSM ranges from 2,000 to 8,000 milligrams a day. But start gradually, he suggests, since in high doses MSM can cause diarrhea and other gastrointestinal problems. When you develop knee pain, take 1,000 milligrams twice a day with food for the first 2 to 3 days. Then each week, add another 1,000 milligrams to your daily intake until the pain subsides, he says. If you develop gastrointestinal problems such as cramping, cut back to a lower dose.

MSM often relieves acute pain in a day or two, Dr. Jacob says. But chronic knee problems such as arthritis will require more prolonged use of the supplement. In fact, it may be weeks or even months before you get relief from certain conditions. It's safe to take MSM for more than 1 year.

Get some kneaded relief. Rub an over-the-counter capsaicin cream such as Zostrix or Capzasin-P onto your sore knee, suggests Paul Blake, M.D., a pain-management expert and outpatient-services director at Meridian Point Rehabilitation Hospital in Scottsdale, Arizona. Capsaicin, an extract from spicy red peppers, is a natural analgesic that gradually can soothe knee aches. But be patient, it may take several days for the cream to do its job.

Since some people are sensitive to the compound, test the cream on a small area of skin to make sure that it's okay for you to use, Dr. Blake says. If the cream seems to irritate your skin, don't use it. And be sure to wash your hands once you've applied the cream. Pepper cream may work wonders on your knee, but it could cause considerable discomfort if you accidentally rub it in your eyes or other sensitive tissues. For most people, it's safe to use this cream indefinitely.

Treat it gingerly. A natural anti-inflammatory, ginger can help relieve knee pain, says Andrew T. Weil, M.D., director of the program in integrative medicine at the University of Arizona College of Medicine in Tucson and author of *Spontaneous Healing* and *8 Weeks to Optimum Health*. Take two

500-milligram capsules of powdered ginger once or twice a day with food. The capsules are available at most health food stores. It's safe to take this until your symptoms subside.

Know your ABCs. Vitamin and mineral supplements strengthen your nervous system, help your body maintain and rebuild cartilage and tendons, and help reduce pain in your knees and other joints, researchers say. Here's what they suggest.

▶ Vitamin A: Take 5,000 IU a day. It helps build cartilage and tendons, Dr. Catanzaro says.

▶ Vitamin B$_6$: Try 50 milligrams a day. B$_6$ helps keep nerves healthy so they'll be less apt to sense out false-alarm pain signals to your brain, Dr. Catanzaro says.

▶ Vitamin C: Take 1 gram four times a day, suggests Luke Bucci, Ph.D., vice president of research at Weider Nutrition International in Salt Lake City and author of *Healing Arthritis the Natural Way*. Animal studies have shown that vitamin C stimulates the growth of cartilage. If taking this much gives you diarrhea, reduce the dosage.

▶ Vitamin E: Try 400 IU daily. Scientists in Germany and Israel have found that regular doses of vitamin E can cut the need for pain-relieving medication by 50 percent in just 2 weeks, Dr. Bucci says. He speculates that the vitamin helps regulate the production of anti-inflammatory prostaglandins, some of the body's natural painkillers.

▶ Niacin: Take 250 milligrams of niacinamide, a form of niacin, three or four times a day, Dr. Bucci suggests. Niacinamide does not cause the flushing, itching, and other side effects that niacin does, but it still promotes blood circulation to the knee. Doses this high, however, must be taken under medical supervision.

Stifle swelling. Bromelain, which is a pineapple extract, and curcumin, the compound in turmeric that gives the spice its yellow color, can help relieve painful swelling of the joint, Dr. Catanzaro says. Take 1,000 milligrams of bromelain and 500 milligrams of curcumin three times a day for 3 weeks to 1 month, then see your health-care practitioner to be reevaluated, he suggests. These substances are available at most health food stores.

Extract it. Grape seed extract is a potent anti-inflammatory that can help relieve knee pain, says Sota Omoigui, M.D., medical director of the L.A. Pain Clinic in Hawthorne, California. The extract, which is available at most health food stores, also blocks the formation of unstable molecules called free radicals that can cause painful damage to cells and other tissues in your body. He suggests taking 50 to 100 milligrams of the extract daily. It's safe to take this until symptoms subside.

PAIN PREVENTERS

Slim down. Small changes in your eating and exercise habits can add up to a big difference in your waistline and can go a long way toward curtailing knee pain, Dr. Metzl says.

"I can't emphasize weight control enough. It's very important," he says. "Losing weight is a very helpful way of preventing knee pain. It probably helps to prevent osteoarthritis. And it certainly allows people to be much more active."

Walking, swimming, and the other activities suggested in this chapter can help you lighten your load. On the dietary side, if you want to lose ½ to 1 pound a week, you have to shave only 150 calories a day from your menu. That's the equivalent of a slice of cheese pizza, a 12-ounce can of root beer, or one beef frankfurter.

Try this simple weight-loss trick: Drink an 8-ounce glass of water about 10 minutes before you eat. That way, your stomach will already have something in it, and you won't have to eat as much to feel full, says Maria Simonson, Sc.D., Ph.D., director of the Health, Weight, and Stress Clinic at the Johns Hopkins Medical Institutions in Baltimore.

Root for yucca. Take 500 milligrams of yucca root four times a day to prevent knee pain, suggests Dr. Catanzaro. Yucca, a medicinal herb, does a couple of things that stop pain before it starts. It helps you maintain strong cartilage, plus it strengthens connective tissue surrounding the joint. It's safe to take this for 3 months, then see your health-care practitioner to be reevaluated. Yucca is available at most health food stores.

Try a little tenderness. If you garden or do other activities that require lots of kneeling, wear knee pads, Dr. Metzl suggests. It will help prevent bursitis, a painful inflammation of the fluid-filled sac above the kneecap.

Leg Pain

It's a wonder your legs don't hurt all the time. Ever since you learned to get up and walk around on them, your legs have been doing a lot of the heavy work for the rest of your body. Aside from carrying your body weight whenever you're upright, your legs—and the veins and muscles that make up your legs—also absorb hundreds of foot-pounds of pressure with every step you take.

Subjected to a lifetime of nonstop labor, your legs are bound to complain once in a while. Usually, it will be after you've walked around too much at the mall, stood in line too long at Walt Disney World, or spent 3 hours crammed into the coach section of an airliner on your way back east to see the grandkids.

Leg pain can be caused by a pinched nerve in your back (sciatica) or from joint ailments like osteoarthritis. But if it's related to the circulatory system, the most likely culprits are varicose veins, phlebitis, and arteriosclerosis (plaque buildup) in the arteries of your legs, which leads to a condition known as intermittent claudication.

VARICOSE VEINS

Genetics plays a big role in why you have varicose veins. If your mother or a grandparent had them, you may have inherited the tendency. You may also get varicose veins, however, if you sit or stand in one position for long periods or are overweight.

The problem lies not so much with the veins but with the valves in the veins that prevent blood from flowing back into your legs on its way to your heart. Being a liquid, blood naturally wants to run down-hill. The force of your heart pumping and the muscles in your legs keep it moving against gravity. When you move your legs, the muscles in your calves massage the veins and milk the blood upward. Doctors refer to this mechanism as the calf pump.

The valves in the veins also keep the blood from dripping back. But if they don't close properly, blood pools up into little lakes, and the veins expand with the added volume.

Initially, all you may get are spider veins—faint red lines along the skin surface—but eventually, these varicosities may grow in size. When that happens, you get a dull, generalized ache in your legs and sometimes a throbbing pain.

For Fast Relief

Use gravity. When your legs feel heavy and achy, put your feet up to create a slope that will make it easier for blood to flow back toward your heart, says Normand Miller, M.D., at the Vascular Center and Bloodflow Laboratory at Mercy Medical Center in Baltimore.

Lie on the floor and put your feet up on the couch or tilt back in a recliner. "Putting your legs up helps to empty the venous system. It gets that stagnant blood out of there," says Dr. Miller. "Just a few minutes of this can help you feel better."

For sleeping at night, you can place bricks or blocks of wood under the posts at the foot of the bed, says Frank Fort, M.D., of the Capital Region Vein Centre in Schenectady, New York. "It doesn't have to be a steep decline. Two to four inches is usually enough."

For Lasting Relief

Shake a leg. The worst thing for your varicose veins is inactivity, says Dr. Fort. Don't spend all day sitting in that chair or lying on the couch. Take a walk, pedal an exercise bike, or do the tango. You have to move around.

"Exercise activates the calf pump and helps build strength in the venous system," he says. "Exercise can only help."

Apply pressure. When your veins are weak and expand easily, you can give them added support by wearing pressure stockings. These elastic stockings put pressure on your tissues and compress those lakes of stagnant blood in your legs.

"The idea is to squeeze those lakes and

turn them into rivers," says Dr. Miller. You can buy pressure stockings in most drugstores and medical supply stores. A general support hose may be enough if your only complaint is fatigue in your legs.

"For most people, a light-support knee-high stocking is enough," he says. "But if a woman chooses to wear support panty hose, that's fine, too."

Note: Only wear these stockings during the day. Take them off at night, but keep your legs elevated for support while you are sleeping.

Phlebitis

There are two types of phlebitis: clotting in the superficial veins of the leg and deep-vein thrombosis, or clotting in the main channels that return blood to your heart.

You're more likely to get superficial phlebitis if you have varicose veins, although men sometimes develop it without a lot of symptoms of varicose veins, says Dr. Fort.

Something as simple as a blow, mosquito bite, or bee sting to the leg can cause a vein to distend or expand. When that happens, blood no longer flows straight and smooth but more slowly and turbulently. Instead of a river, you end up with a small lake of blood. Sometimes, it congeals, hardens, and forms a clot. Inflammation may set in, says Dr. Fort. You may notice a redness and feel a hard cord or bulge beneath your skin, he explains.

"When you press on it, it hurts. It can be real sensitive to the touch," he says. "It may also hurt when you're walking or moving your leg." Even though it can reach the diameter of a garden hose, a superficial clot is not life threatening, he says. Rarely does it travel far along the course of the affected vein.

If you have a tendency to form superficial clots, you may be in danger of having deep-vein thrombosis, which forms a painful type of clot that may move to your lungs. And that is a much more serious matter, says Dr. Fort. See a doctor whenever you experience leg symptoms such as unusual swelling or pain. The doctor can determine which type of clot you may have and can treat you accordingly.

Once you've seen the doctor, you can help ease the pain of phlebitis yourself with these measures.

For Fast Relief

Take a break. If you know you're prone to any type of phlebitis, take precautions. Sitting in one place too long will definitely put you at risk, says Dr. Miller.

(continued on page 342)

Get a Leg Up

Here are some exercises to do a few times a day to activate the calf pump mechanism that milks your blood upward and to improve vein circulation in your legs. Doing the exercises while lying down also enables you to take advantage of gravity. If you have varicose veins, you should do these exercises at least twice a day, but three or four times a day, if possible, says Frank Fort, M.D., of the Capital Region Vein Centre in Schenectady, New York.

First, lie on your back on the floor with your legs straight. Then, lift your legs up and rest them on a box, the edge of a chair, or several piled-up pillows so that your legs are straight and at a 45-degree angle, says Dr. Fort. Your legs should contact the box or chair at midcalf, leaving your feet free to move.

The following three exercises should all be done from this position.

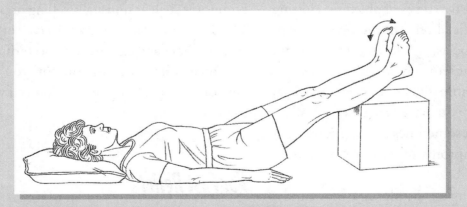

Toe flexion. Flex your toes forward and then backward at a comfortable pace. Repeat this back-and-forth motion for 30 seconds.

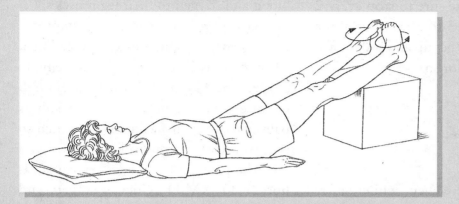

Foot circle. Moving your feet at the ankles, draw a circle in the air with each foot. Draw five clockwise circles with your left foot while drawing five counterclockwise circles with your right foot. Then, reverse the direction of each foot for five circles.

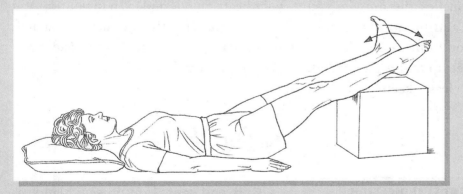

Foot flexion. Flex your feet forward and backward as a way of flexing your calf muscles, alternating so that your right foot is flexed while your left foot is pointed, then switching. Flex 10 times in a period of about 30 seconds.

When you're traveling for long periods, exercise your legs frequently. If you're riding in a car, make sure to stop every 2 hours and walk for 3 to 4 minutes. On a cross-country flight, get up and walk down the aisle every hour or so.

For Lasting Relief

Tap your feet. Even while you're seated, it's a good idea to keep your blood moving, rather than letting it pool in your legs. Lift up on the balls of your feet and flex your calf muscles, says Dr. Fort.

What this does is activate the calf pump in your leg. As you flex the muscle, you squeeze the veins and pump the venous, unoxygenated blood from your legs.

"If you can't get up and walk around, you want to at least keep your feet moving," he says.

INTERMITTENT CLAUDICATION

The word *claudication* describes a limping or lameness in the legs.

People with intermittent claudication have plaque buildup in the arteries of their legs. In other words, they have hardening of the arteries that diminishes the flow of blood and oxygen to their leg muscles.

Usually, you don't feel any symptoms unless you're walking or exercising. Then, when the muscles of your legs require more oxygen and blood, they can't get enough because of the blockages. The result is pain, tension, and weakness—so much so that you have to stop walking. When you rest, the pain soon subsides, explains Elliott Badder, M.D., chief of surgery and member of the Vascular Center and Blood-flow Laboratory at Mercy Medical Center in Baltimore.

If you have intermittent claudication, you likely have plaque buildup around your heart muscle and even in your carotid artery. Consequently, you may have a high risk of having heart attack or stroke. See a doctor, says Dr. Badder.

For Fast Relief

Halt and rest. Intermittent claudication pain occurs because your muscles cannot get the blood and oxygen they need to do what's being asked—climbing a set of stairs or taking a walk. If you stop and rest, you'll lower the muscles' oxygen demand, and the pain will ease in a few minutes, says Dr. Badder.

For Lasting Relief

Snuff the butts. Nicotine in cigarettes is a vasoconstrictor, meaning that it causes your veins and arteries to shrink and constrict. When the pipelines in your legs are already partially blocked, the last thing you need is another impediment to bloodflow, says Dr. Fort. "If you're a smoker, you just have to quit. Otherwise, you won't get any better."

Smoking may be the major reason you're having trouble in the first place. It is a major contributor to plaque buildup in the arteries. Cigarette smoke also contains carbon monoxide. Every time you take a puff, carbon monoxide enters your bloodstream, attaches itself to hemoglobin, and robs the blood of its ability to carry oxygen to your muscles.

"Smoking is just bad news all the way around," says Dr. Badder.

Get in training. If exercise makes your legs hurt, why do it? Because unless you keep at it, you won't get any better, says Dr. Fort. On the other hand, if you work at it, you can vastly increase the distance you can walk before your legs begin to claudi-cate, that is, until the pain makes you stop, he says. Before you start any exercise program, check with your doctor first. Then follow this easy program: Go out for a walk. Walk at a comfortable pace until you claudicate, and then stop and rest. Wait a few moments until the pain disappears, and then start walking again. This time, you'll claudicate sooner.

Repeat the process of walking and resting for a total of 1 hour per day. Don't overdo it. If you have a lot of soreness afterward, shorten the time and start more gradually.

"At the end of 6 weeks, you should be able to increase your walking distance before you experience pain, quite a bit—as much as double the distance," says Dr. Fort.

Walking is probably the easiest exercise to do to train these muscles, but you can also ride a stationary bike or swim. Whatever exercise you choose, you have to do it regularly—at least three or four times a week, says Dr. Badder. "Not only that, you have to do it vigorously enough so that you claudicate," he adds.

Supplement with carnitine. Carnitine, a nutritional supplement, has been used in Europe to treat intermittent claudication. It's thought to improve the efficiency of oxygen-starved muscles so that they can do more with less. In other words, carnitine may improve the aerobic metabolism of the muscle.

If you want to try carnitine, Dr. Fort recommends taking 2 grams twice a day, orally. You can buy carnitine in health food stores and drugstores. Expect to take the supplement for about a month before you start to notice results. Then, keep taking the supplement to prevent leg pain. Don't take carnitine without a doctor's guidance, however.

Tip the vino. The benefits of red wine have become more evident over the last several years, especially where preventing clots is concerned. Certain elements in red wine seem to inhibit plaque buildup. One to two glasses of red wine daily is recommended, unless there's a medical or personal reason you shouldn't drink. To be safe, check with your doctor first, says Dr. Badder.

Get your vitamins. Taking a daily multivitamin along with a vitamin E supplement falls into the category of "it can't hurt you, and it may help," says Dr. Badder. There is some evidence that vitamin E may inhibit atherosclerosis, a form of arteriosclerosis, and that vitamins with antioxidant properties may be helpful.

A typical daily dosage of vitamin E ranges from 200 to 400 IU. There are, of course, many daily multivitamins on the market. Just avoid any that include vitamin K, which can actually promote blood clotting, he says.

"There is some suggestive evidence that vitamins are helpful," says Dr. Badder. "If you want to try them, there's no reason not to."

Muscle Pain

More than 600 muscles are at work in your body, propelling you as you walk, swim, hold a newspaper, sweep a floor, cast a fly rod, or open a window. There are almost 10 muscles, for example, packed into your tongue that allow you to delicately lick a stamp or forcefully blow out a raspberry noise at a friend.

Other muscles are large. Your heaviest muscle—the gluteus maximus—literally brings up your rear, where it helps you extend your hips and gives you a built-in cushion to sit upon.

Starting at the age of 30 or so, however, you naturally start losing some of the muscle that carries you through a lifetime of motion. Though about a third of your weight was muscle when you were young, by the time you reach 75, it accounts for only about 15 percent of your weight.

Your muscles may become more achy after exertion because the system of blood vessels that keeps them nourished also decreases, says Willibald Nagler, M.D., physiatrist in chief and chairperson of rehabilitation medicine at the Cornell campus of the New York Presbyterian Hospital in New York City. Blood vessels carry to muscles the oxygen that they require to work properly. And as you use your muscles, they produce waste products that are also carried away by blood vessels.

So when your muscles ache from, say, vacuuming the stairs or chasing the grandkids around the backyard, they may be hurting from a lack of oxygen and a buildup of wastes, in addition to tiny tears that can form in them after exercise, says Dr. Nagler.

Even though your muscles are going through changes, you shouldn't retire them from all activity to protect them from pain. Exercise can help keep them strong, stretching can make them more flexible, and some basic remedies can reduce the aches that find their way to them.

For Fast Relief

Turn up the heat. When a muscle protests that you've been gardening, golfing, or doing anything else too much, put some moist heat on it, suggests William Grana, M.D., clinical professor in the department of orthopedics at the University of Oklahoma in Oklahoma City. Heat boosts the circulation of blood to the achy muscle, which will bring it more oxygen and flush out the wastes it needs to send away.

Just wet a towel with warm water, wring it out, then place it over your sore spot for about 20 minutes three or four times a day.

For Lasting Relief

Squeeze 'em to ease 'em. When you massage your achy muscles, you provide relief in several ways, says Patricia Benjamin, Ph.D., dean of the Chicago School of Massage Therapy and coauthor of *Tappan's Handbook of Healing Massage Techniques.* As you press them, you increase circulation to the muscles and squeeze out those waste products that they produced while working, she says. Also, massage helps you feel better by creating warmth in the area and relieving muscle tension.

Use lotion as you massage yourself, so that your hands will slide over your skin better. Grasp the sore area firmly and rub your hand along it in a gliding motion, squeezing the muscle as you move along. It's a little like gripping a tube of toothpaste and pressing the contents toward the opening, says Dr. Benjamin.

Regardless of which muscle is sore, massage it toward the center of your body to help circulation in the veins. For example, if you're massaging your upper arm, slide your hand toward your shoulder; if it's your leg, rub upward toward your abdomen. You can also knead your muscles as you do this, says Dr. Benjamin. Firmly press your fingers and thumbs into the area as if you were forming clay or dough.

These motions shouldn't hurt but may create a good type of soreness.

Give your muscles a break. If you enjoy a regular activity that makes your

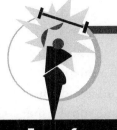

PUNCTURE YOUR MUSCLE PAIN

Acupuncture is one of the favorite forms of muscle pain relief for Richard Linchitz, M.D., a physician with the Pain Alleviation Center in Jericho, New York. While the regular kind can work well for these aches, he's especially enthusiastic about a style called tendinomuscular acupuncture, which he practices.

Both forms of the oriental healing art involve sticking thin needles into specific spots on the body to affect the flow of energy along theoretical pathways in the body called meridians. This form, however, concentrates on the tendinomuscular meridians, which lie closer to the surface of the skin, says Dr. Linchitz. "I can't say enough positive about it—it's an extraordinarily effective treatment for muscle pains and aches."

Usually, people who try it need a few sessions of acupuncture, though they often find significant relief after their first visits. The earlier you have acupuncture done after you start aching, the better it works, he says.

muscles sore, such as bicycling or swimming, certainly don't stop doing that activity, but do give yourself plenty of time to recover before the next session, says

Richard Linchitz, M.D., a physician with the Pain Alleviation Center in Jericho, New York.

Between each burst of the same type of

exertion, take at least a 48-hour break, Dr. Linchitz says. In the meantime, you can mix in exercises that use different muscles.

Rub in the relief. You may find relief in the salves and liniments on many supermarket, drugstore, or health food store shelves.

Some of them have a counterirritant effect, which means they create sensations on your skin that compete for attention with the pain messages your muscles are sending out, says Ronald Lawrence, M.D., Ph.D., assistant clinical professor in the psychiatry department at the University of California, Los Angeles, School of Medicine and a founding member of the International Association for the Study of Pain.

One such product is Tiger Balm, an ointment made in Asia that contains menthol and camphor, which Dr. Lawrence recommends.

Another type of counterirritating cream contains the ingredient capsaicin, which comes from spicy red peppers. Capsaicin also works by depleting a chemical in your body called substance P that helps nerves conduct pain. This takes time, however, so you may need to use a capsaicin cream for several days before it starts to have an effect, Dr. Lawrence cautions.

Try an old country remedy. Lotions and salves containing arnica may also help your muscle pain, Dr. Nagler says. Arnica is a yellow-orange flower that grows in Europe and Western North America and that has long been used as a folk remedy.

You should be able to find arnica products at health food stores and some supermarkets. Some people are allergic to a chemical in the flower, so dab a little on a small patch of skin first. If it gives you a rash, don't use it.

Spell relief with MSM. Dr. Lawrence is a proponent of a nonprescription remedy called methylsulfonylmethane, or MSM—enough so that he helped write a book on it: *The Miracle of MSM.*

This nutritional supplement acts as an analgesic and anti-inflammatory to soothe muscle pain, Dr. Lawrence says. It comes in a lotion or gel form that you can rub on your skin or in pills and powders that you take internally. He recommends either type as effective for muscle pain. Look for MSM in health food stores or drugstores.

PAIN PREVENTERS

Get ready for exertion. "The most important thing for older people is proper warmup," Dr. Linchitz says. "Proper warmup will help prevent a lot of the muscle soreness and muscle problems."

The best way to warm up for any form

of exertion is to start doing the activity slowly and gently, then gradually step up the pace. After about a 10-minute warmup of any light activity, such as walking, you can then stretch the muscles that you're using in the exercise. Don't start stretching "cold," or before you've warmed up, he says.

Good hints to keep in mind are to stretch out as far as you can, in a steady motion without bouncing, then hold the position for 10 to 30 seconds. Repeat each different stretch three to five times. If a muscle hurts, you're stretching it too far. (For more information, see Stretching on page 170.)

Keep yourself going. Mike Mc-Cormick, a certified athletic trainer and partner with Athletico Sports Medicine and Physical Therapy in Chicago, thinks that muscle pain is in part due to electric can openers, automatic breadmakers, and the neighbor's kid who mows lawns.

"Part of the problem is that all the means we've invented to make our lives easier over the last couple of generations have actually hurt us more than helped us, because they made us less active," McCormick says. "People who are stiff and sore think that they should be less active, but the opposite's true. If you're stiff and sore, you should be more active."

With regular exercise, you can delay muscle shrinkage, stiffness, and weakness, Dr. Nagler says, and studies on the issue agree.

According to the National Institute on Aging, as long as you don't have a medical condition that prevents it, you should try to get at least 30 minutes of endurance exercises each day. These include swimming, walking, yard work, or any activity that increases your breathing and pulse rate for an extended period of time.

At least twice a week, you should include exercises that strengthen your muscles, making sure not to work the same muscles 2 days in a row. You can purchase hand and ankle weights from a sporting goods store, or just use cans of food as weights. (For more information, see Strength Training on page 163.)

Neck Pain

An original amid the conventional buildings dotting downtown Seattle, Rainier Tower gets more than a few gawks from first-time visitors. To some, the white 28-story office complex built atop a 12-story pedestal resembles a golf tee precariously balancing a quart of milk.

But in many ways, the pedestal looks precisely like a neck supporting a gigantic head—except this "neck" holds up a 20,000-ton "head." Your neck doesn't support quite that kind of load—a typical head weighs between 10 and 12 pounds. But after a lifetime of twisting, turning, and bending, it certainly can feel as if the seven vertebrae and 32 muscles between your head and shoulders are holding up the equivalent of a massive skyscraper.

"It's a good analogy," says David Bilstrom, M.D., director of the physiatric medical acupuncture program at Christ Hospital and Medical Center in Oak Lawn, Illinois. "There's a lot of weight resting on top of your neck. Even when you're standing or sitting still, the neck is doing a lot. It may look as if nothing is going on. But the body is constantly making small adjustments involving the neck to maintain that posture. So the neck muscles are constantly working. There really is almost no rest for them."

Neck discomfort is one of the most common pains affecting older Americans. By age 65, x-ray studies show that 95 percent of men and 70 percent of women have at least some potentially painful degenerative changes in their necks, says Donald R. Gore, M.D., clinical professor of orthopedic surgery at the Medical College of Wisconsin in Milwaukee.

These changes are, in part, normal. As you age, the disks in your neck, which act like shock absorbers, lose much of their natural strength and elasticity. As a result, the entire structure of your neck can begin to crumble—overtaxing muscles, hindering joint movement, and pinching off nerves. Poor posture, arthritis, osteoporosis, and falls and other accidents can also take their toll on an aging neck.

Seek immediate medical care if your neck pain is accompanied by numbness, tingling, or pain in your arms, hands, or chest, says Mark Gostine, M.D., president of Michigan Pain Consultants, based in Grand Rapids. You also should see a doctor if in addition to a sore neck you develop any muscle weakness or dizziness.

But in most cases, neck pain can be eradicated by one of these natural pain relievers.

For Fast Relief

Press the point. If the pain is caused by muscle tension—as most neck pains are—then try applying constant, mild pressure with your fingertips to the most painful spot for 3 minutes, suggests Stephen Price, D.C., a Los Angeles chiropractor. This technique, called ischemic compression, encourages tense muscles to relax, increases bloodflow to the site, and can quickly subdue your neck pain. Unlike acupressure, which has set pressure points that might not be anywhere near your ache, ischemic compression allows you to attack the site of the pain directly, he says.

Don't press on the spot as hard as you can. Moderate pressure is the key, Dr. Price says. When you first apply pressure, on a scale of 1 to 10, you should press until the pain is about a 5. Once you find the most painful spot, keep your finger still. As the end of the 3 minutes approaches, the pain should dramatically subside. If the pain is in a hard-to-reach spot, ask someone to press on it for you.

For Lasting Relief

Rub it out. A cream containing capsaicin, an extract from spicy red peppers, can soothe most acute pain within minutes after being rubbed on a sore neck, says John Catanzaro, N.D., a naturopathic physician specializing in pain management and director of the Health and Wellness Institute in Seattle. In addition to being a natural painkiller, capsaicin can

GET THE POINT WITH ACUPRESSURE

If you want to try acupressure to relieve neck pain, there are two acupressure points located on each side of your neck, behind your ears at the base of your skull, that can swiftly ease your discomfort, says David Bilstrom, M.D., director of the physiatric medical acupuncture program at Christ Hospital and Medical Center in Oak Lawn, Illinois.

Painful muscle tension is common at these points (Bladder 10, or B10, and Gallbladder 20, or GB20), Dr. Bilstrom says. You can apply pressure to any of these points for up to 1 minute, as needed to relieve neck soreness. Acupressure points are usually more sensitive than the surrounding areas, but to experience results, you need to press hard enough that you get an aching sensation.

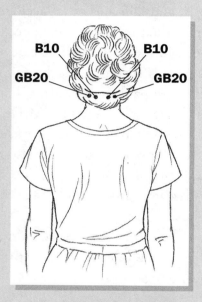

help reduce swelling of aching neck muscles and joints. Zostrix, Capzasin-P, and other products containing the extract are available at many drugstores.

It can be used as needed, but since the compound can cause some people to develop skin rashes, test the cream on a tiny patch of your skin before applying it to a larger area. If the cream seems to irritate your skin, don't use it, he says.

Use only a small amount, about the size of a pea. Be patient; it may take several days for these over-the-counter creams to soothe pain resulting from arthritis. Also, since capsaicin can cause discomfort if it's accidentally rubbed into your eyes, wash your hands carefully after use.

Put a package of peas in place. Chill the pain with frozen peas straight out of your freezer, Dr. Gostine suggests. Unlike chunks of ice, a bag of frozen peas can be precisely molded into the area of your neck that is hurting. Be sure to wrap the bag in a thin towel before applying it to your skin.

You can ice your neck in this way for up to 45 minutes four times a day. Keep two bags of the vegetables handy, he suggests. That way, you can keep one on your neck while the other is cooling in the freezer.

Turn off the heat. Although it may seem soothing, heat is actually bad for a sore neck, Dr. Gostine says. Applying hot packs or warm towels will increase blood-flow to the area, promote swelling, and actually prolong your pain.

"The reason heat feels good when you first use it is that temperature sensations and pain are conducted through the same nerve fibers," he says. "When you apply heat, it obscures the pain because only one sensation can go through that nerve fiber at a time. So heat distracts your attention from the pain for a while, but in the long run, it will exacerbate your discomfort."

Sleep on a slope. If your neck hurts at bedtime, try this: Put two pillows under your head, carefully positioning one on top of the other so that your neck tilts slightly toward the painful side as you sleep, Dr. Gostine says. More than likely, your neck pain will be muted when you awaken the next morning. By the way, this technique is effective no matter if you sleep on your back, side, or stomach, he says.

Floor it. Two simple floor exercises can help relieve your neck pain, Dr. Price says.

Start by lying flat on your back with your knees bent for 1 minute. Relax completely and allow the small of your back to flatten so that it completely touches the floor. Then each day, add 1 more minute to this position until you reach 20 minutes daily. This position will allow gravity to push on your spine and gradually straighten out your posture and take pressure off your neck, he says.

Once you've mastered this stretching exercise, try this: Gently push the back of your head against the floor for the final minute that you are lying there. This isometric exercise will help strengthen your neck muscles and help you hold your head more erect.

"These floor exercises can produce remarkable changes in posture, which then relieve pain in the back and the neck," says Dr. Price. "You're basically trying to undo the ravages of gravity that have built up over the past 60 or 70 years."

Clamp on a collar. Cervical collars that immobilize your neck can help temporarily relieve acute joint pain caused by an accident or a flare-up of arthritis, Dr. Gostine says.

"An acutely sore joint wants to remain quiet. It really doesn't want to be aggravated and put through a full range of motion. So when you have acute neck pain, wearing a collar is a good idea," he says.

But it's not a good idea to immobilize your neck for too long. Wearing a cervical collar for more than a few days can actually weaken your neck muscles, increase your susceptibility to injury, and prolong your pain. So if your neck pain persists for more than 3 days after you begin wearing a collar, see your doctor, Dr. Gostine suggests. Cervical collars are available at medical supply stores and most drugstores.

Give nature a nudge. If you have acute neck pain, try dissolving a Traumeel tablet under your tongue every couple of hours until the pain subsides, Dr. Catan-

zaro recommends. Traumeel is an over-the-counter product made with several homeopathic remedies, such as arnica, calendula, and belladonna, that alternative-medicine experts say relieves muscle and joint pain. Traumeel, which can be purchased at many health food stores and drugstores, is also available as a cream that can be rubbed into a sore neck as needed.

Take some turmeric. If you have arthritis in your neck, herbs like turmeric and ginger can help relieve your aches and pains, Dr. Gostine says. These herbs help inhibit the production of leukotrienes, hormonelike substances that trigger swelling of muscle and other tissues surrounding the neck joints. He recommends taking 1 to 2 grams of each herb daily. It's safe to take these until your pain subsides. Turmeric and ginger are available at most health food stores.

Gulp glucosamine. Studies suggest that glucosamine, a sugar that is one of the body's natural building blocks, helps repair painful joints, including those in the neck, Dr. Gostine says. He recommends taking 1,500 milligrams of glucosamine a day. Keep in mind that it can take several weeks for this natural remedy to build up in your body and begin working. It's safe to take this until your neck pain diminishes.

Load up on antioxidants. Antioxidant vitamins help prevent the painful deterioration of joints in your neck and other parts of your body, Dr. Gostine says. He recommends supplementing your diet with 1,000 milligrams of vitamin C and 400 IU of vitamin E daily.

Just the flax, ma'am. Just 2 teaspoons of flaxseed oil a day may be enough to corral your neck pain, Dr. Gostine says. Flaxseed is loaded with alpha-linolenic acid, the plant version of the omega-3 fatty acids found in fish that help prevent painful swelling in the joints. Researchers suspect that flaxseed oil is a potent pain reliever because, unlike other oils, it lingers in the body. The oil uses this extra time well—its beneficial compounds trickle into your bones and soothe painful neck joints. You can take this until your pain goes away.

Flaxseed oil can be mixed with orange juice and other cold beverages. You can find it at most health food stores. Flaxseed oil goes rancid quickly, so buy refrigerated oil and keep it in the fridge at home.

PAIN PREVENTERS

Take five. Holding your neck in one position for a long period of time—even when you're just sitting in a chair watching television—can trigger pain. So every 20 to 30 minutes, be sure to stretch your neck a bit, Dr. Price says. Slowly turn your head to the left, keeping your chin level, until you feel a mild stretch or tug from the muscles in your neck. Hold that position for a count of 30. Then, slowly turn your head forward, relax for a count of 30, and repeat this stretch on your right side.

Note: You don't have to look completely over your shoulder as some exercise books recommend. Stretching your neck muscles too much—particularly if you haven't regularly stretched them in 10 to 20 years—can do more harm than good. So whatever stretch you do, do it only to a point where you feel a mild tugging, Dr. Price says.

"How long you stretch a muscle is much more important than how hard you stretch it," he says. "A comfortable, but not overreaching, stretch will produce a more supple neck and lessen your chances of injury."

Arm yourself. In a chair without armrests, you're more apt to let your hands dangle at your sides while your sitting, Dr. Bilstrom says. That puts a lot of stress on your upper back and neck. So whenever possible, sit in a chair that has armrests. More than likely, you'll naturally rest your arms on the sides of the chair and slash your risk of developing sore neck muscles.

Likewise, try to pick a chair that allows

(continued on page 358)

MAKE A FEW REST STOPS

When you travel, stretching every 20 minutes may not be practical. But you should stretch your neck at least every couple of hours, says David Bilstrom, M.D., director of the physiatric medical acupuncture program at Christ Hospital and Medical Center in Oak Lawn, Illinois. The following stretches can help keep your neck pain-free on the road and can be useful additions to any neck exercises you do at home. For each exercise, do 5 repetitions, then increase over 1 to 2 weeks to a maximum of 10 repetitions. If any of these exercises causes you pain, stop doing it.

Neck flexion/extension. Sit in a sturdy chair, keeping your neck, shoulders, and trunk straight. Lower your chin slowly to your chest, keeping your mouth closed. Then, moving gently to the point of pain, bring your head as far back as possible to look up at the ceiling.

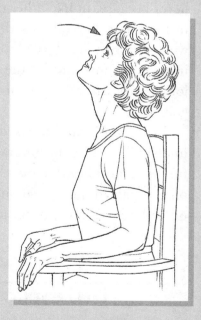

To intensify the stretch, put your palm on the back of your head. Then, for a count of 10, push your head against it so that you feel light pressure but no strain. Slowly drop your head forward and there will be a reflex relaxation of the muscles, which will allow more efficient stretching.

You can also do this with the muscles on the side of your head. Place the palm of your right hand on the right side of your head, gently push your head against it for a count of 10, then tilt your head to the left side. The muscle on the left side of your head will reflexively relax so that you'll get a better stretch. Do this two times on each side of your head.

Head tilt. Stand with your feet shoulder-width apart and clasp your hands behind your back. Slowly lower your head toward your left shoulder until you just begin feeling the muscles on the right side of your neck stretch. Hold that position for a count of five. Then, slowly raise your head back to its normal position and repeat to the right side.

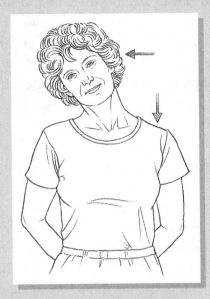

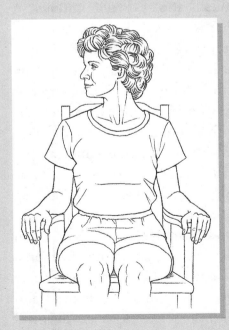

Neck rotation. Sitting in a chair, keep your neck, shoulders, and trunk straight. Turn your head slowly to the right and then left, moving gently to the point of pain. Then relax.

you to rest your arms with your elbows bent at a comfortable 90-degree angle. If the armrests are too high or too low for you, the chair can overtax the muscles in your shoulders and neck and eventually cause pain, he says.

Back up your neck. Good posture can help prevent neck pain, Dr. Bilstrom says. "It's hard to support the neck, but you can do a better job of supporting it by controlling what is going on in the lower part of your body. If you're sitting so that your knees and hips are all bent at 90 degrees, that's going to put your entire body into a position that doesn't overwork the neck."

Sit so that your buttocks point to where the seat and the backrest meet, he suggests. Sit comfortably erect, with your feet flat on the floor. If you're sitting in a straight-back chair, consider using a pillow that fits between the small of your back and the chair to help provide support for your lower spine.

As for standing, many older people believe squeezing or pulling their shoulders together is the best way to stand up straight. But if you do that, it will push your head in front of your shoulders and actually put more pressure on your neck, Dr. Price says. You'll be less prone to neck pain if you *relax* your shoulders as you stand. That will help straighten out your neck and keep your head aligned between your shoulders.

Skip the spin cycle. Wheels, gears, and planets are all things that are supposed to spin. Your neck isn't. Rolling or revolving your neck in a circular motion to "loosen" it up can actually cause painful disk damage and pinched nerves, Dr. Gostine says.

"You may have been able to get away with rolling your neck around when you were in high school, because your disks were supple, your muscle tissue was fairly elastic, and you didn't have arthritis. But as you get older, putting that type of force on the neck is unwise."

Purchase the perfect pillow. A pillow that is too small or too large can trigger neck pain because neither will support your head properly as you sleep, says Dr. Bilstrom. So how to find one that is just right? Consider getting an orthopedic pillow with a cutout in the middle. This U-shaped pillow will cradle your head and offer more side support for your neck, he says. Orthopedic pillows are available at most medical supply stores.

Roll your own. Instead of a pillow, you also might consider doing this: Fashion a towel into a tight roll, secure it with safety pins, then tuck it under your head and sleep on it, Dr. Price suggests. This roll helps keep your head in a more neck-friendly position as you snooze.

Take off the shoulder strap. Carrying a heavy suitcase, purse, or gym bag on one shoulder can trigger neck pain, Dr. Price says. If you can, get a suitcase or handcart with wheels so you can pull your luggage along behind you when you travel. Instead of a shoulder-strap purse, use a handbag that you can tuck under your arm.

Or switch to a fanny pack, which fits around your waist and doesn't put any strain on your neck at all. But just to be safe, consider wearing the pack backward so that it rests on your lower back instead of on your front, Dr. Bilstrom suggests. Carrying a hefty fanny pack on the front side of your body can pull your pelvis forward, increasing the pressure on your entire spine, including your neck. When you need something, you can easily swing the pack around to your front, get the item, then swing the pack back again.

If you must use a shoulder strap, put it over your head so that the strap rests on the opposite shoulder from the bag, Dr. Bilstrom says. That will help distribute the weight of the bag more evenly and at least lessen the strain on your neck and shoulder muscles.

Don't put the caller on hold. Avoid propping a phone receiver up between your neck and shoulder, Dr. Price says. It can strain the muscles of your neck and cause pain. Instead, always hold the receiver in one hand so that your elbow is supported by a table or armrest. If you spend a lot of time on the telephone, consider getting a speakerphone or headset, he suggests.

Osteoporosis

Osteoporosis is like high blood pressure. You may not know you have it unless you get checked out. And on its own, it can be painless, but complications arising from it can be painful indeed.

With osteoporosis, you may fracture bones after a fall that years earlier wouldn't have fazed you. Or you may develop tiny microfractures in your vertebrae, the bones that form your spine. As vertebrae fracture, the spine starts to crumble. "That can cause chronic pain for several reasons related to the poor alignment of the spine resulting from vertebral fractures," says Ethel Siris, M.D., director of the Toni Stabile Center for the Prevention and Treatment of Osteoporosis at Columbia-Presbyterian Medical Center in New York City. But osteoporosis doesn't have to reach this painful late stage.

This is one condition for which you're best off using conventional medicine *and* self-help measures like exercise and nutrition. On the conventional side, one test you'll need from your doctor is a bone-density measure called DEXA. If you get a DEXA test and know your bone density, it will help you and your doctor figure out the best course of action. In some cases, hormone-replacement therapy or medications that inhibit bone breakdown, such as alendronate sodium (Fosamax), raloxifene hydrochloride (Evista), or calcitonin (Calcimar), may be what you need. If your bones are still pretty strong, exercise and good nutrition may suffice.

If you're a woman, keep in mind that you could lose 15 percent or more of your bone mass in the 5 to 10 years after menopause. Bone loss continues, but more slowly, after age 65 in both men and

BONES BEFORE AND AFTER

Once osteoporosis sets in, a healthy bone can start to appear more honeycombed, and the integrity of the bone wears away.

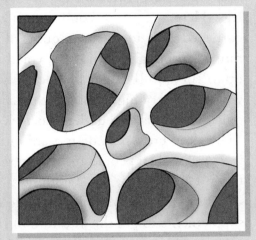

Normal bone

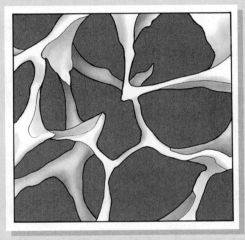

Bone with osteoporosis

women. At any age, there are things that you can do to minimize potential pain by minimizing your risk of painful fractures.

For Fast Relief

Ask your doc what's up. If you have pain, you should see your doctor to deter-

mine if you have a fracture or pinched nerves, Dr. Siris says. Then, here's what your doctor might recommend.

▶ Rest them bones. Microfractures do not require that you be immobilized, but you'll have less pain if you find comfortable sitting and lying positions and rest up for a few days. "The pain will almost always dramatically lessen over time," she says.

▶ Use heat to melt pain. Heat seems to work well for temporarily relieving the back pain associated with microfractures, Dr. Siris says. Use a heating pad or, after a few days of rest, a whirlpool bath.

▶ Get braced. You may need to see an orthopedic specialist for a brace that helps to stabilize your back, she says. Such a brace may not be a natural remedy, but in the long run, it may be a better pain reliever than the drugs you might end up taking because you didn't opt for a brace.

For Lasting Relief

Get enough of the sunshine vitamin. Vitamin D is essential for healthy bones. It allows our bodies to absorb the calcium we eat, stimulates the formation of bone tissue, and regulates the amount of bone we break down, says Michael Gloth, M.D., associate professor of medicine in the division of geriatric medicine at Johns Hopkins University and chief of geriatrics at Union Memorial Hospital, both in Baltimore.

Some people develop osteoporosis because of a vitamin D deficiency, he says. The deficiency causes a gland called the parathyroid to crank up production of hormones that take calcium out of bones. Getting enough vitamin D prevents this.

Some people, especially homebound elderly, become so deficient in vitamin D that they develop osteomalacia, the adult form of rickets, a softening of the bones that causes deep, intense pain, often in the legs. Here again, the condition is easily corrected with adequate amounts of vitamin D, although in this case, you'll need up to 100,000 IU a day for about a week, which is a very high amount that should only be administered under a doctor's care. "This deep bone pain disappears within a few weeks when people are getting the vitamin D they need," Dr. Gloth says.

Most sun-deprived older people need supplements to get the 400 to 800 IU of vitamin D they need. Dr. Gloth has also found that mild vitamin D deficiency can cause intense muscle pain with minimal pressure and that this pain disappears when vitamin D levels get back to normal. "This is something to consider if someone hurts badly in their muscles when they are rolled over in bed," he says.

Bone up on calcium. Calcium helps hormones and bone-strengthening drugs work better, and in people age 65 or older, it plays a crucial role in the maintenance of bone mass, says Roberta Bourgon, N.D., a naturopathic physician at the Wellness Center in Billings, Montana. Aim for

1,000 to 1,500 milligrams a day from foods and supplements. Take calcium supplements in divided doses between meals with vitamin D. And take your last supplement of the day near bedtime, she says. This helps to keep blood levels of calcium high at night, when your parathyroid gland "samples" the blood and decides how much hormone to secrete. So it helps keep the gland from breaking down bone at night.

Pay close attention to other nutrients. Other nutrients besides calcium and vitamin D play important, often unappreciated roles in bone health, Dr. Bourgon says. For instance, vitamin K is needed for the first phase of bone production. Vitamin C is needed to form and strengthen the structural proteins found in bone. Trace minerals such as copper, zinc, manganese, magnesium, and silicon also play vital roles in the production of bone. You're assured of getting a good array of these nutrients by eating a varied diet that includes whole grains and lots of fruits, vegetables, seeds, and nuts.

Keep moving. Bone actually benefits from being slightly stressed, Dr. Gloth says. The stress induces the bone tissue to lay down more bone. You can stress your bones a number of ways. Weight-bearing exercise such as walking maintains bone. Of course, if you're a jogger, continue what you're doing. Same with strength training or weight lifting, if you can manage it.

Dr. Siris notes, however, that the more strenuous activities are geared for prevention. If you've already had fractures, you should consider walking or water activities.

"I tell people that the best exercise for them is something they like and will do," she says. For older people, walking may be the best option. Water workouts can also help since the water itself provides resistance that your muscles need to work against.

Tai chi, a Chinese form of martial art used for exercise, is a good choice for people concerned about osteoporosis, because its gentle, slow movements improve balance and increase muscle mass, Dr. Bourgon says. Yoga can also produce some of the same benefits. Exercise also guards against falls, because you have enough muscle to regain your balance.

Pain Preventers

Wear sensible shoes. Topple off a high heel, and you could have a broken ankle, wrist, even hip. It's not worth it, Dr. Siris says. You're best off with flat, well-cushioned shoes that provide traction outdoors but that don't "grab" the carpet inside.

"Un-booby-trap" the house. Don't use throw rugs unless they have skid-proof backings. Install a grab bar in the bathroom. Get hard-to-open windows fixed so that you don't fracture bones yanking them open. Install good lighting at stairs and walkways, inside and outside your home.

Travel with care. Airports seem out to get people with osteoporosis, Dr. Siris says. "This is the time to request a wheelchair, get help with your luggage, and watch where you walk," she says. Some of her patients have broken bones tripping over luggage; others have toppled over while negotiating the "gangplank" to the plane.

Move with prudence. The same basic moves that help prevent back injuries can safeguard people with osteoporosis, Dr. Siris says. Always bend at your knees, not your waist. When you're carrying things, keep them close to your body. Try not to twist and lift at the same time. If you think some object may be too heavy for you to lift, don't even attempt it. Get help.

Prostate Pain

Men usually get prostate pain from infection, inflammation, and trauma. The pain usually occurs in the lower back, pelvis, and perineum, the area between the anus and the scrotum. Just think of the area as the place on which you sit.

The conditions that cause prostate pain are acute and chronic prostatitis (inflammation of the prostate), noninfectious prostatitis, and prostatodynia—a word that simply means "pain in the prostate." Strangely enough, prostate cancer rarely causes pain, nor does benign prostatic hyperplasia (noncancerous enlargement of the prostate).

Acute prostatitis comes on as a gnawing, aching pain in your back and rectal area. The prostate is swollen. You may have a frequent, urgent need to urinate, but a weak urine stream when you do go. You also may be fatigued because your body is trying to fight off the infection, says Willard DeBraber, D.O., a urologist in Muskegon, Michigan. If you have these complaints, you'll need to see a doctor for evaluation and possible antibiotics.

Chronic prostatitis is much more subtle and intermittent. The pain is more of a discomfort or tenderness in the perineum. The pain may flare up and then disappear for a time, only to recur soon after.

Some causes of prostatitis are unknown or unidentified, although acute and chronic forms are often caused by a bacterial infection due to backup of urine in the prostate ducts. Meanwhile, noninfectious prostatitis is mysterious in that bacteria are not detectable in urine or prostate fluid, but the body is producing infection-fighting cells as it does with other forms of prostatitis. This form of prostatitis causes the same type of pain as in acute or chronic types.

In any case, you should see your doctor, who will likely order up some antibiotics to treat the problem. If the medication does not relieve the symptoms of noninfectious prostatitis, he will suggest other treatment.

Prostatodynia has similar symptoms to prostatitis but without evidence that anything is physically wrong, says Dr. DeBraber. "It's like a pain in the neck. It probably has to do a lot with muscle tension, spasms, and stress. Things are just really tight down there, and it hurts. You probably also have problems with urination." Urologists may use alpha-blockers—prescribed oral medication—to relax the muscles in and around the prostate, which will reduce difficulty in urination associated with prostatodynia.

After you get a diagnosis and any necessary medication, there are also nonprescription things that you can do yourself to pacify a painful prostate.

For Fast Relief

Take a warm bath. When it hurts where you sit, then where you need to sit is in a tub of warm (but not hot) water for about 20 minutes. These warm sitz baths, as they are known, relax muscles, increase circulation, and generally relieve some of the discomfort, says Jean Fourcroy, M.D., Ph.D., a urologist in Bethesda, Maryland. "Heat and sitz baths are simple ways to relieve pain down there. I would recommend doing them as needed."

For Lasting Relief

Have sex. About half the fluid in semen is contributed by the prostate. When you ejaculate by masturbating or having sex, you clean out the ducts of the prostate and remove fluid containing the infection, says Dr. DeBraber. Therefore, he recommends ejaculating two or three times per week.

"I tell guys, 'Hey, make sure you keep those tubes cleaned out,'" he says. "Some say, 'That sounds fine. Talk to my wife.'"

Avoid trouble foods. Hot and spicy foods as well as alcohol and caffeine seem to exacerbate prostate pain, especially if there's inflammation involved. The reason may be that the nerves in that area are just more sensitive or that spicy foods cause abdominal gas and bloating, says Dr. Fourcroy. "We really don't know why, but avoiding these foods and drinks do seem to help."

Intermittent prostate pain also may be caused by allergic reactions to what you're eating or drinking, says Dr. DeBraber. After a heavy meal and a few beers, some guys have an aching, tender prostate and perhaps a problem with urination.

"Allergic prostatitis isn't that common, but it does happen to some guys," says Dr. DeBraber. "You should pay attention to cause and effect. If you eat or drink something and then you feel pain down there, don't consume it."

Get stress relief. When Dr. De-Braber diagnoses prostatodynia, one of the first things that crosses his mind is mental stress. Some guys under stress experience prostate and perineal pain. It may be because of muscle tightness and spasms, which can be relieved by alpha-blockers, warm baths, and stress management.

"I'll examine these guys and then ask them, 'Are you under a lot of stress?' And they'll say, 'Yeah, doc. How did you know?'" he recalls. "I'm urologist, not a psychologist, but I tell these patients to find a way to deal with the stress. 'Take a vacation. Talk with a counselor. Find a way to deal with the stress.'"

PAIN PREVENTERS

Relax when you relieve yourself. Forcing yourself to urinate quickly is a good way to set yourself up for prostate infections and inflammation, says Dr. Fourcroy. When you urinate, you have to contract your bladder and relax your urethra in synchrony. But when you're in a hurry, you may not properly relax your urethra. Your bladder contracts, and some urine gets pushed up into the little ducts of your prostate.

"When you do that, you have a sputtering of urine rather than a stream coming out," says Dr. Fourcroy. The advice here, then, is to simply take your time.

"Relax and enjoy it," she says. "You don't want to force urine out. Nor do you want to suddenly shut off the flow because you're in a hurry."

Drink lots of water. It never hurts to drink a lot of water when you're dealing with any kind of infection of the urinary tract. Water dilutes the urine and makes it less acidic and salty, say Dr. DeBraber. "Water keeps everything flowing down there, and that's good."

Shingles and Nerve Pain

Your grandchildren may never have to worry about shingles.

Like smallpox, this nasty viral vestige of the childhood disease chickenpox is almost certainly destined for history's dustbin.

"Historically, shingles may well be known as a disease of the twentieth century. The children who are being vaccinated for chickenpox now won't ever get it or perhaps even know much about it," says Seth Waldman, M.D., chief of pain medicine at the Hospital for Special Surgery in New York City.

But for those of us born decades before the advent of the vaccine, who endured chickenpox as an obligatory rite of passage, shingles remains a threat. Considered to be one of the most tenacious sources of pain known to man, shingles affects about one in five adults, most commonly after the age of 50, and the risk of developing it increases with age. In fact, researchers at Harvard Medical School found that people over age 64 are six times more likely to develop shingles than those younger than 25. Up to half of all Americans over age 80 can expect to have at least one outbreak.

A Pox upon You

Shingles and chickenpox, as you probably know, are caused by the same virus. When you got chickenpox as a child, your immune system was able to destroy most but not all of the virus. So although you recovered, some of the virus was

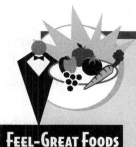

SIZZLING SPICE STIFLES SHINGLES STING

A diet rich in cayenne pepper—a spicy red pepper—may help speed pain relief when you have shingles, says Allan Magaziner, D.O., a nutritional-medicine specialist in Cherry Hill, New Jersey, and author of *The Complete Idiot's Guide to Living Longer and Healthier*. In fact, capsaicin, an extract from cayenne, is an active ingredient in over-the-counter lotions, such as Capzasin-P, that are used to treat shingles pain.

Cayenne pepper enriches the flavor of many dishes. On a typical day, for instance, you could sprinkle it on scrambled eggs for breakfast, mix it into soup and a tuna sandwich for lunch, and for dinner, marinate a pork chop in a sauce made with cayenne, wine, vinegar, paprika, and crushed garlic.

still hiding in your body's nerve cells. Decades later, certain factors—doctors suspect that stress, illness, and weakened immunity all have roles—triggers the long-dormant virus to reactivate and travel along the nerve fibers that extend to your skin. As the virus moves along these fibers, it can cause pain, tingling, or numbness.

When the virus reaches the skin, it causes a rash and blisters, known as shingles. The rash and blisters usually appear on the chest or back. But shingles also can pop up on your face, around an eye, down an arm or leg, or even inside your mouth. The rash and blisters almost always occur on just one side of the body. Symptoms resembling the flu, such as headache, nausea, and fever, commonly accompany an outbreak.

POST-POX PAIN

Usually, shingles and its accompanying pain disappear within a month. But in some cases, the pain lingers on long after the rash has faded. This manifestation of shingles, known as postherpetic neuralgia (PHN), is caused when nerve fibers in the infected area are damaged, says Sota Omoigui, M.D., medical director of the L.A. Pain Clinic in Hawthorne, California. A few people, for instance, develop extreme skin sensitivity to the point that clothing or even a slight change in temperature can trigger sharp, jabbing, or burning pain. PHN pain is often difficult to relieve or forecast.

"It can be a frustrating problem for both doctor and patient. This is one of the most difficult medical problems around. No one can predict whether a person with this problem is going to be better in 2 months or 2 years," says Jose Angel, M.D., director of the pain-management center at the University of Colorado Health Sciences Center in Denver.

Prescription drugs such as antidepressants and anticonvulsants are commonly prescribed to ease the pain of shingles and PHN, Dr. Angel says. But the best way to prevent prolonged pain from shingles is early treatment with antiviral drugs, such as acyclovir (Zovirax), which block reproduction of the virus and minimize nerve damage. Contact your doctor immediately if you develop a rash or an unexplainable burning, localized pain.

But even antiviral medications probably won't suppress all of the pain caused by shingles, Dr. Angel says. If you're suffering from shingle and nerve pain, these ideas may help.

For Fast Relief

Soak up the pain. Twice a day, apply a compress made with the astringent solution Domeboro and cool water to your shingles outbreak, Dr. Omoigui suggests. As it evaporates, the compress dries out the rash and draws pain-producing hormones known as prostaglandins out of the fluid inside the blisters. Follow the instructions on the package.

For Lasting Relief

Be a wort hog. St. John's wort, an herbal remedy, can help dampen nerve pain caused by shingles, Dr. Omoigui says. The herb also has antiviral properties that can lessen the severity of the disease. At the

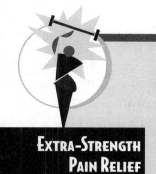

VITAMIN INJECTIONS SHORTEN SHINGLES DISCOMFORT

Injections of the B vitamins thiamin and B_{12} are the fastest and easiest way to get rid of acute shingles, says Allan Magaziner, D.O., a nutritional-medicine specialist in Cherry Hill, New Jersey, and author of *The Complete Idiot's Guide to Living Longer and Healthier*. These vitamins help soothe the inflamed nerves that are affected by the disease.

Although thiamin and vitamin B_{12} are found in many foods, including grains like oats, barley, and whole-grain cereals, injections are necessary in order to get adequate doses of these vitamins into your body quickly. Once they are in your system, these B vitamins can lead the charge to fend off shingles and its accompanying pain. When you are diagnosed, ask your doctor if this approach is appropriate for you, Dr. Magaziner suggests.

first sign of outbreak, he recommends that you begin taking 200 to 300 milligrams of St. John's wort two or three times daily until the pain is gone.

Reach for supplemental relief. Vitamin and mineral supplements can help control shingles and may stem its pain, says David Edelberg, M.D., founder of the American Whole Health Center in Chicago. He suggests taking 2,000 milligrams of vitamin C twice a day, 400 IU of vitamin E twice a day, and 1,000 milligrams of citrus bioflavonoids twice a day until the shingles outbreak is gone. Citrus bioflavonoids are available in most health food stores. If taking this much vitamin C gives you diarrhea, reduce the dosage.

Let like cure like. A small homeopathic dose of Herpes Zoster, the virus that causes shingles, can bolster your immune system, prevent lingering pain, and reduce the recurrence of the disease, says Cynthia Mervis Watson, M.D., a family-practice physician in Santa Monica, California, who specializes in herbal therapy and homeopathy. Take a 30X dose once or twice a day until the pain disappears. Be aware that it may take several days for this remedy to take effect, so don't give up on it just because it doesn't provide immediate relief. Herpes Zoster is available by prescription through a homeopathic physician.

Clutch an olive branch. Olive leaf extract is a powerful antiviral that can halt the progression of shingles and alleviate pain, Dr. Watson says. Begin taking 500 milligrams three times a day as soon as possible after you are diagnosed and until the shingles outbreak is gone. Like vitamins and minerals, olive leaf extract helps your immune system pounce on the virus early, diminishing both the rash and your

discomfort. Olive leaf extract is available at most health food stores.

Chill out your mind. A double dose of imagery can have a profound effect on shingles pain, says Dennis Gersten, M.D., a psychiatrist and medical director of the Gersten Institute for Higher Medicine in Cardiff-by-the-Sea, California, and author of *Are You Getting Enlightened or Losing Your Mind?* Whenever you feel the pain intensifying, take a couple of deep breaths and do this two-part imagery sequence.

First, imagine that you are holding a ball of mercury (the silvery liquid found in thermometers) in your hands that can draw pain out of your body like a magnet. Then, imagine that the pain caused by shingles is being gobbled up by this ball. Let the ball, which is now full of pain, pour out of your fingertips, and watch it roll out of sight.

Once you've done that, picture yourself in a wintry, extremely cold spot, like Norway or the North Pole. All of your body is covered with clothing except for the area affected by shingles. As the −60°F cold penetrates the exposed rash, imagine that it begins to kill off the virus causing the outbreak and eradicates your pain. Do this imagery sequence for 1 minute, as needed, Dr. Gersten says.

Unwind. Yoga can help relieve stress and anxiety that you may be feeling when you have shingles, and it can have a profound effect on your pain levels, says Judith Lasater, P.T., Ph.D., a physical therapist in San Francisco and author of *Relax and Renew*.

"Yoga lowers your blood pressure, improves circulation, improves immune function, and relieves muscle tension. All of those things are going to help you feel less pain and help you deal with pain better when you do feel it," she says.

As soon as you find out you have shingles, begin practicing the following basic relaxation pose for 20 minutes daily, she says. This pose also can be used to relieve cancer pain and surgical pain.

Sit on the floor. Turn to one side and lean on your elbow and forearm as you slide onto your side. Then, roll onto your back and lie with your arms out to your sides and your legs comfortably spread. (If you have difficulty lowering yourself to the floor, try leaning on a stable chair or another piece of furniture for support, Dr. Lasater suggests. You also can do this position on your bed, sofa, or reclining chair.) Rest your head and knees on a couple of rolled-up towels or blankets. Once you're in a comfortable position, cover your eyes with an eye bag, cloth, or other covering.

Swallow, and relax your jaw. Let your cheeks feel hollow and loose. Relax your tongue. Allow your fingers to curl naturally as you relax your hands with your palms facing up. Let your legs roll outward. Allow the entire back of your body to feel at ease and in complete contact with the floor.

Imagine that your arms and legs are getting longer and heavier. Picture the large muscles of your legs, buttocks, and trunk dropping away from the bones. Then, imagine the smaller muscles of your arms, neck, and head moving away from the bones. Let the bones themselves feel heavy and the skin loose all over your body. Notice that the abdominal organs seem to nestle gently back into your body. Savor the silence, she suggests.

When you're ready, take a long, slow, gentle inhalation through your nose, then slowly, gently exhale through your mouth. Make sure that you feel your belly rise as you inhale to ensure that you're breathing with your diaphragm. Breathe normally for two or three breaths, then take another deep breath. Feel your diaphragm, lungs, ribs, and the muscles of respiration contracting to squeeze the breath out in a steady stream. Repeat the cycle of two or three normal breaths followed by a deep one.

Do a total of 30 complete in-out breaths before coming out of your pose, Dr. Lasater suggests. Sit up and take several breaths before standing up and resuming your normal activities.

Rub it out. If pain persists after the rash disappears, try rubbing an over-the-counter capsaicin lotion, such as Capzasin-P, on the affected area, Dr. Angel says. Capsaicin, an extract from spicy red peppers, is a natural analgesic that usually begins soothing shingles pain within 2 to 4 weeks.

But to be effective, the rash must be completely healed and the recommended regimen—applying the lotion three or four times daily—must be followed zealously. Otherwise, the pain may recur, sometimes within days.

Capsaicin can cause a burning sensation on the skin and can irritate the eyes. So wear rubber gloves when applying the ointment, and be sure to wash your hands thoroughly after use, Dr. Omoigui urges.

Sinusitis

Nicholas Villarruel came down with a very sudden and *very* unusual sinus ailment one July day. According to news accounts, he was working in a Denver factory that produces triggers that make automobile air bags inflate, when a machine blew up, shooting a small explosive trigger up into his sinus.

Fortunately, a surgeon—with bomb-squad personnel on hand—was able to carefully remove the device without setting off an explosion, which almost certainly would have made Villarruel's bad day even worse.

Though the sinus problems we encounter are rarely so dramatic, they can range in severity from an uncomfortable nuisance to a serious health threat. When your sinuses are working smoothly, they may play several roles in keeping you comfortable, though their exact job is still unclear.

Doctors think that these air-filled pockets behind your face give resonance to your voice and reduce the weight of your skull as well as provide a filter to catch dust and other airborne irritants. Normally, tiny hairs called cilia sweep a constant flow of mucus from your sinuses into your nasal passage through a drainage hole as narrow as a pencil lead. This sticky fluid traps pollutants in your nasal passage, then is harmlessly swallowed and digested in your stomach.

This process grinds to a halt, however, when the lining of your sinus or nasal passage becomes inflamed and cuts off the flow of mucus and air, which is a condition called sinusitis. Commonly, a viral infection, such as the flu or a common cold,

Name That Sinus Pain

Sinus pain or headache may vary in its location, depending on which sinus cavity or group of sinuses is involved.

Ethmoid sinus pain usually develops between 4:00 and 6:00 A.M., or as soon as you awaken in the morning, and usually disappears several hours later only to return at about the same time the next morning. It may occasionally return in the evening for several hours as well.

Ethmoid headache or pain is usually around your eyes, in your forehead, behind an eye, or between your eyes. Pain or tenderness to palpation or finger pressure may sometimes be noted at the inner side of your eye or at the base of your nose where it joins your cheek or brow.

Frontal sinus pain or headache is somewhat similar to ethmoid pain, but usually more intense. It begins midmorning, usually around 10:00 A.M., increases toward the middle of the day, and nearly always disappears by midafternoon.

Maxillary sinus pain or headache is mostly in your cheeks and is sometimes accompanied by discomfort in a nearby upper tooth. It may also occur in your nose where it joins your cheek or in your temple area, your eye, your ear, your jaw, or the back of your head on the same side as the affected sinus. Walking down steps or stepping off a curb may occasion-

triggers it. Other causes include allergies, air pollution, and changes in air pressure from a coming storm or an airplane ride. The result is the same: Your sinuses get blocked and become a breeding ground for infection and pain.

"It's very simple—if there's a plug in the hole, the sinus won't drain, and that can cause pain to occur," says Wellington Tichenor, M.D., a New York City internist and allergist specializing in the treatment of sinusitis.

ally cause cheek discomfort and sometimes a sensation of fluid or pus moving around within the cheek sinus.

Sphenoid sinus headache may refer pain to the top, sides, or back of your head and frequently behind an eye. The pain feels worse during midday or early afternoon.

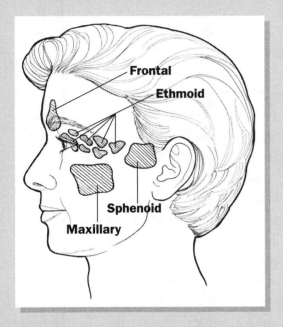

Sinus cavities are located around the eyes and cheeks as shown here.

Chronic sinusitis affects 30 million to 40 million Americans. An even greater number may experience acute or subacute sinus infections each year, but fortunately, older people appear to be less susceptible, says Lee Williams, M.D., associate pro-fessor of otolaryngology at Johns Hopkins University and author of *The Sinusitis Help Book.*

Depending on which sinus is affected and the nature of its involvement, you might feel a headache well away from the problem area, or sometimes localized pain and tenderness to finger pressure directly over the sinus itself, Dr. Williams says. Sinus pain may occasionally radiate to an eye, an ear, or an upper tooth.

Sinusitis can be acute, with symptoms such as pain, nasal congestion, fever, and thick drainage from your nose over the course of 2 to 8 weeks. Chronic sinusitis, with many of the same symptoms as well as sore throat, malaise, and poor sense of smell, can linger on for months.

Since the sinuses are crowded tightly near your eyes and brain, it's important to control infection in that area before it spreads. See a doctor if you notice swelling around your eye, greenish mucus from your nose, or pain that lasts for more than 14 days after a cold starts. You may need antibiotics and other prescription drugs to clear up your sinuses, or even surgery if your problems are severe enough.

There are also a number of ways to ease sinus pain in your own home with simple remedies.

For Fast Relief

Flush them out. Doctors commonly recommend that you rinse out your nasal passages with salt water to clear out debris and infection when you have sinusitis and to help the area stay healthy the rest of the time.

"It's a very good home cure—I have literally thousands of patients doing it," says Michael Kaliner, M.D., medical director of the Institute for Asthma and Allergy in Washington, D.C. "Most patients believe when they start doing it that this is something they should have been doing all their lives."

Mix up a solution of ¼ teaspoon of salt and ¼ teaspoon of baking soda in 8 ounces of warm water (or you could use bottled water and noniodized salt, along with a pinch of baking soda).

Bend forward, with your head over the sink. With a bulb syringe, available at drugstores, squirt this solution up one nostril, then the other, until all 8 ounces have been used. It may leak out your other nostril or down the back of your throat (if it does, just spit it out), but "the critical thing is that it goes in the nose and comes out someplace," Dr. Kaliner says. You should do this twice a day, once in the morning and once at night, during a bout of sinusitis. As a preventive measure, do this once or twice a day. Be sure to clean out the bulb with water after each use.

Alternatively, you can pump a saline spray, also available at drugstores, up into your nose, he adds.

For Lasting Relief

Make it like a sauna in there. Another way to clean out your nasal passages is to breathe steam through your nose, Dr. Kaliner says.

There are several ways to get your sinuses steaming. An inexpensive method is to boil a pot of water, take it off the stove, and inhale the steam through your nose, he says. Make sure that you approach the rising steam cautiously, however, and don't let it scald you.

Other ways to breathe in steam are to lean over a facial sauna device or simply take a hot, steamy shower.

Don't get dried out. To keep your sinuses draining well, don't allow yourself to get dehydrated. Make certain that you drink plenty of fluids—6 to 8 full glasses a day, Dr. Williams says. This will help the mucous membranes lining your sinuses and nasal passages to stay moist, which in turn will make them more resistant to infection and sinus flare-ups.

Try a souper remedy. According to Dr. Tichenor, Mom may have been on to something when she ladled out bowls of hot chicken soup to treat your childhood colds. There is some evidence that it can help move mucus in your sinuses better than an ordinary hot fluid, though it's unclear how it works. So go ahead and make yourself a bowl when you're hungry.

Towel off. Another way to improve sinus drainage, which may also reduce your pain, is to apply warm, moist heat to your face, Dr. Williams says.

For example, soak a damp washcloth or folded towel in hot water from the spigot, wring it out, then lay it over your nose, face, and cheeks. Make certain that the washcloth isn't hot enough to burn you. Reapply as soon as it begins to cool, and continue doing this for 5 to 10 minutes several times a day. Lying down with a dry towel over your face after the procedure keeps the area from cooling off too rapidly.

Don't take pain lying down. Sleeping elevated on a 7-inch-high sleeping wedge with a pillow on top of that will improve drainage and limit swelling in your sinuses, thereby reducing pain, Dr. Williams says. These wedges are available in some medical supply and department store catalogs, and most drugstores will order one for you.

It's better to lie on your "good side," with your affected sinus "up" in order to reduce swelling and improve its drainage, he says.

Make Pressure Work for You

You may hold the solution to your sinus troubles in your own fingertips.

Patrick LaRiccia, M.D., a physician and registered acupuncturist who works as director of the Acupuncture Pain Clinic at Presbyterian Medical Center of Philadelphia, says that you can use acupressure techniques at home to treat your sinusitis pain. This remedy simply requires that you prod particular points on your body with your fingers.

Most acupressure points occur in symmetrical pairs—that is, one point is on the left side of your body, and the other is in the same location on the right side of your body. Both points in a pair should be pressed simultaneously when possible. Working both sides this way balances your body and increases acupressure's effectiveness.

For sinus relief, press down with the pads of your fingertips for about a minute each on points ST2, ST3, GB14, and LI20 (see illustration). Use firm pressure, but not so much that it hurts, Dr. LaRiccia says. You can also use a similar pressure on LI4 and LI11 on your hands and arms, and ST36 on your leg.

You can use these acupressure techniques three or four times a day, as necessary, Dr. LaRiccia says.

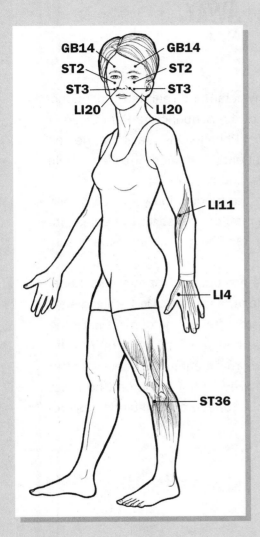

GB14 GB14
ST2 ST2
ST3 ST3
LI20 LI20
LI11
LI4
ST36

Pressing the acupressure points shown here may help you reduce sinus pain. According to acupressure specialists, these points are connected to energy channels, or meridians, that flow from the major organs. In this illustration, GB stands for the Gallbladder meridian, LI represents the Large Intestine meridian, and ST stands for the Stomach meridian.

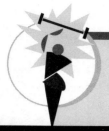

POKE THE PROBLEM AWAY

Patrick LaRiccia, M.D., a physician and registered acupuncturist who works as director of the Acupuncture Pain Clinic at Presbyterian Medical Center of Philadelphia, says that he has used acupuncture to cure patients' allergies or at least help them manage them with less medication.

When used in addition to the medication your doctor prescribes, this ancient Oriental method of inserting needles into specific parts of the body can also help you handle a sinus infection easier, he says.

To treat sinus problems, the acupuncturist may insert needles into the patient's face, legs, and arms. Dr. LaRiccia says that while all acupuncturists are different, he doesn't stick the needles in very deeply, just a couple of millimeters into the skin. Patients should notice improvement in their sinuses after a few acupuncture sessions or even that same day, he says. Even if you feel better, continue to take any antibiotics as prescribed by your doctor.

PAIN PREVENTERS

Inflate your sinuses. Some people may experience sinus pain and ear discomfort at high altitudes, including when flying and especially when descending in a plane. This happens particularly if they have chronic sinus blockage or chronic Eustachian tube blockage. In such instances, inflating your ears and sinuses repeatedly during flight will prevent a partial vacuum in your ears or sinuses and possibly save you considerable discomfort.

To ward off this pain, Dr. Williams recommends that you do the following exercise. Three times a minute during takeoff and ascent, close your mouth, pinch your nostrils shut, and swallow. Then, immediately force air into your sinuses and ears by blowing your nose with your nostrils still pinched shut. If you blow immediately after you swallow, you don't have to blow hard to fill those cavities with air. A loud squeaking sound means that things were badly blocked, making it even more important to keep doing it.

After the plane levels off, do this three times an hour during the entire flight until you start descending. Then, once again start puffing air up into your ears, nose, and sinuses three times a minute once you start your descent to land. Continue to do this until you land and for a while afterward if your ears or sinuses still feel blocked. You should not do this with a fresh cold, nor should you fly with a cold. If you do this procedure with a fresh cold, you could force infection into your ears or deeper into your sinuses.

Surgical Pain

God only knows how many ways doctors have tried to eradicate surgical pain. For thousands of years, the best they could offer was a glass of wine, a sip of brandy, or a bit of opium. Then in the 1840s, a few bold physicians began successfully anesthetizing their surgical patients.

"We Have Conquered Pain," one London newspaper called this breakthrough. And thanks to it, these days most of us take it for granted that we won't feel pain *during* surgery. But postoperative pain remains defiant, challenging doctors and intimidating many of the more than seven million Americans over age 65 who undergo invasive procedures each year.

"Most people, particularly those who are older, equate surgery with pain," says Sota Omoigui, M.D., medical director of the L.A. Pain Clinic in Hawthorne, California. "And probably with good reason, since up until a few years ago most people in the hospital were undermedicated for pain."

Substantial improvements in anesthesia, surgical techniques, and pain medications have sharply whittled down the number of older Americans who experience moderate to severe discomfort following surgery, says Seth Waldman, M.D., chief of pain medicine at the Hospital for Special Surgery in New York City. But there also are plenty of things that you can do for yourself before and after your operation to derail discomfort.

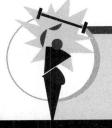

TOUCH TAMES SURGICAL PAIN

Healing touch therapies such as Therapeutic Touch or Reiki—an Asian technique that involves the channeling of healing energies through hand placements—are powerful ways to promote relaxation and enhance recovery, says Andrew T. Weil, M.D., director of the program in integrative medicine at the University of Arizona College of Medicine in Tucson and author of *Spontaneous Healing* and *8 Weeks to Optimum Health*. In fact, a number of studies have documented Therapeutic Touch's ability to relieve pain, boost immunity, and speed healing of surgical wounds.

"I would encourage trying at least one session of these noninvasive therapies," he says. "If you can, schedule a daily treatment for 2 to 3 days before and after your operation."

Some hospitals offer these treatments. But in other instances, you may have to locate an independent practitioner.

BEFORE SURGERY: BE PREPARED

A growing body of research suggests that patients who take active roles in preparing for surgery experience faster healing, reduced postoperative pain, less need for medication, and shorter hospital stays, says Andrew T. Weil, M.D., director of the program in integrative medicine at the University of Arizona College of Medicine in Tucson and author of *Spontaneous Healing* and *8 Weeks to Optimum Health*. Here are a few ways you can prepare for surgery that may lessen your pain afterward.

For Fast Relief

Listen to positive vibes. Ask your surgeon if you can listen to an audiotape of positive affirmations during the operation, Dr. Weil suggests.

A growing number of health professionals, including Dr. Weil, believe that even under anesthesia, people can hear what is going on around them and are in a highly suggestible state of consciousness.

A number of studies support this idea, including one at Beth Israel Medical Center in New York City that shows that patients who heard positive affirmations on tape while they were under anesthesia required 50 percent less postoperative medication than a control group.

Steven Fahrion, Ph.D., director of research at the Life Sciences Institute of Mind-Body Health in Topeka, Kansas, another proponent of this technique, says the results have startled many of his colleagues. "We've had several surgeons literally say, 'I've never seen one of my patients recover this well.' So we've come to believe in the use of positive-affirmation tapes before, during, and even after surgery," he says.

Several companies produce positive-affirmation audiotapes for use during hospital stays, including the Audio Prescriptives Foundation, 70 Maple Avenue, Katonah, NY 10536-3721; and Interstate Industries, P.O. Box 505, Lovingston, VA 22949-0505.

You also can record a custom tape yourself, Dr. Fahrion says. The statements should be positive. They should describe what you want to happen or how you want to feel after the surgery. You might, for instance, record phrases such as "I am pain-free," "I feel relaxed," "I feel good," or "After this operation, I will feel comfortable and will heal very quickly."

If you are given permission to do this, make sure that you have an autoreverse cassette player with earphones so you'll be able to continuously listen to the affirmations during the operation without disturbing the surgical team, Dr. Weil urges.

For Lasting Relief

Know what to expect. Before your operation, ask your surgeon or anesthesiologist for videotapes, pamphlets, and other materials that explain what to expect before, during, and after surgery. In particular, ask about the pain you might anticipate feeling as you recover, suggests Heike Mahler, Ph.D., a psychologist at the University of California, San Diego.

UNDER THE KNIFE

More than seven million Americans over age 65 undergo surgery each year. Here's a look at the five most common surgical procedures done on older men and women. How much pain you may feel following one of these procedures depends on several factors, including the severity of your condition before your operation, the extent of your surgery, and your self-help strategies.

MEN

- Prostate removal
- Cardiac catheterization
- Heart bypass
- Pacemaker insertion or replacement
- Biopsy of the digestive tract

WOMEN

- Cardiac catheterization
- Surgery to correct bone fracture
- Joint and hip replacement
- Biopsy of the digestive tract
- Pacemaker insertion or replacement

"People who are well-informed about the sensations to expect after surgery may interpret the process as less threatening. As a result, it doesn't feel as bad. It isn't perceived as being as painful," Dr. Mahler says.

Take Arnica before and after. If possible, begin taking Arnica 30C three times a day a couple of days prior to your surgery, suggests says Cynthia Mervis Watson, M.D., a family-practice physician in Santa Monica, California, who specializes in herbal therapy and homeopathy. Arnica, a homeopathic remedy, will help reduce swelling and soreness after your operation. To accelerate your healing, take one 200C dose of Arnica as soon as possible after surgery. Arnica is available at many health food stores.

Head it off at the pass. A posse of herbal remedies can corral surgical pain, says John Catanzaro, N.D., a naturopathic physician specializing in pain management and director of the Health and Wellness Institute in Seattle. If possible, 2 to 3 days before your operation, begin taking the following herbs three or four times daily: 200 milligrams of frankincense, 100 milligrams of devil's claw, and 100 milligrams of prickly ash. In addition, take 1,500 milligrams of glucosamine sulfate, an amino acid that may be a potent pain reliever, once a day. Also take 1,000 milligrams of the mineral supplement methylsulfonylmethane (MSM) two times a day starting at least 2 weeks before surgery. This combination, which also can be used after surgery for as long as pain persists, has analgesic effects that dull pain, speed healing, and reduce swelling, says Dr. Catanzaro. Glucosa-

mine and these herbs and supplements are sold in most health food stores and many drugstores.

Picture a happy ending. Guided imagery has proved especially useful for those facing surgery, Dr. Weil says. In a study involving 130 colorectal surgery patients at the Cleveland Clinic, those who listened to guided-imagery tapes for 3 days prior to and 6 days after surgery described their pain to be half as severe, used 37 percent less pain medication, and were released from the hospital almost 2 days sooner.

"My experience with this mind/body approach has convinced me that no physical ailment is beyond its reach," Dr. Weil says. "I would advise anyone who is preparing for surgery to practice guided imagery regularly."

The night before your operation, imagine getting ready for your surgery. Picture being given medicine to relax you. Then imagine going into the operating room, where a skilled surgeon, an anesthesiologist, and highly trained nurses are waiting for you. Picture yourself peacefully falling asleep as the general anesthetic is given to you, says Dennis Gersten, M.D., a psychiatrist and medical director of the Gersten Institute for Higher Medicine in Cardiff-by-the-Sea, California, and author of *Are You Getting Enlightened or Losing Your Mind?* Then, imagine your surgery proceeding remarkably well. There is little bleeding, and you are sewn back up without any problems. The operation is a great success. Finally, take a moment to picture yourself in the recovery room, slowly becoming more alert. You may feel some discomfort, but you are relaxed and able to cope with it quite easily.

Repeat this imagery on the day of your surgery 30 minutes before you leave your room for the operation, Dr. Gersten suggests. This should be followed by 30 minutes of focusing just on your breathing.

Take hands-on control. Thermal biofeedback, a simplified and literally hands-on version of a high-tech stress-reduction method, can help alleviate surgical pain, Dr. Fahrion says. Developed at the Menninger Clinic in Topeka, it's based on the premise that when a person is under stress such as an impending surgery, the body restricts blood-flow to the extremities, decreasing their temperature to below the usual 98.6°F. But warming your hands with thermal biofeedback can quash the production of stress hormones, reduce muscle tension, and produce other physical changes that can diminish pain by at least 33 percent, he says.

The only things you'll need to get started are an oral thermometer and your hands. If possible, practice thermal biofeedback for about 10 minutes a day for about a week prior to your surgery, Dr. Fahrion suggests. It will help you familiarize yourself with the technique and help prepare your body for the upcoming stress of the operation. But even if you undergo an unexpected procedure, practicing thermal biofeedback after surgery can help dampen pain, he says.

Sit or lie in a comfortable position and wrap your hands around the thermometer. Rest your hands on your lap and focus your mind on any sensation that you feel in your fingers. Do you feel a tingling or pulsing in your fingertips? That's a signal that your hands are warming. It's okay to take an occasional glance at the thermometer, but don't strive to raise your hand temperature. That will occur naturally. If you get distracted, refocus your attention on your hands.

The goal is to raise your finger temperature to 97°F and hold it there for about 10 minutes. As you become more accustomed to the sensations in your hands, you should be able to do this technique without using the thermometer, Dr. Fahrion says. After surgery, you can use thermal biofeedback as needed to help you cope with anxiety and pain.

AFTER SURGERY: TAKE CHARGE

In most cases, anti-inflammatory medications and narcotics are indispensable al-

INNOVATIVE PROGRAM HELPS
NEW YORKER GLIDE THROUGH SURGERY

The night before his quadruple-bypass surgery, just about the time when most people would be asking for a sedative, Anthony Jablonski was getting a healthy dose of reflexology.

"It was soothing, it was calming," says the 74-year-old, recalling how a nurse used the ancient pressure-point technique to wilt his presurgery jitters. "It felt as if I were on a glider. I felt a swaying, swinging motion while she was rubbing my feet. It felt great."

Reflexology and other alternative treatments certainly aren't standard preoperative procedures at most hospitals, but maybe they should be, says Jery Whitworth, R.N., executive director of the department of Complementary Medical Services at Columbia-Presbyterian Medical Center in New York City, where Jablonski was treated.

lies in the days following surgery. So don't try to be a hero, Dr. Omoigui urges. Allowing your pain to creep up to an intolerable level isn't wise because you'll need more medication to relieve your discomfort. And the more medication you need,

the greater your risk of side effects like nausea and drowsiness. Plus, unrelieved surgical pain can make it difficult to sit up, walk, and do other daily activities that will speed your recovery.

So the best thing you can do to muzzle

"Even in the intensive-care unit, we have seen marked decrease in pain perception with just a 15-minute session of reflexology," she says. "Of course, that's just anecdotal evidence that needs further study. But to the average person, research doesn't matter. They just want relief."

Although most people are receptive to these therapies, some older participants cringe when techniques like yoga, reflexology, or meditation are mentioned, Whitworth says.

But Jablonski, a retired New York Transit Authority executive, dove into the program with few reservations. "I wasn't skeptical at all. I figured I didn't have anything to lose, but a lot to gain, so why not go through with it," he says.

In addition to reflexology, he listened to relaxation tapes before, during, and after his operation.

"I'd recommend this program to anybody because it calmed me down and helped me get through the whole procedure," he says. "Before I knew it, I was on my way home."

discomfort after an operation is to take your pain medication on a regular schedule as prescribed by your doctor, usually every 4 to 6 hours, Dr. Omoigui says. But there are also plenty of things you can do to help yourself. The following nondrug strategies can help reduce the dosage, limit the side effects, and, in some cases, prolong the effects of your pain medication after surgery. Don't take any herbal preparations or reduce your pain medication without checking with your doctor first.

For Fast Relief

Brighten your day. After surgery, whenever you feel uncomfortable, picture your pain as an ominous, black rain cloud. Then, imagine this cloud slowly dispersing wider and wider across the sky. Visualize it gradually losing its shape and changing colors from black to pink to white. Then, when you're ready, let this white cloud—and your pain—drift away. Allow yourself to marvel at the most beautiful, cloudless blue sky you've ever seen. Just doing this imagery for 30 seconds at a time can help ease your discomfort, Dr. Fahrion says.

For Lasting Relief

Let grapes stomp it. Grape seed extract, available at most health food stores, is a potent postoperative pain reliever, Dr. Omoigui says. The extract helps reduce swelling after surgery and blocks the formation of free radicals, rogue cells that slow healing and prolong pain. He suggests taking 50 to 100 milligrams daily while you're recovering.

Bet on bromelain. Bromelain, an enzyme extracted from pineapple, is another natural anti-inflammatory substance that can relieve pain after surgery, Dr. Omoigui says. He recommends taking 500 milk-clotting units (mcu) of the enzyme four times a day while recuperating. Bromelain is available at most health food stores.

Caution: Avoid taking bromelain before your operation since it is a blood thinner that can cause excessive bleeding during surgery.

Take the A train. DL-phenylalanine (DLPA), an amino acid, dampens pain by altering nerve signals to the brain, says Allan Magaziner, D.O., a nutritional-medicine specialist in Cherry Hill, New Jersey, and author of *The Complete Idiot's Guide to Living Longer and Healthier.* He suggests taking 1,000 milligrams twice daily after your surgery for as long as you have pain. DLPA capsules are available at many health food stores. Don't take DLPA without a doctor's guidance, however.

PART FOUR

Pain Makers—Everyday Aches

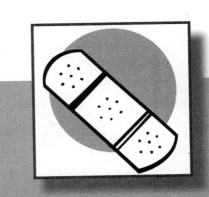

Soothing the Smallest Aches

Everyday pains tend to be what doctors call acute: They come on sudden and sharp, but they don't last very long. Touch a hot pan on the stove, and you get an acute everyday pain. Pretty mundane, as pain goes.

But you do a lot in a day, and those little aches and ouches can add up. And if you're already dealing with other types of pain—say, from arthritis—then the little pains get lumped in with the bigger pains, and before you know it, pain is dragging you down.

We think it's important to know how to control all types of pain, even the ordinary, everyday stuff. And that's what you'll find in this section—techniques for controlling or eliminating everyday aches and pains.

In these chapters, you'll find cures and advice you might never have considered before, drawing from disciplines your doctor may not know about. Of course, we're also recommending in this section that you follow your physician's advice in any kind of injury or illness that sends you to the doctor's office. Taking a medication for an infection or getting a few stitches to close a cut may be your first and best course of action to ease pain and accelerate healing. Yet a good home remedy may make recuperation that much easier.

Any ache—no matter how small—is still an ache. If it keeps you from paying attention to your grandchild or enjoying your food when you're going out to dinner with friends, it shouldn't be ignored. Everyday pains are much more than just nuisances when they interfere with living. This section is all about ways to clear up that interference.

Airplane Ear

For some people, fear of flying boils down to fear of flier's ear. Just about the time when the canned voice on the crackling speaker tells you to fasten your seat belt and make sure that your seat and tray table are upright and locked, a number of people who share your pressurized cabin are going to begin experiencing dreads of all kinds. Among those dreads is anticipation of ear pain.

If you're among those who experience this pain, you may have discovered that it takes more than a few good gulps or yawns to clear your ears. Sometimes, ear pain builds steadily as the flight descends. After deplaning, your ears may still be painful and clogged, and your hearing less than perfect. Sometimes, it can even take a day or two before the pain and clogged-up feeling clears out of your ears and you can breathe a sigh of relief . . . until the next plane flight.

What's the culprit here?

The primary source of this ear pain is a buildup of pressure in the middle-ear space (between your eardrum and inner ear) that is caused by a malfunctioning of the Eustachian tube, according to Jack A. Shohet, M.D., assistant clinical professor of neurotology and skull-base surgery at the University of California, Irvine. The Eustachian tube—named after the sixteenth-century Italian Eustachio, who first started probing this part of the ear—equalizes the pressure between the outside environment and the middle-ear space. It is somewhat straight, rather than winding, but it has a narrow opening that opens and closes every time you swallow or move your jaw in a certain way, according to Dr. Shohet.

This tube is not the tidiest of little passages. As long as it's carrying appropriate amounts of clear air or clean mucus, your Eustachian tube causes no problems. But if something blocks its tiny opening, like mucus or swelling from a cold or allergy, the air pressure can't be equalized between the outside environment and the middle-ear space, he says. When the pressure can't be equalized, it causes severe pain and can even result in a ruptured eardrum.

Ergo, the agony of airplane ear. When the plane descends and there is a quick altitude change, the pressure builds rapidly. Your Eustachian tubes start to groan under the pressure, and that complaint comes through loud and clear as ear pain.

You should avoid flying if you have a cold or allergies, Dr. Shohet cautions. The lining of your Eustachian tubes is probably swollen, and there is a greater risk for significant ear pain and even eardrum perforation, he says.

Knowing the cause won't tell you the cure. But here are a few tactical flight plans you can make to help hold off airplane ear before, during, and after takeoff and landing.

For Fast Relief

Try a "blow-pop." Any time you feel your ears begin to clog, there's a quick way to head off trouble. Take a breath, pinch your nostrils, close your mouth, then gently force your breath toward your ears, suggests James Reibel, M.D., assistant professor of otolaryngology at the University of Virginia Health Sciences Center in Charlottesville. If all goes well, you'll feel a slight tickling inside your ears, followed by a slight pop as the pressure is relieved. The gentle blowing can equalize pressure across your eardrums, temporarily relieving the pain and correcting your muffled hearing. Just remember to blow gently. Forcing too much air into your tubes can make your ears hurt even more.

Note: You should not do this procedure with a fresh cold; you could force infection into your ears or deeper into your sinuses.

For Lasting Relief

Chew some papaya. Chewable papaya-enzyme tablets, sold at drugstores and health food stores, can reduce swelling in your middle ears and thin your mucus, according to Murray Grossan, M.D., an oto-laryngologist at Cedars-Sinai Medical Center in Los Angeles. The beneficial effects of this enzyme will help your Eustachian tubes to function better, he says.

The chewable tablet is most effective if you keep it in your mouth between your cheek and gums. Chew on the tablet long enough to soften it and release some of the papaya enzyme, then hold it between your cheek and gums while it dissolves. You can use these tablets one to four times a day, according to Dr. Grossan—so just take them along on any plane flight and use them when you need them.

Reach for the roof. To help clear those Eustachian tubes, touch your tongue to the roof of your mouth and swallow, suggests Dr. Grossan. This technique should unplug your ears and bring your hearing back to normal.

PAIN PREVENTERS

Carry candy and gum. When you suck on hard candy or chew on bubble gum, you have to swallow often. And every time you do, you automatically force small amounts of air into your Eustachian tubes, reducing pain. This action also helps fluids drain from your ears, says Don R. Powell, Ph.D., founder and president of the American Institute for Preventive Medicine in Farmington Hills, Michigan.

Drink lots of hot tea. The warm fluid can help promote drainage, says Dr. Grossan. The tannic acid from the tea may also reduce swelling. When the flight attendant comes by with drinks, ask for two cups of tea instead of just one. They're usually happy to oblige.

Do some cold coping. If you have a cold and you have to fly, you may be writing a recipe for misery. If possible, postpone the flight, especially if you already have an earache with the cold, suggests Dr. Reibel. But if you have to fly, drink plenty of fluids, both to help cure the cold and to help prevent ear infection. Also, be sure to use oral decongestants beforehand and take them along on your flight, he recommends.

Bedsores

Bedsores are sneak attackers, literally catching unsuspecting victims while they're down.

Bedsores, or pressure ulcers, occur when a person lies in bed or sits in a chair for long periods of time without shifting his body weight, says Dee Anna Glaser, M.D., associate professor of dermatology at St. Louis University School of Medicine.

"Because you're immobile, there is constant pressure or rubbing of weight-bearing parts of the body—such as the buttocks, hips, shoulders, back, and even feet—against the surface of the bed or chair," she explains. "Eventually, the constant pressure or rubbing cuts off the necessary nutrients and oxygen to the skin for too long of a period of time, then the skin's tissue dies and a sore develops."

If you have bedsores or you're caring for someone who is immobilized and therefore at risk for pressure ulcers, you should know it's possible to ease and even prevent the pain of these sneaky attackers. Here are some techniques to try.

For Fast Relief

Don't stay in one place. To keep bedsores from developing or to ease the pain of existing ones, change sleeping positions every 2 hours, suggests Lon Christianson, M.D., a dermatologist for the Dermatology Clinic Limited in Fargo, North Dakota. "The bedsores are caused by either prolonged direct pressure on one body part or the friction between that body part and

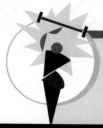

COMFORT FROM COMFREY

When it comes to pressure ulcers, a little herbal medicine can succeed as well as conventional remedies, says Andrew T. Weil, M.D., director of the program in integrative medicine at the University of Arizona College of Medicine in Tucson and author of *Spontaneous Healing* and *8 Weeks to Optimum Health*. He recommends an herbal poultice for wounds that are slow to heal, such as bedsores. The active ingredient in the poultice is comfrey root, which can be bought in bulk from many herb suppliers or found as dried chips in most health food stores.

In a blender, grind the herb into a powder. Then mix it with aloe vera gel to make a paste. Gently put the paste on the cleaned and disinfected bedsore and cover it with a clean gauze bandage. Dr. Weil recommends changing the poultice once a day and washing the wound out with hydrogen peroxide until it heals. Do not use the poultice on deep or infected wounds because it can promote surface healing too quickly and prevent healing of underlying tissue.

the sleeping surface itself. To lessen your odds of developing bedsores, make a conscious effort to share the load on different parts of your body rather than sleeping in the same position all of the time."

For Lasting Relief

Keep it clean. Keep existing bedsores clean and bandaged, says Dr. Christianson, who recommends covering the sores with gauze bandage and microporous tape (such as 3M Transpore Clear tape). To ease the pain that further infection might cause, the bandage should be changed and the area cleaned with sterile water and antibacterial soap at least twice a day. You can find sterilized water in your local drugstore.

Use props. Dr. Christianson also suggests having extra pillows on hand because they can be used to prop up one body part to provide relief elsewhere. "For instance, if you have bedsores or redness and discomfort around your hip, place a pillow under your waist or thighs, and that will take some of the stress off your hip," he says. "Or if you develop bedsores on your heels, which is common, pillows may be placed under your legs from your midcalf to ankle to keep your heels off the bed."

Reach for a doughnut. Who says doughnuts aren't good for you? If bedsores have developed on your buttocks or lower back, you can alleviate some pain by placing either a rubber inflatable or fabric doughnut onto your favorite comfy chair before sitting down, says Dr. Glaser. Another plus? "They're pretty inexpensive and are readily available. They can be found at most drugstores and health-care supply houses," she adds.

Use an egg crate to feel great. Placing an egg crate mattress over your regular mattress can possibly make all the difference in the world, pain-wise. "These mattresses are designed like the crate that eggs come in," says Dr. Christianson, "and they help distribute the pressure on certain body parts, which is good for people with existing bedsores or for less mobile senior citizens who fear developing them." You can find egg crate mattresses in any department or variety store.

Watch what you wear. Some clothing can make an already painful situation even worse, says Dr. Christianson. "For instance, a pair of pajamas might have a seam right where you have an existing bedsore and might rub against the sore every time you shift around in bed, causing you unnecessary pain."

PAIN PREVENTERS

Use lotion as your potion. During the stage when your skin is sore and red just prior to the formation of bedsores, wash the sore and affected areas with a soap that contains emollients, like Dove and Oil of Olay, Dr. Christianson suggests. After washing those areas, he strongly encourages applying petroleum jelly several times per day, if possible.

"Keep the jelly near your bed so that you can apply it before you go to bed," he says. "By applying the jelly or a skin lotion, you are replenishing some lost oils and keeping your skin from drying out. The lubricant may also ease the friction between the weight-bearing joint and the sleeping surface and therefore make you less susceptible to bedsores."

Drink it down. Maintaining proper levels of hydration is important to your skin's overall health. "Your skin tends to break down if you are malnourished or dehydrated, so proper diet is an important component in skin care," says Dr. Glaser. "And keeping good levels of nutrition can be hard for some bedridden seniors, who often lose their appetite and therefore don't get the proper amount of calories and protein every day."

Therefore, three tenets of general nutrition—eating a healthy diet, drinking 8 to 10 glasses of water per day, and getting your recommended dietary allowances of vitamin C (60 milligrams) and zinc (15 milligrams) either through a multivitamin or through diet—are recommended to help your overall health and the health of your skin, says Stephen Schleicher, M.D., codirector of the Dermatology Center in Philadelphia. "These three things should keep seniors healthier and should help the overall integrity of their skin."

Boils

Some people just develop boils. Others don't. It seems like that has always been the way of it: Some women who shave or wax their legs end up with a blocked or damaged hair follicle, and before you know it, a boil develops. Other women can shave or wax their legs regularly and never have a problem with boils.

While boils may seem pretty arbitrary as to whom they infect, there is a rhyme and reason as to how they pop up.

Here's how it happens, says Dee Anna Glaser, M.D., associate professor of dermatology at St. Louis University School of Medicine. Bacteria invade through an opening or break in the skin that can be caused not only by shaving but also by anything causing friction or irritation to the skin. They infect either a blocked oil gland or hair follicle. Then, your body's immune system sends in white blood cells to kill the invaders. The ensuing battle causes inflammation and produces debris (pus). As a result, a pus-filled abscess about the size of a quarter begins to grow beneath the skin surface, rising up red with pain.

While boils can be painful and unsightly, they often can be easily treated in the privacy of your own home. "A steady regimen of applying warm compresses and washing with an antibacterial soap should cause most boils to rupture and then heal before too long," says Dr. Glaser. Antibiotics may be necessary, however.

If a boil doesn't seem to be getting better after 10 days to 2 weeks of treatment, get it looked at by a doctor, says Lon Christianson, M.D., a dermatologist for the Dermatology Clinic Limited in Fargo, North Dakota. "Skin cancers are sometimes misinterpreted by people as being just boils. So, if the same boil or a small group of boils hangs around for 2 weeks, then it's time to see a doctor just to rule out more serious things."

But in most cases, you should be able to banish the pain of a boil with the help of these remedies.

For Fast Relief

Bring things to a head. At the first sign of a boil, apply heat or a hot compress, wrapped in a thin towel, over the boil for 10 to 15 minutes three or four times per day. The heat should help ease the pain immediately and gradually help the boil to drain and disappear. "Applying a heating pad set at a comfortable temperature, a warm washcloth, or a comfortably hot water bottle directly to the boil will eventually force the boil to come to a head, drain, and heal a lot faster," says Stephen Schleicher, M.D., codirector of the Dermatology Center in Philadelphia.

For Lasting Relief

Solve the problem with Silica. Silica is a homeopathic remedy found in health food stores. Look for 12C potency Silica, says Michael Carlston, M.D., assistant clinical professor in the department of family and community medicine at the University of California, San Francisco, School of Medicine. When the boil is red and swollen but there's no pus yet, take one dose of the Silica once or twice a day until the boil comes to a head. Silica may be difficult to find. If you can't locate it, please ask your local health food store for assistance.

Reach for *Rumex*. To help ease the pain of a boil, use the herb *Rumex crispus*, sometimes called yellow dock, which you can find in capsule form at health food stores, says Steven Bailey, N.D., a naturopathic physician at the Northwest Naturopathic Clinic in Portland, Oregon. Take two 100-milligram capsules three times a day until the redness and swelling are gone. If this remedy doesn't work within 2 weeks, it's time to see your doctor.

Bottle up the boil. If you don't have a hot-water bottle to place directly on the boil, then Dr. Christianson suggests that you rinse out a plastic soda bottle with a twist-off top and use that as a refillable hot-water bottle. "For senior citizens, this is an inexpensive way to come up with a hot-water bottle because almost everybody has soda bottles lying around the house," he says. "And the beauty of those plastic bottles is that they'll keep warm liquids pretty warm and cold liquids pretty cold."

Dr. Christianson suggests putting hot tap water in the soda bottle, wrapping the bottle in a thin towel and applying it to the infected area three or four times per day until the boil is completely drained.

PAIN PREVENTERS

Keep it clean. Once opened, the boil will drain pus for 2 to 3 days and then should heal, says Dr. Christianson. Since the pus can be contagious, you should cover the open boil with a 4- by 4-inch gauze bandage and medical tape. The bandage should be changed three times a day. When you do change it, wash the area with an antibacterial soap like Dial, Zest, or Safeguard. This should help keep future boils from spreading or developing.

Don't play Sir Lancelot. The temptation, whether you're age 6 or 76, is to pop the boil with your bare hands or with a sharp pin. Avoid the temptation to do so, says Dr. Christianson. Either method is an easy way to spread the infection or drive the bacteria even deeper into your skin.

Lather up. If you're prone to boils, you should be able to keep them from popping up so frequently by washing your skin with an antibacterial soap. "That won't totally prevent boils," says Dr. Glaser. "But if you seem to be one of those folks who seem to get boils, washing with an antibacterial soap will help to fight that bacteria that could get into a damaged hair follicle or an area of skin with diminished immunity and cause a boil."

Bruises

The vicious edge of a coffee table. A car door swung a little too wide. The neighborhood dog that always greets you a little too enthusiastically. Every day, your body collides with other objects.

There's nothing extraordinary about that—it's all part of life in the proverbial school of hard knocks. But sometimes, those everyday impacts can be great enough to damage blood vessels beneath your skin, tearing vessel walls and allowing blood to leak from them. What you will end up with is a bruise. The area of impact can become swollen and tender and will certainly turn a couple of shades of black and blue—not to mention purple, yellow, and chartreuse—as it heals.

There are several ways in which aging increases your chances of bruising. Blood vessel walls become thinner, making them more easily ruptured. Reduced stores of fat mean that you have less padding to protect your blood vessels from an impact. Hormones that made your skin more elastic, such as estrogen, are on the wane. Cumulative sun damage destroys veil cells, the very cells that help protect your blood vessels, says Melvin Elson, M.D., a dermatologist and director of the Longevity Institute in Nashville, New York, and Miami.

And, not to put too fine a point on it, you become less nimble over the course of time. Your reflexes have lost some of their razor edges, making it hard for you to avoid the collisions you were once able to sidestep.

Hands, forearms, and feet are particu-

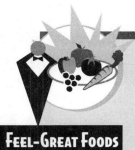

FEEL-GREAT FOODS

CURRY YOUR BRUISE'S FAVOR

The tropical root that turmeric comes from looks a little bland, brown, and boring from the outside. But cut into it, and its rich orange-yellow flesh bursts with color. Its magnificent color is one reason why turmeric the spice is so central to Indian cuisine. Many Indian dishes, and just about every curry, can claim turmeric as an ingredient.

Indian medicine has also used the power of turmeric for centuries because of the spice's great anti-inflammatory properties, says Shiva Barton, N.D., the lead naturopathic physician at Wellspace, a multidisciplinary health-care center in Cambridge, Massachusetts. Consuming turmeric reduces swelling and helps heal bruises. So head down to your nearest Indian restaurant and heap on the curry. Or you can buy turmeric capsules in health food stores. Dr. Barton recommends taking about 400 milligrams three to six times a day.

larly vulnerable to bruising in seniors because they have the least amount of fat, they are used a lot, and they have had the most amount of sun exposure, which thins and damages skin's elasticity, says Richard Roberts, M.D., professor of family medicine at the University of Wisconsin Medical School in Madison.

To be sure, bruising isn't a major agony as pains go. It's just, well, a pain. But it's one you can heal with speed and ease if you follow this advice.

For Fast Relief

Put on some parsley ice cubes.
"When a bruise is fresh, ice is the way to go," Dr. Roberts recommends. "It causes the blood vessels to tighten or narrow in the area, reducing the amount of blood flowing through the injured vessel, and that in turn reduces the amount of bruising and swelling. And it's the swelling that really hurts."

Sharleen Andrews-Miller, a faculty member at the National College of Naturopathic Medicine in Portland, Oregon, and associate director of the college's public clinic, discovered a new way to use an old gypsy remedy for bruising. The gypsies used parsley for its anti-inflammatory and anesthetic properties. You can take 1 cup of fresh parsley and combine it in a food processor with about 2 tablespoons (or 1 ounce) of water until you have a thick slurry like a pesto, she says. Then, pour that into an ice cube tray and put it in the freezer. After the cubes are frozen, you can pop them out and use them to soothe the site of your bruise and keep swelling down.

With older, more delicate skin, people should take care that they don't give themselves frostbite. Don't apply ice directly to the bruise. Wrap it in a clean washcloth or towel and leave it on the bruised area for only 15 to 20 minutes. Apply ice as often as needed.

For Lasting Relief

Warm it up. After 2 to 3 days, once the internal bleeding has pretty much stopped, you can start using topical heat on the bruised area.

"The heat seems to improve the circulation to the area," Dr. Roberts says. "That improved circulation brings the other blood elements that help resolve the bruise quicker, such as white blood cells, whose enzymes dissolve the remnants of blood cells that have leaked beneath the skin." Plus, there's the added comfort of the heat to help alleviate any stiffness you may be feeling in the bruised area.

A towel dampened with warm water can be draped over the area to speed this process. Apply the towel for 10 to 15 minutes as often as needed.

Coat it with vitamin K cream. Applying a cream with vitamin K in it can help ease your pain by speeding your healing. Vitamin K, a vitamin found in leafy green vegetables, promotes blood clotting. Look for a cream containing between 1 and 5 percent vitamin K, Dr. Elson says. Apply it to the bruise twice a day or once at night. Rub a small amount on already moistened skin to help it go on gently. "After the first couple of times you use it, you're going to get benefit almost immediately. Also, the vitamin K is anti-inflammatory, so if you're hurting, it stops the discomfort," he says.

Apply arnica. Arnica, a plant with bright yellow flowers and a bouquet of healing properties, has been used for centuries as a remedy for bruises and sprains. Use an arnica cream or gel, which is available at health food stores and even some drugstores. Rub it in gently two or three times a day, says Shiva Barton, N.D., the lead naturopathic physician at Wellspace, a multidisciplinary health-care center in Cambridge, Massachusetts. But don't apply it to an open wound and don't take it internally.

Pad it up. Most people do a pretty good job of not bumping into a bruise and irritating it. But sometimes, a bruise is on a part of the body, such as the hand, that is pretty susceptible to getting knocked around. To avoid the pain of reinjury, you can take the added precaution of dressing the bruise with an elastic sports bandage or self-adhesive bandage. Be sure to dress the bruise loosely so that circulation is not disrupted. "The padding helps if you do accidentally bump it, but I think equally important is that the bandage reminds you to be a little more careful or mindful of the bruise," says Dr. Barton.

Pursue a pineapple cure. Bromelain, an enzyme from the pineapple plant, is another ancient remedy for bruising. Found in health food stores as tablets, bromelain should be taken in dosages of 300 milligrams three to six times a day. It's anti-inflammatory and helps with healing, Dr. Barton says.

Burns

Nothing screams for your attention as much as the pain of a burn, and as you get older, that pain becomes an even more important signal. With age, skin becomes thinner, and a burn—say, a scald from hot tea spilling on your forearm—will reach much deeper tissue and do more damage than it would have when you were in your twenties.

In addition, growing older means that your general rate of healing will be slower, leaving more time for the burn to become infected.

For these reasons, even small burns on older people can be very serious and should be looked at by a doctor, notes Robert Sheridan, M.D., a surgeon at the burn and trauma unit at Massachusetts General Hospital and the Shriners Burn Hospital, both in Boston.

Age makes you vulnerable to getting burned by leaving you a little less agile and less able to break contact with a flame or hot surface. So while you may have spent a lifetime cooking in a housecoat or robe and dodging the dangers of a dangling sleeve over a hot burner, your age and the declining speed of your reflexes may catch up with you.

First-degree burns, which damage the outer layer of skin, are marked by pain and redness. In second-degree burns, the damage extends below the outer layer of skin and leaves blistering and pain in its wake. Third-degree burns damage the full thickness of the skin—as well as tissue, muscle, and bone below the skin—and leave an open, charred wound.

Follow these tips to quell the pain that accompanies even the least severe burn.

For Fast Relief

Go with a cold flow. Get the burned part of your body in cold water fast to numb the pain and cut down on swelling. For a milder first-degree burn, holding the burned area under the faucet as you run the cold water may be sufficient. For a burn that's really red and shows signs of blistering, use ice. Wrap the ice in a clean towel or washcloth and apply it to the burn. You can even use a bag of frozen vegetables in a pinch, says D'Anne Kleinsmith, M.D., staff dermatologist at William Beaumont Hospital in Royal Oak, Michigan. She recommends taking a bag of frozen peas, wrapping it in a thin towel, and putting that on the burned skin. "The nice thing about that is it will kind of conform to the contour of the skin," she says. Just keep applying the cold water or the ice or the peas until the worst of the pain is gone. Don't keep the ice on for more than 20 minutes without a break, though, or you may damage your skin.

For Lasting Relief

Cleanse the burn. If the burned skin looks as though it is blistering, or if there is an open wound, you'll want to lessen the risk of an even more painful infection by cleaning the area. Wash it gently twice a day with mild soap and water or rinse it with hydrogen peroxide, Dr. Kleinsmith advises. Afterward, apply an antibiotic ointment to the wound.

Opt for aloe. This member of the lily family has been used as a home remedy on burns and other skin problems for centuries. And according to Gloria Graham, M.D., clinical professor of dermatology at the University of North Carolina at Chapel Hill, that's because aloe really works. "It's wonderful for burns. This is what patients have always told me—that aloe vera knocks the pain out right away."

If you're growing your own aloe plant, you can use a leaf from it. Cut the leaf off the plant and squeeze the gooey gel out of the plant onto the burn. You can even keep leaves on hand as you regularly trim your plant, in case you get a burn. They last for several weeks before they dry out, she says. Apply the aloe several times a day, as needed, to keep the damaged skin moist.

If you don't have a plant handy, you can buy aloe vera gel in the drugstore. Be careful though, Dr. Graham advises. Many products say that they have aloe in them but may have only trace amounts or may include a host of other ingredients that may inactivate the aloe. Look for a product that is pure aloe vera, she suggests.

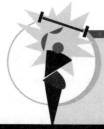

BURN RUBBER

assage for a burn? Wouldn't that hurt? Well, yes, if you touched your burn directly. But a massage on another part of your body could help you bear the pain of your burn. Touch therapy is a very ancient, almost innate form of medicine.

"When you hurt yourself, your instinct is to rub the injured area," says Maria Hernandez-Reif, Ph.D., director of research at the Touch Research Institute at the University of Miami School of Medicine.

Not only is rubbing an instinctive reaction, it's physiologically beneficial, as the institute's research shows. In one study, severely burned patients were massaged on nonburned areas of their bodies just before their bandages and dressings were changed in a very painful procedure. Patients who had massages reported less pain during the dressing procedure.

Bandage the burn. A burned patch of skin has a lot more sensitivity to the environment. A breeze or patch of sunlight might be enough to cause pain. But burns hurt less—and tend to heal a little faster and better—when they are covered. If the burn is small enough and has a regular shape, you can use a commercial adhesive bandage. But if the burn is larger or has an odd shape, or if your skin is sensitive to the glue in commercial bandages, you can create your own bandage with a piece of clean gauze and paper tape, which is more gentle on your skin, Dr. Kleinsmith says. Change your bandage twice daily, when you wash your burn.

"What we're actually finding is that when you do massage the skin, it's more than just a feel-good thing. It sends messages up the spinal cord into the brain and actually leads to the reduction of stress hormones," she says. Those hormones can actually make pain more intense.

If you have a spouse or someone who can give you a massage on a nonburned area of your body, great. Baby oil, wheat germ oil, a favorite type of massage oil, and cocoa butter (often used in burn units) are good lubricants. The massager should use long, gliding types of strokes on the arms or legs, applying moderate pressure—not so light that it tickles, but firm enough that the skin rolls and moves a little under the hands—or knead the muscles.

If no one else is available, you can give yourself a massage. Form each of your hands into the shape of a letter C, Dr. Hernandez-Reif says. Then, use your hands in a gliding back-and-forth motion along the skin of your legs or arms.

Beat blister blues. If your burn is bad enough, a blister will form under the skin and become a pain in its own right. If you can, leave it alone. It will eventually drain and dry out on its own. If it's bothering you, there is another option. "Sometimes, these blisters just bubble up and are quite annoying. It's hard to put clothing on, and you don't want them to break at an inopportune time. So if you want to, sterilize a needle and just drain it," Dr. Kleinsmith says. Just don't peel off the remaining skin of the blister. "You want that skin to stay intact," she advises. Just drain the fluid. Your skin will stay more protected and be less likely to get infected.

Canker Sores

Canker sores are a bit like unwanted relatives. They drop in without warning, and though they usually only hang around for a few days, it seems like forever. While they're around, life is simply uncomfortable.

If you suffered a lot of these sores in the past, you may have noticed that they don't plague you as much as they used to. Consider it one of the benefits of aging: Canker sores just don't crop up much in people over 50, says Roy S. Rogers III, M.D., professor of dermatology at the Mayo Clinic in Rochester, Minnesota.

Many people who complain of canker sores actually have abrasions from ill-fitting dentures or self-inflicted bites, he says, although occasionally someone past 30 will experience a real canker sore outbreak.

When this happens, it usually means that the person is suffering from a vitamin or mineral deficiency, he says, something that's readily remedied.

Despite a great deal of research into the cause of canker sores, the actual trigger mechanism remains elusive. Many doctors think that stress can trip an eruption; others believe that canker sores are a symptom of a compromised immune system. Much research points to acidic irritants like tomatoes, citrus fruits, and nuts.

Canker sores are not contagious, but that doesn't mean they don't warrant serious attention. "If any sore in the mouth persists for longer than 2 weeks, recurs frequently, or is so painful that it's hard to eat or even think about anything else, see your doctor or dentist immediately," says Dr.

Rogers. Otherwise, here are some steps to soothe the sting.

For Fast Relief

Try goldenseal. Goldenseal can help relieve the pain of canker sores and promote healing, says Andrew T. Weil, M.D., director of the program in integrative medicine at the University of Arizona College of Medicine in Tucson and author of *Spontaneous Healing* and *8 Weeks to Optimum Health*. Even though this herb has a strongly bitter taste, goldenseal is a good disinfectant and promotes scab formation of the canker sore.

To relieve canker sore pain, Dr. Weil suggests using goldenseal powder in the form of a rinse. In 1 cup of warm water, mix ¼ teaspoon of salt and ½ teaspoon of goldenseal powder (it will not dissolve completely). Rinse the solution in your mouth for 30 seconds to a minute, then spit it out. You can buy goldenseal powder in bulk or in capsule form at health food stores. And, if you can tolerate it, a pinch of cayenne pepper is a good addition to the solution. Cayenne pepper, a spicy red pepper, increases blood-flow to the area, promotes healing, and contains a powerful topical anesthetic.

For Lasting Relief

Keep it clean. To reduce canker sore irritation and, therefore, pain, use a hydrogen peroxide mouth rinse four times a day, suggests David J. Conover, D.D.S., a dentist who practices in Cincinnati.

A 50-50 solution of hydrogen peroxide and water swished over the sore for 30 to 60 seconds kills bacteria, gently anesthetizes the area, and speeds healing, says Dr. Conover. Avoid swallowing the solution, and rinse your mouth with plain water after using it.

Conventional saltwater rinses do the same thing, he says, but hydrogen peroxide doesn't present an additional health threat to people with high blood pressure or fluid-retention problems the way salt does. To use a saltwater rinse, mix 1 teaspoon of salt to 6 ounces of cool tap water, gargle the solution, and spit it out.

Try alternative antiseptics. Dr. Weil suggests applying tincture of propolis to canker sores. Propolis, the cement made by honeybees to construct their hives, has remarkable antiseptic and healing properties, he says. Be sure to follow the directions on the label. Propolis can cause contact dermatitis.

Tea tree oil is another natural anti-infective that works well on canker sores, says

Dr. Weil. Often called a first-aid kit in a bottle, the clear liquid, which is steam-distilled from the leaves of a common Australian tree, has been known among the aboriginal people for centuries for its healing properties. Moisten a cotton swab with 1 or 2 drops of the oil and apply to the canker sore. Both of these remedies are available in health food stores.

Make it vanish with vitamin E. To increase healing and decrease pain, break open a capsule of vitamin E and rub the vitamin-rich gel directly on the canker with a cotton swab or your clean finger, suggests Craig Zunka, D.D.S., past president of the Holistic Dental Association in Front Royal, Virginia. Do this four times a day for best results.

PAIN PREVENTERS

Cut out certain foods. While no one knows for sure what triggers canker sore pain, a great deal of research points to abrasive, acidic, salty, spicy, and chewy foods, which can irritate the already ulcerated skin.

If you're prone to canker sores, stop eating tomatoes, strawberries, citrus fruits, chocolate, and other acidic foods, and see if that reduces the outbreaks, says Dr. Conover. Different people react to different foods, so you'll need to run a mini-experiment on yourself to determine what your trigger may be, he says.

Dr. Rogers adds that this is not the time to indulge your yen for tortilla chips and salsa. You want to avoid any chance of poking, irritating, or accidentally biting the sore area. Keep from irritating the sore by choosing bland foods (like potatoes), cold drinks, and milkshakes.

Be better with a B-complex. Taking a vitamin B complex will help relieve the pain of a canker sore, says Dr. Weil. Take one 100-milligram capsule once a day or as directed by a physician until the pain subsides.

Cleanse with care. While a canker sore is active, Dr. Conover suggests, take extra care with oral hygiene. Be cautious with toothpicks and toothbrushes, he says. It's easy to reinjure the area, extending the canker sore's unwelcome stay.

Cold Sores

Whether they're called fever blisters or cold sores, those raging bumps that erupt on your lip or the surrounding skin are almost impossible to disguise. But easing the pain that they cause is not impossible at all.

Cold sores are caused by the herpes simplex virus. Once you get infected, the virus is with you for life: It lives in nerve cells where the immune system cannot find it, becoming activated from time to time. One of the blessings of getting older is that over time the virus seems to burn itself out, so you have fewer and fewer outbreaks. But when you do have them, they can be a real, well, pain.

Outbreaks tend to go away on their own in 7 to 10 days, and if you've had them before, you may notice that you get some warning just before cold sores arrive.

That warning usually comes in the form of numbness, tingling, itching, or burning on your lip or on nearby skin. Then, a small cluster of tiny red blisters breaks out, as does often searing pain. Over the next few days, a yellow crust forms on top of the blister, and the pain eventually subsides. Cold sores are highly contagious, and you don't want to spread them by kissing, by sharing food and drink, or by not washing your hands after touching the cold sores.

To speed healing and minimize the pain, try these methods.

For Fast Relief

Eliminate it with L-lysine. To speed the healing of cold sores, take the amino

417

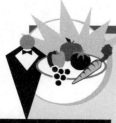

SOOTHE SORES WITH LEMON BALM

When cold sores erupt, lemon balm tea can encourage their retreat, says Marcia Aschendorf, N.D., a naturopathic physician practicing in Cincinnati.

The delightfully fragrant herb is soothing to the soul, but more important, lemon balm has a distinct anti-herpes effect, says Dr. Aschendorf, who notes that this action is currently being borne out by traditional scientific testing.

Also known by herbalists as melissa, lemon balm has been long prized for its medicinal properties; in fact, Charlemagne, king of the Franks in the late eighth and early ninth centuries, ordered lemon balm planted in every monastery garden.

Lemon balm contains flavonoids, polyphenolics, and other compounds that appear to have antiviral properties, says Dr. Aschendorf, who suggests preparing a simple tea by steeping 2 tablespoons of the herb (or a lemon balm tea bag) for 10 to 15 minutes in a cup of boiling water. Then, strain and drink as needed.

acid L-lysine, suggests William S. Eidelman, M.D., a physician specializing in natural medicine who practices in Ojai, California.

He suggests taking 1,500 milligrams of L-lysine three times a day, between meals, until the cold sore is gone. Available in health food stores and drugstores, essential amino acids like L-lysine aid your body's natural healing process, he says.

Although this may seem like a large dose, smaller amounts are far less likely to work, says Dr. Eidelman. Don't take amino acids without a doctor's guidance, however. The use of individual amino acids in large doses is considered experimental, and the long-term effects on health are unknown.

For Lasting Relief

Salve the sore. Natural salves made of aloe vera also speed the healing of cold sores, says Andrew T. Weil, M.D., director of the program in integrative medicine at the University of Arizona College of Medicine in Tucson and author of *Spontaneous Healing* and *8 Weeks to Optimum Health.*

Aloe vera is a traditional herbal remedy noted for its skin-healing properties, he says. Apply the salve according to the product label for as long as you have the canker sore.

Protect the area. When a sore is in full swing, it seems as if even the air around you can irritate it. To avoid that kind of pain, use a cotton swab or your clean finger to daub petroleum jelly over a cold sore to keep it covered and protected, suggests David J. Conover, D.D.S., a dentist who practices in Cincinnati. This creates an effective barrier between the sore and environmental irritants.

Avoid irritating foods. When salty, spicy, or citric foods come into contact with a cold sore, the pain can reach stratospheric levels, says Dr. Conover. To keep pain under control, avoid all of these foods, he advises, opting instead for bland choices.

Try ice. For some people, repeated ice applications reduce pain and dry up the cold sores, says Dr. Weil. Put an ice cube directly on the cold sore for 5 minutes, he suggests, then remove it for 10 minutes. Repeat this process as often as necessary for relief.

Flush with salt water. Flushing the area with a saltwater rinse helps to dry up the cold sore while slightly numbing it, says Dr. Conover.

Mix 1 teaspoon salt with 6 ounces of cool tap water. Fill a plastic needleless syringe with the mixture and direct the rinse over the sore. He suggests doing this two or three times a day, but no more. Too much salt water can irritate the cold sore, making it worse and far more painful.

If you suffer from high blood pressure or fluid retention, you should substitute a rinse made of half hydrogen peroxide and half water, says Dr. Conover. Be sure not to swallow the solution.

Look to licorice. Licorice is an herbal remedy with well-documented wound-healing and pain-soothing components. Dr. Eidelman suggests taking one 200-milligram licorice capsule three times a day.

Look for licorice that has had the glycyrrhizic acid removed; this component can increase blood pressure and cause water retention in some people. Deglycyrrhizinated licorice (DGL) retains all of its healing properties.

PAIN PREVENTERS

Build up immunity. Take zinc to strengthen your immune system and speed cold sore healing, says Dr. Eidelman. He suggests 30-milligram zinc supplements taken three times a day on a permanent basis.

Avoid arginine. To help prevent cold sore recurrences, cut down on or eliminate foods rich in arginine, advises Dr. Weil. The herpes simplex virus thrives on this essential amino acid, which is prevalent in many foods. Chocolate, cola, beer, grain cereals, chicken soup, gelatin, seeds, nuts, and peas are all high sources of arginine.

Cuts

No matter how old you are, your body still has an amazing ability to heal cuts or abrasions. During the first 24 to 48 hours after even a minor cut or scrape, your body marshals forces like Eisenhower commanding the D-Day invasion, throwing everything it has at the injury. Blood clots seal off the wound. Tissues swell up to protect the area. The body's pain chemicals send signals to draw infection-fighting cells to the area. In particular, the pain chemical prostaglandin, a hormone released by the body after a cut, sends out a call for white blood cells to come and battle infection-causing germs.

During the week or two following the injury, the second stage of healing occurs and is marked by cell multiplication and the construction of new capillaries. In the final phase, which can last several weeks after the second phase, connective tissue rebuilds the skin that was cut apart.

As impressive as this show of healing force is, you still need to pay extra attention to cuts and scrapes as you age. These minor injuries tend to occur more often with older people because their skin becomes more fragile. In addition, older skin heals at a slower rate than younger skin—sometimes 20 percent to 60 percent slower. Malnutrition, certain medicines, and systemic disease such as diabetes can delay the body's natural healing response, too.

Topical antibiotics and over-the-counter analgesics play their roles in the battle against pain, of course. But while your body is performing its reconstructive work, there are several drug-free ways you can assist with the healing process and minimize pain while you're at it.

For Fast Relief

Turn to flower power. Calendula, or marigold, is an old folk remedy that has anti-inflammatory and antibacterial properties, according to Shiva Barton, N.D., the lead naturopathic physician at Wellspace, a multidisciplinary health-care center in Cambridge, Massachusetts. Health food stores sell calendula ointment or drops, which can be applied topically to a scrape to aid healing.

For Lasting Relief

Clean it out. Any time you are cut or scraped, gently washing the wound out can help with healing and pain in several ways. First, it can help flush bacteria-friendly particles like dirt or pebbles from the area. "Any foreign body will serve as a focus around which bacteria will be more efficient at attaching themselves and multiplying, growing and causing infection," says James Leyden, M.D., professor of dermatology at the University of Pennsylvania in Philadelphia.

You really only need to use a mild soap and the flushing action of a stream of warm water to cleanse the wound. Bar soap can be used, but mild liquid soaps may be best. "It's a lot harder to overdo it in terms of irritation with liquid soaps than, say, with a bar," he says. Abrasions slow wound healing, so always cleanse gently.

Of course, you can always flush out a wound with substances like peroxide and alcohol. But while their antimicrobial properties will help get rid of bacteria, those same properties can irritate skin cells and will cause additional stinging and pain. Look for an antibiotic product rather than an antimicrobial one. The topical antibiotics don't sting or burn like the antimicrobials, says Dr. Leyden, and they also help prevent the growth of bacteria in the wound.

Cover it up. You may have grown up with the notion that if you get a cut or scrape, you should leave it unbandaged to let the air get at it. That's the wrong tactic, most doctors today say. Bandaging your damaged skin can reduce your pain, especially in the case of a scrape where a wide piece of skin has been torn or shorn off, exposing sensitive nerve endings to the air. "It's the same principle, for instance, if you have a cavity and the dentist squirts air on it; it hurts a lot," Dr. Leyden says.

The added benefit you'll get from using a bandage is a quicker healing time. If you cover a cut, it will take 5 to 7 days to heal—half the time an uncovered cut would take to heal. Covering the cut will help keep it moist, and you won't get a scab. Scabs are part of the reason an uncovered cut takes longer to heal.

Spread on a "bandage." Even if you don't have a bandage handy, you can eliminate this problem by covering up the wound with petroleum jelly, says Nancy Silvis, M.D., assistant professor of clinical medicine/dermatology at the University of Arizona in Tucson. This will create an effective barrier between the air and the nerve endings and, as an added benefit, will help keep the wound moist, which aids healing. Add the jelly, as needed, to keep the wound from drying out.

Flush out with comfrey. Another topical home remedy for cuts and scrapes is comfrey, a plant that has long been used on wounds to help speed healing and reduce inflammation. You can use it in a tealike form, Dr. Barton recommends, but don't drink it. To 1 cup of boiling water, add 1 tablespoon of comfrey leaves and let it steep and cool. Strain the leaves out and flush the wound with the liquid.

Visualize your healing. Sometimes, visualization can help speed the healing process, Dr. Barton states. So close your eyes and imagine that three-stage process of wound healing. "Depending on your temperament," he says, "you could actually visualize the cells growing and closing the wound. Or you can envision some sort of metaphor, like filling in a ditch or water running into a hole and filling it up."

Eye Cysts and Sties

Pimples are for kids. But sometimes, no matter what your age, oil glands can get blocked and cause those nasty blemishes. For the most part, they're unsightly. But when an oil gland in your eyelid gets blocked, that pimple-like formation—doctors call it a hordeolum, cyst, or sty—can be as painful as the longest eyelash that ever lodged itself in your eye.

Normally, bacteria lurk in many places on the skin, and antibodies in tears keep this bacterial population in the eye under control. A cyst or sty forms when that normal balance is disturbed and an oil gland lining the eyelid experiences a bacteria population boom. This causes a block and irritates the gland, explains Wayne Fung, M.D., professor of ophthal-mology at the California Pacific Medical Center in San Francisco and a spokesperson for the American Academy of Ophthalmology.

A sty or cyst starts off with tenderness to the eyelid, so a little pressure over the area is always going to be uncomfortable. "And as the abscess grows, the eyelid begins to swell and becomes more red and more tender," Dr. Fung says.

A sty usually resolves itself by coming to a head and rupturing within several days or weeks. In rare cases, a sty stays around longer and may require a surgical incision and drainage. There are several strategies you can pursue to help you say bye to the sty and so long to the pain it causes.

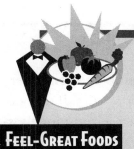

YOU SAY POTATO?

If applying a wet washcloth to ease the pain and speed the resolution of a cyst or sty seems like a messy, sodden proposition, let a potato do the work, recommends Wayne Fung, M.D., professor of ophthalmology at the California Pacific Medical Center in San Francisco and a spokesperson for the American Academy of Ophthalmology. Put a regular potato in the microwave on high for 1 to 2 minutes (be sure to puncture the skin several times with a fork so that the potato doesn't burst). The potato should be warm but not cooked. Wrap the potato with a thin cloth or towel and hold that against your eye for 3 to 5 minutes. It won't drip like a wet cloth, and the potato will retain heat longer.

For Fast Relief

Compress with heat. The best thing that you can do for a sty is to apply warmth to it, Dr. Fung recommends. If you start applying warmth at the very beginning, there is a good chance that you can head the sty off before it grows to even more painful proportions.

Take a washcloth soaked in very warm water and place it over the infected area for 30 seconds at a time. Do this at least four times a day, Dr. Fung suggests. The more often you do it, the greater the chance that you're going to help open that stopped-up gland and the more soothing it will feel. You'll get the added bonus of the heat's helping to trigger your body's own immune response to the bacterial infection that caused the problem in the first place.

For Lasting Relief

Massage it. While you don't want to pop a sty, try to hasten its draining with light, gentle stroking of the closed eyelid where the sty has formed. This gentle massage may help unblock the oil gland, suggests Silvia Orengo-Nania, M.D., assistant professor of ophthalmology at Baylor College of Medicine in Houston. First, apply a warm, wet washcloth for 2 to 3 minutes. Then, use a second, clean washcloth to massage your eyelid for another minute or two.

Use your glasses. When you have a full-blown sty, you'll only cause yourself more discomfort if you continue wearing contact lenses. "With a sty, the lid will become swollen. Hence, putting a contact in or taking it out becomes more difficult," Dr. Fung warns. If you normally wear contact lenses, avoid causing additional irritation to your eyelid by switching to eyeglasses until the sty goes away.

PAIN PREVENTERS

Boost your immune system. Very rarely, people get recurring sties. If they do, they may want to give their immune systems a boost, suggests George Dever, O.D., an optometric physician and herbalist in Seattle. "You have to realize that a sty is caused by either an increase in bacteria population or, more likely, a decrease in immune function," he says.

Adding more vitamin C to your diet may be a wise precaution. Try 2,000 milligrams in the fall and winter and 1,000 milligrams in the spring and summer months, as well as what Dr. Dever refers to as the old classics: garlic, onion, and ginger. "You just can't beat those foods for helping the immune system," he says.

Don't try to pop it. You may be tempted to try to pop a pimple that appears on some other part of your face, but don't try to pop a sty because you could end up with a much worse infection. "The body wants to isolate this infection," Dr. Fung says, "so it constructs kind of a protective barrier around this abscess. If you squeeze it, then you could break that barrier down and spread the infection into the soft tissue of the eye or the outer lid."

Eschew moisturizers. If you're having a flaky skin problem around the edges of your lids, you don't want to use a moisturizer, warns Kathleen Lamping, M.D., associate clinical professor of ophthalmology at Case Western Reserve University in Cleveland. That might make your sty problems worse by clogging oil glands. In fact, you should never apply moisturizer to the lash line, but on the lids themselves is okay.

Keep your cosmetics to yourself. Trading eye cosmetics, especially the moist kinds such as mascara, can help pass around bacteria and other types of germs that can cause sties and other types of eye infections. Just don't do it, advises Monica L. Monica, M.D., Ph.D., a spokesperson for the American Academy of Ophthalmology. Buy new liquid eye cosmetics like mascara after a sty or every 3 to 4 months, as bacteria can grow in moisture.

Eye Pain

Eyes are mysterious little orbs. When they're afflicted with a serious disease, you'll rarely feel pain. But get a speck of dust trapped underneath your lid, and it feels as though a gravel truck has dumped its load onto your eyeball.

No matter what your age, most eye pain stems from a couple of common causes. Physical irritants such as dust, pollen, makeup, and even your own errant eyelashes cause the bulk of eye irritation. Eyestrain—such as when you drive for long periods or spend long hours staring at computer monitors or TV screens—can cause eye pain as well. And any of the above can dry out your eyes, causing further scratchiness and pain.

While it's important to see your doctor regularly to ward off the painless problems that can lead to serious eye conditions, most of your day-to-day eye pains can be cleared up with these simple solutions.

For Fast Relief

Make yourself moister. As you age, it becomes harder for your body to retain fluids and keep your body well-lubricated. Dry eyes account for a large part of eye pain, and it's something you can eliminate fairly easily, says Monica L. Monica, M.D., Ph.D., a spokesperson for the American Academy of Ophthalmology.

Try over-the-counter artificial-tear products, such as Tears Naturale. Apply them as often as you need. "People under-utilize tears. They figure if they use them in the morning and at the end of the day, that's okay," says Dr. Monica. "Actually, in some cases you may need them every 10 minutes or every few hours. It just depends."

Artificial tears come in different thicknesses. They also come with and without preservatives. Obviously, tears with preservatives will last longer, but many people are allergic to preservatives, and an allergy could only compound eye pain.

Brands of preservative-free lubricants include Bion Tears, Refresh, and Thera Tears. "Try a variety and find out which are most comfortable for you," advises Robert Snyder, M.D., chairperson of the department of ophthalmology at the University of Arizona in Tucson.

For Lasting Relief

Bag your eyes. You can relieve general eye achiness by applying a warm or cool compress to your closed eyes, suggests George Dever, O.D., an optometric physician and herbalist in Seattle. Often, he finds, tea bags warmed or cooled in hot or cold water are an excellent way to do this. The tea bags are just the right size to rest over your eyes. He recommends trying chamomile, eyebright, or peppermint tea.

Tape it shut at night. Sometimes, eyes dry out at night when you're asleep. This can happen because of lagophthalmos, a condition in which your eyelid doesn't completely close during the night and, therefore, allows air to evaporate your eyes' moisture. If someone tells you that they saw you asleep with your lids cracked open, or if your dry eyes are really severe in the morning, this could be your problem. Try taping your eyes shut, Dr. Monica suggests. Use a little bit of Transpore tape or paper tape across your lids from your brows to the lower rims of your eye sockets, making sure it crosses your closed lids.

Open some ointment. If pain from dry eyes is quite severe, Dr. Dever recommends using an ophthalmic ointment, such as Hypotears PF, before you go to sleep. These ointments come in small tubes and can be found in the eye-care departments of most drugstores. It can be applied to each eye by pulling the lower lid downward and putting ¼ inch of ointment in the space created between the lid and eyeball. This ointment allows the tissues to heal and prevents tears from evaporating too quickly.

Caution: The ointment will smear over your cornea (the front part of your eyeball that helps focus your vision) and interfere with your vision, so it is best to put it in at night when you are ready to go to sleep.

For less severe dry-eye conditions, lubricating drops are effective.

DON'T TURN A BLIND EYE TO THIS PAIN

Everyday eye pain is usually minor, but most serious eye diseases come on silently, involving retinal and optic fibers rather than pain fibers, which is why it is so important to see an eye doctor on a regular basis. A person with no family history of glaucoma should see an eye doctor every 1 to 2 years, recommends Kathleen Lamping, M.D., associate clinical professor of ophthalmology at Case Western Reserve University in Cleveland. If you do have a family history of glaucoma, see the doctor once a year.

The one disease of this type that does cause pain is a special type of glaucoma that is called angle-closure glaucoma and that can be devastating for your vision. Angle-closure glaucoma causes a sharp pain that is often associated with blurred vision and colored halos.

Flush out the offender. If you get dust, an eyelash, or some other, undetermined foreign particle in your eye, don't rub it. The particle could wind up scratching your cornea and causing you plenty of long-term irritation. Instead, irrigate your eye immediately. If you have nothing but your hands and water, you can cup the water in your hands and open your eye in the water, Dr. Dever says. As wet as you may get, you can also invert a cup of water over your eye and blink so the water gets into your eye. "I would use warm water so that the eye's not shocked by the cold," he advises.

If you have saline solution or artificial tears, use those in place of water, Dr. Monica says. Tilt your head to the side

"Sometimes it feels like a toothache, or people tend to confuse it with a gastrointestinal problem because the pain is so severe that they are throwing up," says Silvia Orengo-Nania, M.D., assistant professor of ophthalmology at Baylor College of Medicine in Houston.

In addition to these confusing symptoms, angle-closure glaucoma pain occurs most often at night, after the pupil has gone through a mid-dilated state at dusk, with the pain peaking around 10:00 or 11:00 P.M.—a time when people may be prone to waiting until the morning to get help. Don't, says Dr. Orengo-Nania.

"Angle-closure glaucoma is something that people tend to ignore," she says. "And if they had treated it earlier, it could have saved their vision." If you have any of the symptoms above, call your doctor right away.

and flood your eye to remove the offending particle.

Even after you think you've gotten the speck out, don't rub your eye, says Silvia Orengo-Nania, M.D., assistant professor of ophthalmology at Baylor College of Medicine in Houston. If you think the foreign body is gone but your eye still feels a little sore or irritated, try using artificial tears to soothe your eye until the irritation goes away.

Ice the orb. If you've been hit or poked in the eye, it's always a good idea to have your injury checked out by a doctor, especially if your vision changes or you develop flashing lights or floaters, light sensitivity or eye pain, or if your eyelid has been torn or damaged. If you simply bump into a door and bruise yourself and have no other symptoms, wrap a cold compress in a thin towel and hold it against your eyebrow for 10 minutes to help ease pain and swelling.

PAIN PREVENTERS

Give your eyes a break. If you have dry eyes or you are not using the appropriate eyeglass prescription, your eyes can begin to hurt in a dull, achy way if they are used intensely for prolonged periods, such as when you've reached the juicy part of that bestseller or when you're watching the late show. Take a rest every hour by looking away from what you're concentrating on and focusing on something at a different distance from you, Dr. Snyder recommends.

"If you have dry eyes, often the staring at the computer screen and the intense sort of concentration can make them worse because you don't blink as much. The computer screen position may force you to maintain a higher gaze position, with elevated lids, than you're used to," he says. Consider repositioning your computer monitor and taking frequent "look-away" breaks.

Make your environment eye-friendly. If you live in a dry climate, you may be dealing with eye pain from dry eyes constantly. Try adding some moisture to your environment by running a humidifier in your house, Dr. Snyder says.

Be wary of how good contacts feel. Contacts, especially, thin, extended-wear contacts, can be very seductive because they help you see while they hardly feel as though they are there. This often leads people to use them for longer than their intended use.

"They feel good, people forget, and then they end up having the same pair in their eyes too long," Dr. Monica says. Wearing them too long can ultimately cause an ulcer on the surface of the eye and pain. So follow your contact instructions faithfully.

Fissures

As pain-related problems go, anal fissures are shrouded in mystery but, in reality, are not so hard to understand. Basically, a fissure is a variety of cut or tear, one that occurs in the thin skin of the anal canal as it is stretched beyond its normal capacity. Stretched too far, the skin will create a miniature chasm that exposes thousands of nerve endings, which in turn send you sharp pain signals.

In the anus, the most common cause of fissures is the passing of a large, hard stool, says J. Byron Gathright Jr., M.D., professor of surgery at Tulane University in New Orleans and former president of the American Society of Colon and Rectal Surgery.

If you have fissures, you know these little sores can make your life miserable. They burn, they hurt, and sometimes they bleed. And because they occur in a place

that's not very polite to talk about, it can be hard to get good advice for treating them and easing pain. This chapter should save you the embarrassment of having to ask. But if these symptoms persist beyond a couple of weeks, cautions Dr. Gathright, you should see a doctor who actually looks at the area in question.

For Fast Relief

Soothe with a sitz. Draw yourself a soothing bath, filling it only 3 to 4 inches high with water. Add ¼ cup of Epsom salts and sit with your knees raised—this position allows the fissure to better come in contact with the water. Sitz yourself for 15 to 20 minutes two or three times per day to ease your pain, says Joseph Andrews, M.D., a gastroenterologist from Wilkes-Barre, Pennsylvania. The combination of the warm water and Epsom salts will help soothe the pain and hasten healing. But be sure to rinse off with plain water before towel drying.

For Lasting Relief

Wipe with witch hazel. If you are suffering from an acute case of anal fissures, Dr. Gathright suggests using either cotton balls or toilet paper moistened with the herb witch hazel to clean your anal area after bowel movements. Sprinkle witch hazel on to the toilet paper yourself, or buy prepackaged medicated pads with witch hazel already in them. Both are available at most drugstores and will help you avoid the pain and irritation that wiping with dry toilet paper can cause, he says.

Reach for some ice. Apply ice or a cold pack covered in a thin towel to the area 5 minutes at a time several times per day to help ease your pain, says John J. O'Connor, M.D., Ph.D., chairperson of the colon-and-rectal-surgery section of the Suburban Hospital in Rockville, Maryland. He says to apply the ice however it's easiest for you but recommends that you lie on your side. Ice applications should be limited to 5 minutes or so; otherwise, you might impair the circulation to the affected area, which would impede the healing process.

Be gentle. Overzealous wiping can impede the healing process of your fissures, says Dr. O'Connor. So wipe gently and don't skimp when buying toilet paper. Treat yourself to a nice, soft, cushiony brand. Just make sure that it's white and unscented. Colored or scented toilet paper contains dyes or perfumes that will only irritate fissures and cause itching.

Steer clear of spicy foods. While no food will cause anal fissures, some foods may irritate the anal canal as they pass through your bowels. "Things that normally cause you heartburn, such as hot and spicy foods, will cause you pain as they pass through your bowels, particularly if you're suffering from fissures," says Dr. Andrews.

PAIN PREVENTERS

Fill up on fiber. The anal opening isn't meant to accommodate large, hard stools.

Rock-hard stools can tug and tear at the anal canal, which can result in anal fissures. The solution is to make sure that your diet is high in fiber, which will produce softer bowel movements.

The Daily Value for fiber is 25 grams. Eating more fruits, vegetables, and whole grains will certainly help in that regard, says Dr. Gathright. Such diet changes will help stools to pass more easily without causing further irritation to existing fissures. A high-fiber diet will also prevent future fissures from forming.

Drink up. Fluids also help you keep your bowel movements soft, which can help minimize fissure pain and prevent future fissures. Drink a glass of prune juice a day, and on top of that take in the recommended six to eight glasses of water, says Dr. Gathright.

Fractures

Bones don't have nerves. They don't feel a thing.

But just try telling your body that if you break a bone. The problem is, every bone is surrounded by hordes of tiny sensors—better known as nerves—that *do* feel a thing. They feel lots of things, in fact, from the moment a bone is fractured.

Even worse for some people is the annoyance, clumsiness, and itchiness of wearing a cast. While casts have improved a lot during the past couple of decades and are now lighter than ever, they're still a lot less convenient, comfortable, and usable than the intact limb with which you were born. Not only that, casts can sabotage your healing in subtle ways.

Just about the time you begin using the phrase "I'm not a kid anymore," you may also be thinking to yourself, "This bone won't heal as fast as my young ones did." That's true, of course; and it's an excellent reason to watch your step on ice, fix the railing on your stairway, and hire someone younger to clean the gutters.

As we age, our bones inevitably become more porous and brittle, which is a polite way of saying that we can't jump around like we used to. Many older people, women especially, are vulnerable to accelerating bone loss—the disease known as osteoporosis—which makes every bone in your body just a little more fragile than it ought to be.

Once a bone is broken, you can't count on it mending as quickly as a 10-year-old's. Needless to say, you're not as active as a 10-year-old either, so you can't help it mend the way you once could. The process is sure to take a while, and slower healing means a longer period of pain or discomfort.

But there is a way you can speed the process. For many kinds of fractures, your doctor is likely to recommend that you take physical therapy or do regular exercise as soon as you can. "That's the new teaching: mobility as fast as possible," says Andrew Palafox, M.D., an orthopedist at Del Norte Orthopaedics in El Paso, Texas.

Several decades ago, the common wisdom was that if you broke a leg or hipbone, you would most likely be given a cast and immobilized for the time it took for the bone to heal. But during the 1970s, researchers concluded that bone heals more quickly if you are up and moving about as soon as possible (within reason, of course).

Walking is especially good, according to Roberto Civitelli, M.D., associate professor of medicine at Washington University in St. Louis. This exercise maintains the right stimulation of bones, he observes.

Of course, if you've broken your leg or hip, walking will be especially painful. And prescription or over-the-counter painkillers may be called for. Here are some tips to help keep you moving while your bones are on the mend.

For Fast Relief

Elevate to alleviate swelling. After you've broken a bone, there's sure to be swelling in the area of the fracture. Keep that part of the body elevated, if you can, to help relieve swelling, which can also help reduce the pain, Dr. Palafox advises.

For Lasting Relief

Ice it down. Near the break, the tissue will be less painful if you can apply ice packs. Even if you're wearing a cast, you can apply an ice pack to the outside and some of the cold will get through, helping to numb the pain, says Dr. Palafox. When you're resting, you can apply an ice pack for 20 minutes on and 20 minutes off, until the pain goes away.

Heat the sore muscles. When you break a bone, the muscles around the fracture are sure to be tense and sore. Use a hot-water bottle or heating pad wrapped in a thin towel to get the muscles to relax, suggests Daniel Baran, M.D., professor of orthopedics, medicine, and cell biology at the University of Massachusetts Medical Center in Worchester. While using ice packs helps to relieve swelling and pain after an injury, using heat helps to relieve muscle spasms around the broken bone.

Ask for Arnica. The homeopathic remedy Arnica can speed wound healing and ease your pain at the same time, says Michael Carlston, M.D., assistant clinical professor in the department of family and community medicine at the University of California, San Francisco, School of Medicine. You can find Arnica in most health food stores and even in some drugstores. Look for Arnica with a potency of 30C, a homeopathic unit of measure. Take one dose of 30C Arnica every 3 to 4 hours for up to 5 days, he says.

Sprinkle a little powder. Itchy skin may not seem like an acute problem when compared to a fractured bone. But when you're wearing a cast, it's downright maddening—particularly for older people, who tend to have more fragile, sensitive skin.

To get some relief, just sprinkle some baby powder, cornstarch, or talcum powder in the space between your skin and the top of your cast, then let it sift down, suggests Dr. Palafox. As the powder reaches your skin, it will provide some relief.

Pain Preventers

Request a recasting. Sometimes, a cast is just too tight. If it's making you mis-erable and you see some swelling around the edge of the cast, be sure to notify your doctor, says Dr. Palafox. It's a quick procedure to cut off the old cast and replace it with a new one.

As the bone knits, take up squeezing. If you've broken your wrist or arm, after the cast is removed you'll need some therapy to prevent loss of muscle mass. A doctor or therapist is likely to recommend exercise to make sure that your muscles don't atrophy or get stiff and sore. As soon as you can use your hand, gently squeeze a tennis ball as frequently as you can. If you can do this for 5 to 10 minutes a day, you'll help to keep your muscles toned up, says Dr. Baran.

Take a calcium supplement. Your bones need calcium to continue their constant process of remodeling and to rebuild after a break. Be sure to take the recommended dietary allowance of 1,000 to 1,500 milligrams of calcium a day in a supplement like calcium citrate.

Incorporate calcium-rich foods into your diet. Foods are another great source of calcium, if you know which ones to choose. The highest amount of easily absorbed calcium can be found in dairy products such as milk and yogurt. An 8-ounce glass of fat-free milk contains 300 milligrams of calcium, and 8 ounces of yogurt has about the same amount. Though you get additional calcium from foods such as turnips and green vegetables, Dr. Civitelli recommends dairy products as the best sources.

Snuff out the cigarettes. "Smoking is not good for fracture healing and for bone health in general," says Dr. Palafox.

While doctors and researchers aren't exactly sure about the mechanism, one theory is that smoking decreases the microcirculation in the body—that is, circulation through the tiny capillaries that carry oxygen-rich, nutrient-rich blood to every part of your body. When microcirculation is reduced by smoking, it means that your bones and tissues aren't getting the support they need from your blood.

Get into the swim of things. When the cast is off, some time in the swimming pool could relieve muscle soreness, says Dr. Civitelli. "Use water exercise if it helps with the pain," he suggests.

Swimming is a comfortable exercise because your body is sustained by the water's buoyancy, so there's not much pressure on your joints. You can exercise with a minimum of pain.

"The most important thing is to try not to become chair-bound," he adds. "Try to be mobile."

Hemorrhoids

Hemorrhoids have the dubious honor of inflicting two very distinct kinds of pain. There's the physical pain, of course. After all, hemorrhoids are swollen veins in your anus caused by excessive muscular straining. Going through childbirth or regularly passing hard stools causes blood vessels to bulge out in the walls of the rectum. Once those vessels are out and in the way, they get irritated by your going to the bathroom, walking, or even just sitting down.

But that's just the half of it. The other side of the pain equation is the pain of embarrassment. Nearly half of all people get hemorrhoids by the age of 50, but no one wants to talk about it with their doctor or pharmacist, and so they consign themselves to suffering in silence. Instead, try these techniques, and you may not have to deal with either type of pain.

For Fast Relief

Take a sitz bath. This soothing remedy involves nothing more than drawing a 3- to 4-inch-deep warm bath, adding 1 cup of Epsom salts, and sitting in it for 15 to 20 minutes several times per day. When you do sit in it, be sure to raise your knees; this helps the sitz bath do its work more effectively, says Joseph Andrews, M.D., a gastroenterologist from Wilkes-Barre, Pennsylvania.

The warm water helps dull the pain while also helping to increase the flow of blood to the area, which can help shrink the swollen veins. The salts draw moisture out of the veins, causing them to shrink, which reduces pain, Dr. Andrews explains. If you have sensitive skin, rinse off with warm water after your sitz bath; otherwise, you don't have to.

For Lasting Relief

Strive for softer stools. The anal opening isn't meant to accommodate large, hard stools. In fact, passing rock-hard stools provides just the kind of strain needed to swell the veins in your rectum. The solution is to make sure that your diet is high in fiber and fluids that will produce softer bowel movements.

Eating more fruits, vegetables, and whole grains and drinking six to eight glasses of water per day is the best at-home remedy for hemorrhoids, says J. Byron Gathright Jr., M.D., professor of surgery at Tulane University in New Orleans and former president of the American Society of Colon and Rectal Surgery.

Another means of boosting your daily fiber intake is by taking a nonprescription fiber supplement such as Metamucil or FiberCon tablets once or twice per day, says Dr. Andrews. Follow the label instructions carefully, and be sure to take the supplements with a full 8-ounce glass of water, he adds.

Try a deep freeze. Tie off four fingers of a rubber glove, fill the remaining finger with water, and put the glove in the freezer. Then, use the icicle that forms as an ice suppository, says Michael Blate, founder of the G-Jo Institute, a natural-health educational organization in Columbus, North Carolina. Here's how.

Insert the frozen finger into your rectum as deep as is comfortable (use a little K-Y jelly as a lubricant, if needed), and hold it in place until the coldness becomes uncomfortable—about 5 minutes, or until the ice melts. Blate recommends applying gloved frozen fingers directly to the affected area several times per day to help ease the pain and swelling that often accompany hemorrhoids.

Treat yourself to some aloe vera. Frequently apply aloe vera gel to the area to ease the pain of hemorrhoids and to promote healing, says Andrew T. Weil, M.D., director of the program in integrative medicine at the University of Arizona College of Medicine in Tucson and author of *Spontaneous Healing* and *8 Weeks to Optimum Health*. You can find pure gel in most health food stores, or simply buy an aloe vera plant, break off one of the leaves,

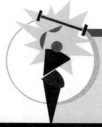

PRESSURE VERSUS PRESSURE

Bearing or pressing down (straining) with abdominal muscles is one of the chief ways hemorrhoids get formed. But you can fight hemorrhoid pain with another type of pressure—acupressure.

Here's how you do it, says Michael Blate, founder of the G-Jo Institute, a natural-health educational organization in Columbus, North Carolina.

Locate the soft hollow just behind your outer anklebone. It's actually between your anklebone and your Achilles tendon (Bladder 60, or B60, for those familiar with acupuncture). To find this point, which Blate refers to as G-Jo Spot 5, take the tip of your thumb or even the eraser tip of a pencil and deeply probe until you find what Blate calls the ouch point. "It will feel like a toothache or pinched nerve when you find it," he says.

Once you've found the point, deeply massage that area for

squeeze out a dab of gel, and apply it with a clean finger.

Work wonders with witch hazel. If you are suffering from acute hemorrhoids, Dr. Gathright suggests using either cotton balls or toilet paper moistened with the herb witch hazel to clean your anal area after bowel movements. The witch hazel causes the blood vessels to shrink down and contract, thus easing your pain. You can ei-

30 seconds using a digging or goading type of massage. Don't be gentle, says Blate, who feels that it must be painful to trigger the point. Then, simply do the same technique on the opposite foot for up to ½ minute.

"If you successfully triggered point number 5, you'll feel a flush of warmth and may start perspiring in several areas, such as the forehead, shoulders, and arms, and then you'll feel a deep sense of relief from the pain of hemorrhoids," he says.

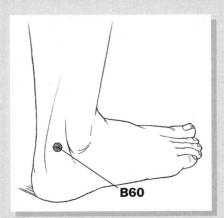

B60

Pressing the acupressure point shown here may help you feel relief from hemorrhoid pain.

ther buy witch hazel and sprinkle it on to the toilet paper yourself or get prepackaged medicated pads with witch hazel already in them. Both are available at most neighborhood drugstores, he says.

PAIN PREVENTERS

Steer clear of certain foods and drinks. There are some foods that won't exactly make your hemorrhoids worse, but that can contribute to your pain by creating further itching or burning as they pass through the bowels. "Foods that don't usually agree with you, such as highly spiced foods, are going to cause you pain as they pass through your anus, particularly if you're suffering from hemorrhoids," says John J. O'Connor, M.D., Ph.D., chairperson of the colon-and-rectal-surgery section of the Suburban Hospital in Rockville, Maryland.

According to Dr. Weil, foods that can cause you trouble include strong spices such as red pepper and mustard. Bothersome drinks include coffee and alcohol. He recommends avoiding these as well as tobacco, which irritates the digestive tract.

Try a little tenderness. Overzealous wiping can impede the healing process of your hemorrhoids, says Dr. O'Connor. So it's extremely important to clean yourself gently and properly. Step one in that process is to choose a brand of toilet paper that won't scratch the already tender area, for obvious reasons. According to Dr. O'Connor, it's just as important to choose white, unscented toilet paper. The scents or dyes that are added to some toilet papers can cause more pain by further irritating an already irritated area. Step two is the use of moistened toilet tissue or cotton balls to wipe the anal area, which provides a more thorough cleaning. But he stresses the importance of drying the area completely to prevent further irritation.

Ingrown Toenail

Ingrown toenails are common in aging feet, but it's not aging that causes them. For most people, it's bad habits: forgetting to trim your toenails regularly, trying to squeeze a few more wearings out of an old pair of shoes.

These and other types of neglect make it easy for toenails to dig into the tender skin on either side, causing pain, redness, and swelling. Pretty soon, what was a minor, avoidable problem becomes a miserable pain that strikes every time you take a step.

When the problem is mild, all you may need to do is soak your foot, making the skin supple enough that you can wedge a bit of dry cotton under the corner of the nail, says Arnold S. Ravick, D.P.M., a podiatrist who practices in Washington, D.C. But if you ignore the problem long enough, the skin around the nail can become infected, and you may end up needing minor surgery to remove the part of the nail that's poking into the skin. Talk about shooting yourself in the foot . . .

Meanwhile, the fact remains that healthy feet shouldn't hurt, regardless of your age, says Dr. Ravick. Ingrown toenails do not have to be a chronic pain. "Treatment for ingrown toenails is fairly straightforward," he says, "but it's easier to avoid them altogether." Here are some ways to do both.

For Fast Relief

Soak in soothing herbs. To relieve the pain of an ingrown toenail, soak your toe

445

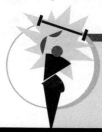

PODIATRISTS KEEP FEET FIT

Ingrown toenail pain can knock you off your feet for days or even weeks. But a podiatrist can get you moving again by providing targeted attention to your painful problem.

Feet, those complex engineering marvels that keep people mobile, change as an inevitable effect of aging. Nails get thicker, skin gets drier, and problems like ingrown toenails increase. After decades of wear and hundreds of thousands of miles, feet can start to break down. Or, they can continue to function remarkably well, but only if they are given proper care.

Podiatrists, who are medical professionals specially trained to care for feet, find themselves in the unique position of helping our aging society stay mobile, says Arnold S. Ravick, D.P.M., a podiatrist who practices in Washington, D.C. Good foot care by doctors of podiatric medicine can keep older people active longer, which in turn can keep them healthier and more capable of caring for themselves, he says.

Apart from solving immediate problems such as ingrown toenails, podiatrists often alert their patients to serious systemic ailments, such as arthritis or diabetes, that first show up as symptoms in the feet.

twice a day for 2 weeks in a warm solution of hypericum and calendula, suggests Isaiah Florence, M.D., director for the Center for Pain Management at Englewood Hospital and Medical Center in New Jersey.

Hypericum, also known as St. John's wort, is a natural substance with germicidal, anti-inflammatory, and antidepressant properties, he says. Calendula, part of the marigold family, is a topical antiseptic and anti-inflammatory. Both are known for their wound-healing action.

Both herbs are available in most health food stores. Mix 1 teaspoon of hypericum tincture and 1 teaspoon of calendula tincture with ½ pint of warm water. Soak your toe for 20 minutes twice a day.

Carefully dry your toe afterward and wedge a piece of sterile cotton underneath the side of your nail to keep it from cutting further into the flesh, says Dr. Florence.

gauze to the thickness of a candlewick and then gently wedging it between your nail and your skin, says Dr. Ravick.

If the nail has punctured the flesh and caused an infection that's red, swollen, and tender, clean the area with hydrogen peroxide and soak the cotton with iodine or an antibacterial ointment like Neosporin, he says. Wrap your toe in a gauze dressing. Follow this treatment for 3 to 5 days; if the infection doesn't clear up, see your podiatrist.

Heat up. Hydrotherapy is another way to immediately reduce the pain of an ingrown toenail, says Dr. Florence.

Soak your foot in warm to hot sudsy water for 30 minutes before you go to bed, he says. Make the water as hot as you can comfortably tolerate and use antibacterial soap.

Dry your toe and then wedge a piece of sterile cotton underneath the side of your nail to keep it from cutting further into the flesh; go to bed with that in place, he says.

For Lasting Relief

Wick away pain. In cases where the ingrown toenail isn't too severe, you can encourage your nail to grow away from the flesh by rolling a small piece of cotton

PAIN PREVENTERS

Trim nails correctly. Proper nail care is the key to correcting—and preventing—ingrown toenails, says K. William Kitzmiller, M.D., a dermatologist and clinical professor of dermatology at the University of Cincinnati.

Cut nails straight across, using sharp nail scissors or clippers. Don't curve the nails to match the shape on the front of your toe. Nails that are trimmed down into the corners are more likely to become ingrown.

If your toenails are thick and difficult to cut, which Dr. Kitzmiller says happens as we age, soak them in warm salt water. Use 1 teaspoon of salt for every pint of warm water, then soak your feet for 5 to 10 minutes to soften the nails.

Don't cut nails too short, he says, and keep nails free of snags by using a fine-textured file or emery board. Your nails should be level with the tops of your toes.

Never try to dig out ingrown toenails yourself, especially if they are infected and sore. Seek treatment from a physician.

Try a U-turn. This is an old folk remedy, but there may be some merit in it. If cutting your nails straight across doesn't keep them from curving into your flesh, try cutting U shapes across the tops so that the sides are slightly longer, suggests Dr. Florence.

Counterpressure from these slight divots causes the nails to grow into the centers and away from the sides.

Wear roomy shoes. Having enough room for your toes prevents the cramping that encourages ingrown toenails to develop, says Dr. Kitzmiller. "You may not think of shoes as preventive devices, but that's exactly what they are—if they fit properly. If they don't, you're at risk for developing a variety of foot problems, especially ingrown toenails."

Avoid shoes that pinch your toes, he says. Stay away from high heels since they force your toes forward, crunching them in the toeboxes.

If your shoes are lined, check to be sure that the linings are intact, says Dr. Kitzmiller. When you've had shoes for a while, the linings can get balled up in the fronts or on the sides and put pressure on your toes.

Have your feet sized whenever you buy shoes, suggests Dr. Ravick. Feet enlarge throughout adulthood, yet people tend to buy the same size shoes year after year. Wearing too-small shoes can cause ingrown toenails and a variety of other foot disorders.

And be sure to measure *both* feet. Your feet can differ from each other by a full size, says Dr. Ravick. If they do, buy for the larger foot.

Insect Bites and Stings

More times than not, uninvited guests such as bees, wasps, mosquitoes, or ticks can't pass up a chance to crash your summer picnic or family camping trip.

"When you head out into the great outdoors, you have to expect to encounter insects," points out Miles Guralnick, an entomologist and president of Vespa Laboratories, a research and manufacturing facility of vaccines for insect-allergic patients in Spring Mills, Pennsylvania. "They just come with the territory."

So what do you do when one of these uninvited guests invades your personal space? Below are some first-aid tips from experts for when one of these critters bites or stings you.

For Fast Relief

Act immediately. The key to effectively limiting the amount of pain you get from a sting is taking quick action, says Guralnick.

The faster you can remove the stinger (if there is one), cleanse the area with soap and water, and then apply some ice, the better your chances of controlling pain and swelling, says Warren R. Heymann, M.D., professor of medicine and head of the division of dermatology for the Cooper Health System in Camden, New Jersey. Here's how to do it.

1. Extract the stinger. Remove the stinger (if there is one) as soon as possible, especially if the culprit was a honeybee,

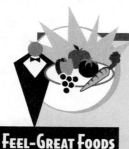

GOT A BITE? PASTE IT

Okay, it's not quite a food, but you do normally put it in your mouth, and you can use it to ease pain from a bite or sting. It's white toothpaste, which often contains a compound (sodium fluoride) that's chemically similar to baking soda, an effective neutralizer for most bites and stings, says Sheila Roit, R.N., a spokesperson for the American Nurses Association in Washington, D.C. The next time you get a bite, apply a dab of toothpaste to the area to relieve the pain, itching, and swelling, she suggests.

which usually leaves its stinger embedded in the skin while it flies away. Otherwise, the venom sac still attached to the honeybee's stinger will continue to pump for 2 to 3 minutes, driving the stinger and its venom deeper into your skin, Guralnick says. Scraping the stinger out is the best approach. Using the back of your thumbnail, a nail file, or even the edge of a credit card, gently scrape along the skin under the stinger and flick it out, without squeezing the venom sac.

2. Cleanse the area. Many stinging and biting insects are scavengers, so they often have undesirable bacteria that they can transmit to you, says Dr. Heymann. Wash the area with water and antibacterial soap or with an antiseptic.

Removing ticks and treating tick bites requires a bit more work, Dr. Heymann says. Because a tick's bite is generally painless, if you've been in wooded areas, it is important to check for ticks and remove them promptly and carefully. Here's how.

1. Use extrafine-tipped tweezers and grasp the tick as close to your skin as possible. Applying steady, firm pressure, pull the tick away from your skin, being careful not to squeeze or twist the tick. (This helps keep it intact. If it ruptures, the bacteria it carries will spread.)
2. After the tick is out, wash the bite with soap and water, disinfect the area with rubbing alcohol, and apply a topical first-aid antibiotic ointment. To make sure you didn't pick up Lyme disease, watch the bite carefully for the next couple of days and keep tabs on it for about a month. If a rash appears or if you develop flulike fever or muscle aches without a runny nose or sore throat, see your doctor.

For Lasting Relief

Put the pain on ice. Place an ice pack wrapped in a thin cloth, or even an ice cube, directly on the sting or insect bite to cut down the swelling and keep the venom from spreading, says Dr. Heymann. Be careful not to keep the ice on for more than 20 minutes to prevent damaging your skin.

Reach for baking soda. Mix baking soda and water until it forms a paste. Apply that paste for 15 to 20 minutes to relieve the swelling and itching that accompanies a bee sting, says Sheila Roit, R.N., a spokesperson for the American Nurses Association in Washington, D.C. Apply as needed. As an alkaline substance, baking soda helps neutralize acidic things like insect bite venom.

Neutralize the sting. If baking soda offers no relief, then your insect probably had alkaline-based venom, such as wasp venom, and you should try dabbing lemon juice or vinegar on the sting to soothe the pain, Roit says.

Try some salt water. To decrease the itching that can accompany a fly or mosquito bite, put ½ tablespoon of salt into a 6-ounce container of warm water, says Claude A. Frazier, M.D., an allergist from Asheville, North Carolina, and author of *Insects and What to Do about Them.* Wash the bite area with the salt water three or four times per day and the bite will eventually dry up.

Give Epsom salts a try. Dissolve 1 tablespoon of Epsom salts in 1 quart of hot water. Let it cool, dip a cloth into the mixture, wring it out, and then apply the compress to the skin for 15 to 20 minutes three or four times per day to ease the itch of the bite, says Dr. Frazier.

Circle it. If you happen to get a tick bite, circle the area with a permanent magic marker and watch the area like a hawk for 48 to 72 hours, says Roit. If nothing happens, you are okay. But if the area swells up, go to your doctor as soon as possible to get checked out for Lyme disease and other tick-borne illnesses.

PAIN PREVENTERS

Use common scents. Don't wear any perfume, cologne, scented body lotion, aftershave, or scented antiperspirant if you are going outside for a prolonged period of time during bug season, says Roit. Ticks, bees, and mosquitoes are all attracted to such smells, making you a more likely target.

Try bath oils. Certain bath oils and body lotions, such as Avon's Skin-So-Soft, have a repellent effect because of their high levels of alcohol, says Dr. Heymann.

Wear white. Stinging insects prefer dark colors, says Guralnick. That's why beekeepers wear khaki, white, or light colors.

Keep your skin covered. Wear long sleeves and pants, if you can, and tuck your pant legs into your boots or socks, Dr. Frazier says. The more skin you can keep covered, the more you'll minimize your chances of getting bitten or stung at all, he adds.

Drink carefully. When you are at a picnic or an outdoor party, peer in your sugary refreshments before drinking. Many bee stings occur when people sip their sodas or iced teas and get stung by an annoyed bee who is drinking from the cans or cups.

Walk smart. Bees love lawns with clover. Wear shoes or sandals in the grass to prevent a painful sting to your foot.

Intercourse Pain

There are people in their nineties and over 100 who are still having sexual relationships.

Sex is, can be, and should be a normal part of life for any adult, says Loren G. Lipson, M.D., associate professor of medicine and chief of the division of geriatric medicine at the University of Southern California in Los Angeles. What may not be normal are the occasional pains that intercourse may cause women. It's estimated that pain with intercourse, called dyspareunia, is something 10 percent of women discuss with their doctors at their yearly gynecological exams. About two-thirds of that group are older women who have experienced menopause.

Certain causes of intercourse pain are age-related. As a woman goes through menopause, her levels of the female hormone estrogen drop. That, in turn, changes her vagina's ability to lubricate itself. At the same time, it decreases the elasticity and the thickness of vaginal tissue. These changes make the vagina less able to stretch during intercourse and very often lead to irritation and pain. Sometimes, other age-related disorders such as arthritis can also make having sex a painful ordeal rather than a pleasure.

Other types of pain during intercourse may stem from infections of the vagina or bladder or from allergic reactions of the genital skin to an irritant.

If you are having painful intercourse, talk it over with your gynecologist, especially if your pain is accompanied by any

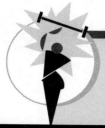

GET PHYSICAL

Occasionally, your pelvic-floor muscles—at the very bottom of your pelvis, near your genitals—function improperly, tensing up and making intercourse difficult. This can happen as part of a cycle that begins when you experience pain from an infection or irritation but the pain continues even after the infection or irritation has gone away.

"Even something as simple as having a vaginal infection can get you into a cycle of having pain," states Gretchen Lentz, M.D., assistant professor in the obstetrics/gynecology department at the University of Washington in Seattle. A physical therapist may be able to help you learn to locate and to contract and release those muscles so that you can relax them and have less pain when you want to have sex. Your doctor can refer you to a physical therapist in your area.

sudden and severe change in bowel habits, blood in your stool or urine, or bleeding after intercourse. These are all symptoms of more serious problems, including certain types of cancer.

Otherwise, turn down the lights and try some of these strategies for pain relief.

For Fast Relief

Use a lubricant. To eliminate the most common cause of intercourse pain, vaginal dryness, you can buy any number of over-the-counter lubricants, says Thomas F.

Purdon, M.D., associate professor and vice chairperson of the department of obstetrics and gynecology at the University of Arizona in Tucson. He recommends looking for water-soluble products such as K-Y Long-Lasting, Replens, and Astroglide. "Some of them have the ability to stay around for several days because they cling to the vaginal wall, so you don't need to necessarily replace them every day," he says. As to the amount you need and how often you need it, that's up to you.

For Lasting Relief

Extend foreplay. As you age, it takes longer for your sexual parts to become stimulated enough to provide ample lubrication for sex. Long, leisurely periods of foreplay can help. "It takes older women—and men—longer to respond sexually, so longer foreplay will allow for more adequate lubrication," says Gretchen Lentz, M.D., assistant professor in the obstetrics/gynecology department at the University of Washington in Seattle. Focus on being intimate with your partner without actually having intercourse. Spend 15 to 20 minutes kissing, touching, holding one another. By then, your body should be ready for intercourse—and you may be

pleasantly surprised to find that it doesn't hurt all that much anymore.

Ease up on the athletics. What you once may have done with acrobatic ease during sex may not be so comfortable as you age. "As we get older, many things happen in our physiology," Dr. Lipson says. "Our tendons are less able to stretch, our joints are less able to accommodate, so that can lead to difficulties having sex, particularly if there is a lot of activity involved." Experiment with less rough sex and fewer contorted positions, but do try different ways of sexual expression.

Change your position. When a woman is experiencing pain upon penetration, it may be wise to experiment with other positions where the woman has more of the ability to guide what is happening. "If she's having pain, sometimes it's nice if the woman can be on top. She can control the depth of penetration that way, and sometimes that will lessen pain. Or they can just try other positions to find one that is comfortable," says Dr. Lentz.

PAIN PREVENTERS

Have a warmup session. Physicians often don't take it into account, but arthritis can contribute to making sex painful, says Dr. Lipson. Intercourse may be quite painful and difficult for men or women who have lower-back arthritis or arthritis of the hips or the knees. "What we've found is having them take a warm bath or a shower before intercourse may sort of loosen things and make things less painful," he recommends.

Be alert to your medications. Some medications, such as antidepressants and high blood pressure medicine, can have a drying effect on the mucous membranes of your body, from your mouth to your vagina. If you're having a problem with vaginal dryness, don't stop taking your medication, but talk to your doctor or pharmacist about this side effect. There may very well be an alternative medicine that can be prescribed.

Remove skin irritants. Occasionally, the outer skin of the genitals can flare up in an extremely painful way during the friction of intercourse. Often, this is contact dermatitis and can be traced back to something in your environment, most often laundry detergent, fabric softeners, or soap—sometimes even harsh toilet paper—

that is irritating your skin, Dr. Lentz says. You can try to uncover the culprit by changing brands of suspected products and noting if there is any improvement. The best overall strategy is to choose the mildest products you can—mild soaps, nonscented toilet paper, and natural fibers such as cotton for your underwear.

Dump the douches. Doctors have been trying for years to make women aware of the fact that they don't need to douche. The vagina is a self-cleansing environment. In fact, douching can irritate the delicate vaginal environment, leading to infection and making sex more painful, says Dr. Lentz.

Break abstinence carefully. Intercourse may be painful if you simply haven't done it in a while. "The postmenopausal vagina can shrink if it's not being used," Dr. Lentz says. That coupled with less elasticity due to decreased estrogen can make starting and enjoying a new sexual relationship difficult. In extreme cases, you may need to see a doctor who can use a dilator to help loosen things up. Typically, if you go slowly and use plenty of lubricant, you will minimize the pain.

Jammed Finger

If you've ever jammed or injured a finger, you know how difficult life can be without full digital dexterity. Simple activities like opening doors and cupboards, fishing change out of a pocket or coin purse, leafing through a book, even dialing a phone can all become wincing exercises in patience and pain.

But a jammed finger doesn't have to leave you in a jam, says Jerome McAndrews, D.C., spokesperson for the American Chiropractic Association. Any impact injury of the musculoskeletal system can traumatize a joint, but timely treatment can prevent long-term damage. Conversely, ignoring an injury can cause the bones of your finger to stay slightly out of alignment. This can lead to the formation of scar tissue in the injured area, resulting in stiffness and chronic pain, he says. The discomfort in the jammed joint can take months to disappear.

Many simple treatments can alleviate pain, provided they are administered within 72 hours of the injury. We quizzed the experts and came up with the following tips to ease your discomfort. It is best to do them as soon as possible after the injury, our experts advise.

For Fast Relief

Attempt a personal alignment. To ease a jammed finger in the moments immediately following the injury, grab it with your thumb and index finger and pull on it gently for 5 seconds, let it rest for 5 seconds, then pull on it again for 5 seconds, suggests David Bilstrom, M.D., director of the physiatric medical acupuncture program at Christ Hospital and Medical Center in Oak Lawn, Illinois. This will stretch compressed tissue, allow squished-out joint fluids to flow back, and pull the joint into better alignment.

Don't do more than one set, however, or else you may cause more harm than good, according to Dr. Bilstrom, who says an ice pack should be placed on the injured area right after this stretch.

For Lasting Relief

Ice it. When you first jam a finger, you want to reduce inflammation and swelling, says Dr. McAndrews, and an ice pack is the best way to do that. Ice also numbs the area, cutting the initial pain. Ice the injury as soon as possible—this is a case where minutes really do count. Wrap crushed ice cubes in a washcloth and hold the ice pack on for 20 minutes, off for 20 minutes, then on again for 20 minutes until the pain subsides.

Continue to use an ice pack, 20 minutes on, 20 minutes off, as often as you can for the first 24 hours after the injury, Dr. Bilstrom adds.

"The more inflammation that occurs, the longer it will take for the healing process to take hold," says Dr. McAndrews, "so get ice on your finger right away."

Then apply heat. The day after the jam, you want to stimulate circulation so that the blood clears away debris from the injured tissue, says Dr. McAndrews. He suggests placing your finger in a dish of warm water for up to 20 minutes. Another option is to soak a washcloth in comfortably hot water, wring it out, and apply it over the injury for 20 minutes. Take care that the cloth isn't too hot.

Give it a rest. If a jammed finger is especially painful, use a splint to keep it from moving, says Fatima Hakeem, P.T., a physical therapist at Woman's Hospital of Texas in Houston. Resting the finger this way helps you avoid an overuse injury, which is sometimes caused by pushing yourself in spite of the pain. Limiting your finger's movement forces it to rest, thereby accelerating the healing process.

She suggests wrapping the injured finger to the adjoining finger with medical tape. Keep the tape a little loose so that the blood flows freely to both fingers. If you

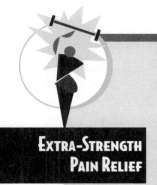

PINNING DOWN PAIN

Acupuncture—the ancient Chinese practice of piercing parts of the body with fine needles to treat disease and relieve pain—is a very effective treatment for jammed fingers, says David Bilstrom, M.D., director of the physiatric medical acupuncture program at Christ Hospital and Medical Center in Oak Lawn, Illinois. "If you can get to an acupuncturist within the first 36 hours, you may need only one treatment to completely eradicate pain, swelling, and stiffness," he says. The placement and location of the needles may vary from practitioner to practitioner. But typically, needles aren't placed directly into areas that are red and swollen.

feel any numbness or tingling or see any discoloration in the finger, the tape is too tight.

Help it with Hypericum. Hypericum is a homeopathic remedy with painkilling properties and is particularly good for injuries where there are high concentrations of nerve endings, says Isaiah Florence, M.D., director for the Center for Pain Management at Englewood Hospital and Medical Center in New Jersey. Readily available in health food stores, where it is sold primarily as a treatment for depression, Hypericum possesses anti-inflammatory properties, much like an over-the-counter analgesic.

For a jammed finger, he recommends a 30C dose of Hypericum every 2 hours for

STRIKE UP THE BAND

Just like any other muscles, finger muscles need to be worked after an injury to regain full function. A rubber band is a fine tool for keeping finger joints supple, says Fatima Hakeem, P.T., a physical therapist at Woman's Hospital of Texas in Houston. Here's a simple exercise that you can try at home.

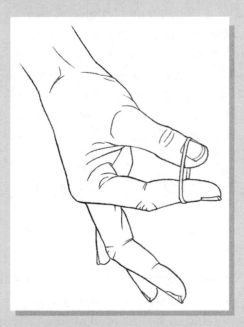

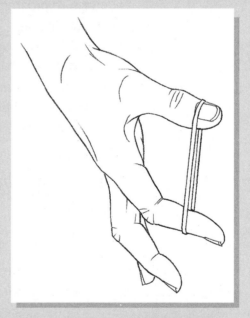

Loop a rubber band between your thumb and the jammed finger. The band should have enough tension that it pulls your finger toward your thumb.

Pull apart your finger and thumb until you feel resistance; repeat 10 times. As the exercise becomes too easy, choose a shorter or thicker rubber band.

3 days. If the injury isn't markedly better in that time, see your physician because you might have a fracture or something more serious than a jammed finger, he says.

Stop stiffness. Once the immediate pain and inflammation of a jammed finger fade away (usually in 2 to 3 days), joint stiffness can remain, says Hakeem, who recommends at-home physical therapy to keep your fingers flexible.

Combine relaxing warmth and hand-strengthening flexibility exercises. Knead bread dough on a weekly basis, says Hakeem. Play with Silly Putty or Play-Doh. Or try a Ther-a-ball, a hand-workout ball specially designed so that you can heat it in the microwave and squeeze it while it's warm. Ther-a-balls are readily available at medical supply stores.

Muscle Cramps

Muscle cramps rank up there as possibly one of the most mysterious muscle-related maladies of all time. Researchers know why we feel pain during a cramp, of course, but there are a number of different explanations as to what triggers the cramp in the first place.

Some experts theorize that as we age, we spend less time exercising. Over time, our muscles become less flexible, so that when we do use them, they cramp up more. Other researchers suspect that dehydration or a lack of electrolytes, essential chemicals that muscles need to stay healthy, may be the problem. Or, another explanation blames cramps on poor blood circulation.

Whatever the cause, one thing is for sure. Cramps grow more common as you age. These involuntary contractions of a muscle—almost always in your calf and sometimes in your foot—can sometimes be painful enough to wake you from sleep and are powerful enough that even after they are gone, you may still feel soreness.

While muscle experts still aren't sure what causes the cramps, they have plenty of ideas for getting rid them. Here's what can help.

For Fast Relief

Grab your toes. Gently pull your toes toward your knee until you feel the cramp subside. If you have a cramp in your leg, this is the fastest and most effective way to get rid of it, says George J.

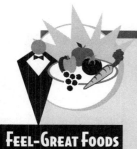

PAIN RELIEF WITH A TWIST

Losing too much salt through sweat may cause cramping along with other symptoms, such as headache and nausea. The solution is pretzels.

Pretzels provide the magical combination of salt and carbohydrate. Plus, they are easy to carry with you and easy to eat during exercise. Chomp on a couple of salted sticks every ½ hour of exercise and wash them down with a few gulps of sports drink or water.

Eating pretzels is better than the old-time method of taking salt tablets, because salt tablets can easily pump too much sodium into your system at once, says Bob Murray, Ph.D., director of the Gatorade Exercise Physiology Lab in Barrington, Illinois.

Caranasos, M.D., professor of medicine and chief of the division of internal medicine at the University of Florida in Gainesville.

After pulling back on your foot, massage the muscle with your hands and then walk around, which provides the best of both worlds: a natural massage and semi-stretch of the muscle.

For Lasting Relief

Check your medicine chest. Various prescription medications, including nifedipine (Adalat) and terbutaline (Brethine), may cause cramps. So talk to your physician if the cramps persist, Dr. Caranasos advises.

CRAMP-FREE LEGS

Massage can help stop cramps, especially in the calves, where muscle cramps are most common, say health-care experts.

Do both of the following massages first on your right leg, then repeat them on your left leg.

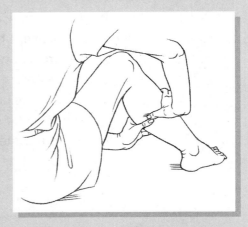

Calf massage. Sit with your lower leg at a 45-degree angle to the floor, and use your thumbs and fingers of both hands to squeeze, stroke, shake, and knead the calf muscle.

Skip the hospital corners. Untuck your sheets at the foot of your bed so that you can sleep with your toes pointed up, suggests Dr. Caranasos. Tight sheets can keep your feet pointed toward the foot of the bed all night, triggering leg cramps.

Replenish what you lost. Some researchers suspect that cramps may be

Quadriceps massage. Sit in a chair and use your thumbs and fingers of both hands to shake, squeeze, and knead the back of your thigh. Then, use your fingers and thumbs to stroke your upper leg lengthwise toward your knee, working your way from the left side of your thigh to the right. Finally, press your thumbs into the top of your thigh, pushing your thumbs toward your knee.

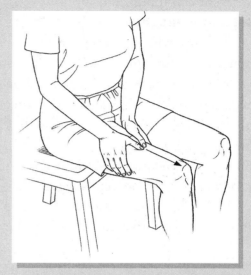

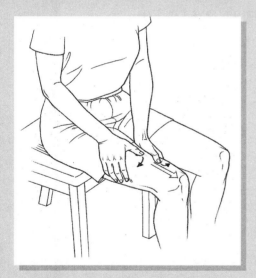

Finish by pressing your thumbs in a circular pattern along the length of your thigh, alternating one thumb and then the other. Work from the top of your thigh down toward your knee.

caused by too-vigorous exercise, which may upset the balance of electrolytes in your system. Within ½ hour of finishing your workout, have a sports drink that contains both carbohydrate and protein, says Richard Brown, Ph.D., an exercise physiologist and coach in Eugene, Oregon, and author of *10-Minute L.E.A.P.: Lifetime Ex-*

ercise Adherence Plan. This may help your muscles recover faster from exercise and may prevent cramping later.

Get more magnesium. No one has proven for sure whether magnesium supplements work for muscle cramps in humans. So far, the research has been done on rats. Rats fed a magnesium-poor diet cramped more easily than those with a magnesium-rich diet.

Take a calcium and magnesium supplement before you go to sleep, suggests Andrew T. Weil, M.D., director of the program in integrative medicine at the University of Arizona College of Medicine in Tucson and author of *Spontaneous Healing* and *8 Weeks to Optimum Health*. The supplement should contain 1,000 milligrams of each mineral.

People with heart or kidney problems, however, should check with their doctors before taking supplemental magnesium. Supplemental magnesium may cause diarrhea in some people.

Take a bath before bed. The warm water will increase bloodflow to your muscles and possibly decrease the likelihood of cramping, says Dr. Weil.

Plantar Warts

Imagine walking around with a stone in your shoe. Sharp, stabbing pain every time you walk—that's the pain of plantar warts.

Noncancerous growths on the bottom of the foot (or plantar surface), plantar warts are caused by a specific bug known as the human papillomavirus (HPV).

"Like every virus, warts are self-limiting, which means they'll go away on their own eventually," says Arnold S. Ravick, D.P.M., a podiatrist who practices in Washington, D.C. Unfortunately, nobody knows how long "eventually" might be, he says—some people could have plantar warts for years, and they may spread in number and size.

Plantar warts are usually larger than they look because most of each wart lies below the skin surface. The pressure of walking flattens the warts and pushes them back into the skin, causing inflammation and pain. If left untreated, plantar warts can grow to an inch or more in circumference, and they can spread into multiple-wart clusters called mosaic warts.

As with any other virus, plantar warts are infectious. They're spread by touching, scratching, even by contact with skin shed from another wart. Plantar warts also bleed occasionally, another way they spread. You can acquire warts through person-to-person contact or indirectly from places like a public-shower floor.

As people age, susceptibility seems to increase, presumably because the immune system is not as strong. Some people may be more likely to suffer from warts if they are taking medication after liver or kidney transplants. Using steroids for a long pe-

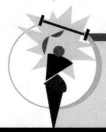

VISUALIZE WART REMOVAL

Can you think away a plantar wart? Many doctors and alternative health providers believe that you can by using visualization, the practice of creating an image in your mind's eye, then concentrating on it for therapeutic effect.

Several recent studies have shown that visualization can help patients eradicate warts, says Isaiah Florence, M.D., director for the Center for Pain Management at Englewood Hospital and Medical Center in New Jersey. Positive, focused thought seems to stimulate the immune system, which helps the body fight wart-causing viruses.

The most powerful form of visualization imbues the patient with a sense of empowerment, says Andrew T. Weil, M.D., director of the program in integrative medicine at the University of Arizona College of Medicine in Tucson and author of *Spontaneous Healing* and *8 Weeks to Optimum Health*. He suggests spending a few minutes each day, preferably when you rise and again when you go to sleep, thinking of the wart surrounded with healing white light

Or, devise an image that's especially meaningful to you. Dr. Weil says that one man he knows got rid of a troublesome wart by imagining a steam shovel scraping away at it morning and night. "Working with mental imagery this way is a good technique for mobilizing your body's healing powers," he says.

riod of time can also increase your vulnerability.

Because the bulk of each wart lies below the surface, plantar warts are difficult to treat, says Dr. Ravick. Doctors apply acid to them, freeze them off, or use an electric cautery to burn them.

Laser surgery is another choice. It does not require anesthesia, it's not very invasive, and there's almost no pain with the newest lasers.

For Fast Relief

Change shoes. Shoes that constrict your feet add to the pain of plantar warts, says Dr. Ravick.

Your first line of defense is to find shoes that minimize pressure. Stay away from high heels or pointed toeboxes. Go for softer, flexible shoes with cushioned insoles. Laced shoes are a smart choice, he says, because they usually provide more cushioning and distribute your weight more evenly across your feet.

Warts thrive in humid environments, so pick shoes made of material that won't make your feet sweat. Air out your shoes between wearings, says Dr. Ravick, noting that it's not a good idea to wear the same pair of shoes every day.

For Lasting Relief

Try tea tree and thyme. Equal parts undiluted tea tree oil and thyme oil is an herbal remedy for plantar warts that you can try at home, says David Edelberg, M.D., founder of the American Whole Health Center in Chicago. You can find these oils in health food stores.

Rub this combination into the wart every day for at least 21 days. It may take up to 3 months to see results, he says, noting that it takes time to kill the virus.

These herbs are known for their antiseptic and healing properties. "Since both are essential oils, they absorb into the skin and won't leave you feeling greasy," says Dr. Edelberg. Since the virus can live in spent skin cells, swab out the insides of your shoes with this compound, then let them air dry.

PAIN PREVENTERS

Don't expose yourself. Wear shower thongs, slippers, or pool shoes when you're in a public area, such as showers or even hotel rooms, says Dr. Ravick. Don't go barefoot. If you do, wash your feet thoroughly with a disinfectant soap after being in an area where the virus can be spread.

Sciatica

Over a lifetime, 40 percent of us will experience sciatica attacks. The attacks vary greatly in their severity, from minor discomfort such as a tingling in the toes or an ache in the calf that abates over time to recurrent attacks over many years that make it hard to walk or even stand up.

Sciatica is generally defined as pain along one or both of the sciatic nerves, the longest nerves in the human body, which run from the lower spine, down the backs of the thighs and legs to the heels of the feet. The sciatic nerves are created by the meeting of several nerve roots that start from the vertebrae of the lower spine. That's a lot of nerve, so it's little wonder that it is a common site for pain.

According to Douglas Shepard, M.D., a physician in Baltimore, sciatica often results when a ruptured or slipped disk in the spine presses on one of the nerve roots. These nerve roots control the sensation in your lower extremities, and before you know it, the pain spreads down your leg and into your feet.

But that's just one of the causes of sciatica, says Dr. Shepard. Bone spurs can also press on the nerve roots, causing the same pain. Or it can just be due to inflammation of the overlying muscles in your lower back. So it's important to see a doctor so you can get an accurate diagnosis and establish what's causing the pain.

That done, try these doctor-approved methods to fight back against the pain that sciatica causes, and get back to living your normal everyday life.

CRUNCH A BUNCH

Abdominal exercises such as crunches keep your abdominal muscles strong, which can help ease sciatica. If you're under a doctor's care for sciatica, get the doctor's okay before you begin exercising.

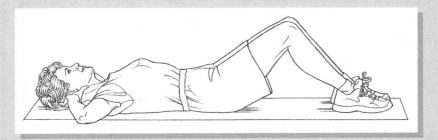

Lie down on your back on the floor with both feet on the floor and your knees bent. Place your hands behind your head with your fingertips cupped behind your ears and your elbows pointing out to the sides.

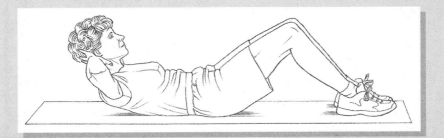

Raise your head and shoulders off the floor as high as you can while keeping your lower back on the floor. Hold for 1 second, then repeat. Make sure not to touch your chin to your chest. You should feel the muscles in your abdomen doing all the work. If you feel your neck straining, you are lifting too high.

Sciatica Soothers

Keeping your leg muscles, especially your hamstrings, loose and flexible is an important piece in the puzzle of fighting back pain, including sciatica. People diagnosed with sciatica should do a set or two of hamstring stretches every day, if possible, says James N. Dillard, M.D., D.C., a pain-management expert and instructor at the Columbia University College of Physicians and Surgeons in New York City.

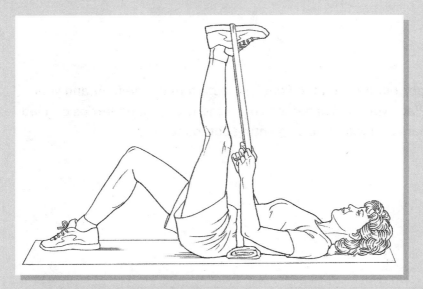

Hamstring stretch #1. Lie on your back on the floor or a bed with a rolled-up towel under the small of your back. Bend your knees at a 90-degree angle and put your feet flat on the floor or bed. Loop a belt around the instep of your left foot, holding on to both ends. Slowly straighten and raise your left leg upward, as shown, as far as you can without pain. Hold for 10 seconds, then lower your leg and repeat with your right leg. Do 5 to 10 repetitions with each leg.

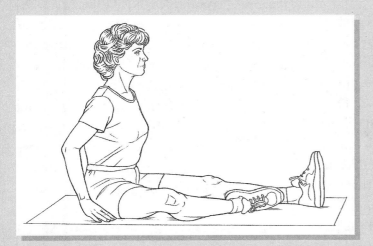

Hamstring stretch #2. Sit on the floor with both legs straight. Bend your right knee and draw your right leg in so that the sole of your foot is against the inside of your left calf. Your left knee should be slightly flexed, and your upper body should be upright (your back should be straight, with your arms in front of your body).

Keeping your back straight, bend over at the hips and reach for the toes on your left foot. Your legs should stay on the ground, with your left knee unlocked, and you should feel a pull in your hamstrings. Hold the stretch, relax, and return to the starting position. Do the stretch two or three times, then repeat with your left leg bent.

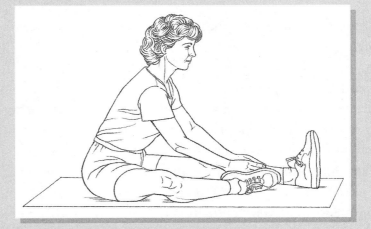

For Fast Relief

Do the opposite. When you feel sciatica pain in one of your legs, your natural reaction is probably to sit down and put that leg up on a footstool. Do the opposite of that, says Jerome McAndrews, D.C., spokesperson for the American Chiropractic Association. Put the unaffected leg up on the stool and rest the pained leg flat on the floor. Why? Because that will stretch out the pain-free leg, which then causes the painful leg to relax and the pain to subside. He says that you should feel relief almost immediately.

For Lasting Relief

Rest, but not too much. Doctors used to prescribe lots of bed rest for back-related pain. Not anymore. According to Dr. Shepard, studies have found that bed rest for more than 4 days can actually interfere with recovery from back pains such as sciatica. The longer you stay in bed, the weaker your muscles become, including the muscles that support your back. He recommends that you gradually return to your normal activities after just a couple of days of bed rest.

Keep moving. "The best advice that I can give is to stay in motion, within reason," says James N. Dillard, M.D., D.C., a pain-management expert and instructor at the Columbia University College of Physicians and Surgeons in New York City. After 4 days, the longer you lie in bed, the worse off you're going to be. Walk, exercise, stretch—even if you have to start very slowly. All these things will do much more good in the long run than days and days of bed rest, he says.

Develop a fetal attraction. When you move around in your sleep, you often inadvertently trigger sciatic pain. But you'll have a better chance of sleeping like a baby if you sleep in the fetal position during sciatica, says Dr. Shepard. Sleeping in this position will keep your hips flexed. This is a better sleeping position because it will keep you from sliding around in the bed and rotating your hips, which puts added pressure on your back.

Don't stay in one place. If you have sciatica and must perform a task that requires you to sit for long stretches of time, take a break and walk around every hour, says Dr. McAndrews. The same applies for long-distance driving. Pull over at a rest stop and walk around the parking lot before continuing on your way.

PAIN PREVENTERS

Start with low-impact exercise. To keep the pain of sciatica from getting an even tighter grip on you, get yourself on an exercise program. Try some low-impact activities such as swimming, riding a stationary bike, or walking. These will improve circulation and build overall muscle strength and flexibility in your legs and back, says Dr. Shepard.

If you're not in the habit of exercising, he recommends first talking with your physician and then gradually building up to the point where you're working out at your own pace for 30 to 45 minutes three to five times per week. Staying in good overall shape is a great first step for people of any age to avoid back problems like sciatica. Once you have sciatica, exercise is important not only to help your back but also to keep other muscles from atrophying.

Lift safely. If you have to lift a heavy object and fear triggering another attack, lift from a squatting position, holding the object close to your body. Rely on your hips and thighs rather than your back to do the work, says Dr. McAndrews.

Warm up. Whether planting petunias or hitting the lanes to go bowling, people with sciatica or other types of lower-back pain should make it a habit to warm up or stretch first in order to get their blood pumping and raise their heart rates. Five minutes of walking in place is all it takes to get blood flowing and prevent injury, says Dr. Dillard.

"It seems obvious, but you'd be surprised how many people aggravate their backs by doing a sudden activity without walking first or doing something to warm up and loosen their muscles," he says.

Stay trim. Carrying extra weight in your belly puts extra stress on your spine. The last thing a person with sciatica needs is any additional stress on his back and spine, says Dr. McAndrews.

Get your wallet out. Most men unknowingly contribute to sciatic pain by virtue of carrying big old wallets in their back pockets. When they sit, the wallets press right on their sciatic nerves, Dr. Shepard explains. Years of this sort of thing can lead to sciatic pain. So, whenever you sit down, take out your wallet. Or consider carrying it in a vest or front pocket.

Shinsplints

Exactly how shin pain ever got the name shinsplints is somewhat of a mystery.

Most doctors and those in the sports-medicine profession hate the term because it refers to an ambiguous symptom rather than a definable ailment and because no one seems to know where the term came from.

Doctors prefer two much less friendly, but more specific, terms. So when you march into a doctor's office and say that you think you have shinsplints, your doctor's brain will translate your complaint into one of the following diagnoses.

Tibial periostitis. This term means that the spot where your muscle attaches to your leg bone, called the periosteum, is inflamed. Whatever words they use, the condition is what most people really mean when they say they have shinsplints. It's the mildest of the two types of shin pain. And you can usually continue to exercise with a nonimpact activity, such as swimming or cycling, while you heal, says Michael Fredericson, M.D., assistant professor of physical medicine and rehabilitation and head track-and-cross-country-team physician at Stanford University.

Stress fracture. This means you have a small crack in your tibia, one of the two major bones in your lower leg. Such a crack may have been caused by an out-of-control case of periostitis, or it may have been caused by direct trauma to your bone, says Dr. Fredericson. If you have a stress fracture, the best way to beat that pain is to stop jarring activities such as running (and depending on the severity, stop all activities) for 4 to 8 weeks while your bone heals.

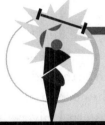

SHINSPLINT RELIEF YOU KNEAD

Ever hear the phrase "hurts so good"? Well, whoever said it first was probably getting a shin or calf massage. If you have shin pain, you might consider one, too.

The deep kneading done by massage therapists and physical therapists can sting—okay, even hurt a little—during the process. But you'll feel wonderfully better when it's over. The massage will loosen tight muscles and break up knots, helping your shins to heal.

Here's what to expect.

"I have found that it helps to work the calf as well as the muscles of the shin," says Aimee Louise, a personal trainer, certified sports-massage therapist, and owner of Simply Fit Wellness Center in Phoenixville, Pennsylvania, whose clientele includes the members of Villanova University's women's running teams. "Usually, I use deeper techniques, really dig in there with my thumbs. A little deep friction—digging around with my thumbs in a circular back-and-forth motion—is great right on the shin. It really gets the blood flowing in the area. And, actually, a foot massage can do wonders for shinsplints as well."

Athletic trainers and physical therapists use slightly different massage techniques than massage therapists. Because many athletic trainers do very slow, long massage to heal shinsplints, their touch may not hurt quite as much. But expect to be on the table longer, as they very gradually deepen the strokes.

Runners, dancers, and other athletes who do sports that jar the lower legs are most likely to get shinsplints. But they can happen as you age, too. If you're a woman and you've had problems with low bone-mineral density (a history of irregular periods can be a sign of this problem), you may get shin pain. If you haven't exercised lately and suddenly take up walking or running, your undertrained leg muscles may lodge a formal protest in the form of shinsplints. If you already walk regularly but one day find yourself with shin pain, the condition may be a result of walking on particularly unyielding surfaces (such as concrete) or walking in shoes that don't provide enough cushion. Also, if you have a tendency toward tight calf muscles or you roll your feet inward when you walk or run, this, too, can also predispose you to the problem.

For safety's sake, you should talk to your doctor if you have any type of leg pain that doesn't go away after a couple of days. If it turns out that you have regular old shinsplints, try the following remedies.

For Fast Relief

Give yourself an ice massage. Put water in a paper cup, place a popsicle stick in it, and freeze. Peel away the paper cup and rub the "ice pop" over your shin before and after exercise, says Steve Cohen, a surgical physician assistant in orthopedics and assistant professor of physician assistant studies at Nova Southeastern University Medical Center in Fort Lauderdale.

Don't hold the ice in one place for too long, as this may cause damage to your skin, he adds. Massage with the ice for 15 to 20 minutes before and after exercising. You can safely do this every day until your pain is gone. This works because the cold reduces the painful inflammation.

For Lasting Relief

Get off your feet. Maybe you've heard this old doctor's joke. A patient walks into the doctor's office and says, "Hey, doc, it hurts when I touch my arm." So the doctor says, "Okay, then don't touch your arm."

The advice to stop running, dancing, or whatever other activity makes your shins hurt probably seems about as endearing as that joke. It's not really the advice you want to hear. But it is one of the fastest ways to pain relief. It's so important that when Cohen wants someone to take a break from exercise, he writes it on a prescription pad.

Resting for anywhere from a few days to a few weeks will allow those inflamed

GET FLEXIBLE

Part of the cause of your shinsplints is a tight calf muscle. To loosen your calf, try this stretch. Stand on the bottom step of a staircase with your knees bent and your right heel hanging off the step. Drop your right heel below the level of the step, then shift your weight so it's over that heel. Hold the stretch for 20 to 30 seconds, then repeat with your left heel.

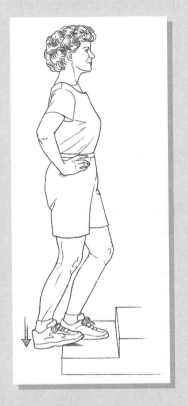

The most important thing to remember when doing this stretch is to keep your knees bent. The simple movement of bending your knees—instead of keeping your legs straight, as many people tend to do—isolates the posterior tibialis muscle, says Rochel Rittgers, head athletic trainer and director of the sports-medicine curriculum at Augustana College in Rock Island, Illinois. This muscle is commonly involved in shinsplints, Rittgers explains.

Do this stretch about 10 minutes into a walk or run—that way, your muscles will be warmed up, making them more flexible and easier to stretch.

muscles to heal. Rest for as long as it takes the pain to subside, says Dr. Fredericson. During your break, you can keep fit by engaging in any activities that don't stress your lower legs. You might try water aerobics, swimming, or cycling.

Then, as you get back into exercising, do so very gradually. Follow the tried-and-true advice of not increasing mileage by more than 10 percent a week and not increasing the intensity of your workout too rapidly, Dr. Fredericson advises. And listen to your body. If you start to feel shin pain, cut back your training, he adds. For 3 to 4 months, avoid hills and stay off hard roads such as those made of concrete.

PAIN PREVENTERS

Strengthen your shins. Strong anterior tibialis muscles in the fronts of your legs can protect you from shinsplints. To strengthen them, stand facing a wall with your toes about 5 inches away from it. (You can place your palms lightly against the wall for support if you need to.) Keep your feet shoulder-width apart as you try to lift your toes and the balls of your feet off the floor and balance on your heels for about 3 seconds. Be sure not to lock your knees, Rittgers says. If balance is a problem, do this exercise while sitting.

Strengthen your feet. Strong feet are important. The bottom of your foot supports your ankle, where a muscle called the posterior tibialis—which is commonly involved in shinsplints—attaches, says Rittgers. In addition to walking barefoot as much as you can, here are some foot-strengthening exercises to do while sitting down.

❯ Dump some marbles onto a towel on the floor and use your toes to pick them up one at a time and put them in a bucket.

❯ Place a towel flat on the floor, just in front of your bare feet. Use your toes to drag the towel under your foot.

Drink plenty of milk. Because stress fractures may in part be caused by poor bone-mineral density, getting more calcium might help. Make sure to drink at least one glass of milk a day or take a daily calcium supplement.

Doctors recommend at least 1,000 milligrams of calcium every day for people over 65. To reach this goal through diet alone, drink 2½ to 3 glasses (8 ounces each) of fat-free milk a day and eat a healthy, balanced diet. If you take supplemental calcium, take a 500- to 600-milligram capsule twice a day for best absorption, Dr. Fredericson says.

Sore Throat

Your nose and throat are the main battlegrounds of your body. When germs get into your nose (and aren't sneezed or blown out), your body's defenses marshal their forces in an area at the top of your throat. There, they wage an all-out war against the invaders. While this war kills the bad guys, it also makes the glands at the top of your throat swell, and that swelling makes your throat hurt.

Colds and flu, both caused by viruses, are the most common causes of sore throat in people age 60 and older, says Robert A. Bonomo, M.D., a geriatrics and infectious-disease specialist at the University Hospitals of Cleveland and the Veteran's Affairs Medical Center in Cleveland.

"Since sore throats in adults are usually colds, they usually go away in 3 to 5 days, even if you do absolutely nothing," says Allen Perkins, M.D., associate professor and residency director in the department of family practice at the University of South Alabama in Mobile.

Still, you don't need to put up with the pain for that long. Here's how to soothe it away.

For Fast Relief

Use honey to take the sting out. Try this throat-soothing honey-citrus tea suggested by Dr. Perkins. It works in numerous ways. First, the fluids themselves soothe your throat. Second, the honey

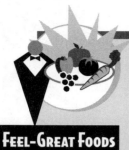

THE ICE CREAM SOLUTION

If you had your tonsils out as a child, you may remember that the one bright moment amidst all the misery was that you got all the ice cream you could eat. Ice cream works as well now to soothe sore throats as it did then. Chiefly because it's cold, of course—real cold. The coldness numbs your throat and shrinks swollen tissues, says Allen Perkins, M.D., associate professor and residency director in the department of family practice at the University of South Alabama in Mobile. It's the perfect prescription.

An added bonus is that it may also give you a strengthening boost of calcium. If you're trying to watch your weight or avoid high-fat foods, try low-fat ice cream or frozen yogurt.

helps coat your throat. Here's all you need to do.

Place three decaffeinated tea bags and one cinnamon stick in a 1-quart teapot. Add boiling water and steep for 3 to 5 minutes. Remove the cinnamon stick and tea bags. Stir in 1 cup of grapefruit juice and ¼ cup of honey. Drink as needed throughout the day. This tea can be served hot or iced.

For Lasting Relief

Suck on some candy. Most of the soothing magic from all the throat lozenges you see at the store doesn't come from fancy ingredients like menthol or secret herbs. It comes from sugar. Plain, sweet sugar. Sweet tastes draw fluid into your throat and leave behind a soothing syrupy coating, making pain melt away, explains Dr. Perkins. And sucking on candy creates lots of saliva, which also helps. So hard candy will soothe away pain about as well as any "medicinal" lozenge. If you are on a limited-sugar diet, sugarless candies containing sorbitol offer the same effect. But be careful: Too much sorbitol may cause diarrhea, he warns.

Go hot and cold. When you have a sore throat, you need to drink a lot of fluids to keep yourself well-hydrated (which keeps those scratchy tissues soothed and lubricated). Drink as many fluids as possible. You simply can't overdo it.

The problem is that if your throat is sore enough, it hurts to swallow just about anything—that is, unless you make your liquids either very hot (but not scalding) or very cold, says Dr. Perkins. Ice-cold drinks will shrink and numb swollen tissues, soothing away pain. So they are your first line of defense against pain. Hot drinks, on the other hand, can sneak by your throat's pain receptors undetected. So you can drink hot tea without discomfort, but anything room temperature or lukewarm is going to hurt when you swallow.

Try eucalyptus. The oil from this herb cools inflamed tissues, while its tannins provide a soothing astringent, explains herbalist James A. Duke, Ph.D., author of *The Green Pharmacy*. You'll find eucalyptus in most health food stores. Put in a few teaspoons of the crushed, dried herb per cup of boiling water. Steep for 5 minutes, then strain before sipping.

Experiment with licorice. The Finns eat a foul-tasting cough drop made from licorice whenever they get sick, and they swear by it. Of course, they've developed a taste for the stuff, and with practice, you can, too.

Many studies have documented the immunity-boosting effects of licorice—the herb, not the chewy candy. Use 5 to 7 teaspoons of dried licorice root pieces per 3 cups of water. Put the herb in the water and bring it to a boil, says Dr. Duke. Simmer until half the water has boiled away, then strain. Drink once a day until your sore throat goes away.

Pacify pain with papaya. Sold in drugstores and health food stores, papaya-enzyme tablets can soothe away pain, reduce swollen tissues, and thin mucus so that the tiny hairs in your nose (called cilia) can beat better, helping your throat to heal, says Murray Grossan, M.D., an otolaryngologist at Cedars-Sinai Medical Center in Los Angeles.

Chew on a tablet and then hold it between your cheek and gums while it dissolves. Do this one to four times a day.

PAIN PREVENTERS

Stay away from caffeine. When you have a sore throat, part of the problem is that you're lacking in fluids, which only worsens that dry, scratchy feeling. You need all the fluids you can get. So cut yourself off from coffee, colas, teas, and any other beverages containing caffeine or alcohol. Both are diuretics, which rob you of the fluid you need. Instead of coffee or soda, stick to herbal or decaffeinated tea and water, says Dr. Perkins.

Get a flu shot. Once you hit age 65, doctors recommend that you get a flu shot every winter to avoid one of the most common causes of sore throat—influenza. Doctors recommend that people age 55 and older get flu shots if they have a medical condition such as diabetes or any type of lung disease. Dr. Bonomo also recommends getting the pneumococcal vaccine injection every 4 to 6 years to prevent pneumococcal pneumonia.

Sprains

You might suppose that sprains are mainly the scourge of the young and restless, but the truth is that sprains become more common as you get older.

When you turn your ankle or twist your elbow the wrong way, you violently stretch and sometimes tear ligaments, tendons, and even muscles near your joint. Initially, this trauma creates swelling and sometimes bruising. But even as that swelling and bruising subside, pain can still linger for months and even years. That's because these now overstretched ligaments no longer do as good a job of holding your bones in their proper alignment. This allows joints to sometimes scrape together.

As you age, your muscle fibers often shrink in size and number, affecting your coordination and balance. All it takes is one slight misstep—it could happen when you're just walking across a room—and you have a sprain as bad as any that a kid might suffer while bounding down a rocky hill or sliding recklessly into third base.

Even though aging can increase your risk of sprain, that doesn't mean that you're destined to limp through the rest of your life, says Michael Fredericson, M.D., assistant professor of physical medicine and rehabilitation and head track-and-cross-country-team physician at Stanford University in Palo Alto, California. For the most part, your muscle fibers shrink from lack of use. If you keep your muscle fibers healthy and busy by keeping up your exercise routines throughout life, sprains won't become an inevitable part of aging.

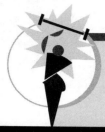

WOBBLE YOUR WAY TO WELLNESS

If you go to a physical therapist to rehabilitate a sprained ankle, you may eventually use something called a wobble board. Basically, it's a flat board that's glued to a round ball. With someone nearby to support you, you stand on top of it and try to keep your balance as the board moves under your feet.

This balance exercise helps strengthen the tendons and ligaments around your ankles, which prevents pain by keeping your bones aligned. The activity also helps speed up nerve connections so that you'll feel your foot turning and take corrective action sooner, preventing future sprains.

You can do a similar balancing act by taking yoga or tai chi, says Steve Cohen, a surgical physician assistant in orthopedics and assistant professor of physician assistant studies at Nova Southeastern University Medical Center in Fort Lauderdale. Both disciplines encourage you to stand on one foot a lot of the time, which is wonderful exercise for your ankle, he says. Once you can stand on one foot for a minute or longer, you are well on your way to strengthening the joint and limiting the potential for reinjury.

For Fast Relief

Pack it in ice as soon as possible. To reduce pain, you need to prevent swelling. Once the swelling sets in, it's difficult to get it to subside, says Dr. Fredericson. So your very first defense should be to ice your sore joint as soon as the injury occurs. Use gel ice packs, a bag of frozen vegetables, or a cup of frozen ice.

Wrap the ice pack in a thin towel and keep it on the injured area for 20 minutes. Remove it for 10 minutes and then ice the injury again for 20 minutes, suggests Steve Cohen, a surgical physician assistant in orthopedics and assistant professor of physician assistant studies at Nova Southeastern University Medical Center in Fort Lauderdale. Keep up this 20-minutes-on, 10-minutes-off icing regimen for as much as you can the first day. It will make a huge difference in the days to come.

For Lasting Relief

Wrap it up. During the first few days, keep the injured area wrapped in an elastic bandage as much as possible, especially while you are sleeping (and, therefore, not icing). This compression will give you some support if you need to walk around on a sprained foot or ankle. But it will also prevent pain by reducing the amount of fluid that accumulates in the area, says Dr. Fredericson. Be careful not to wrap the bandage too tightly—loosen it if your joint becomes painful or numb. Be especially careful when wrapping your knee.

Prop it up. Try to keep the injured joint higher than your heart by propping your leg up with pillows, for example, or wearing your arm in a sling, says Cohen. This will also keep fluid from accumulating.

Get better with bromelain. This isn't a drug; it's a natural anti-inflammatory enzyme found in the core of pineapples. You'd have to eat a lot of pineapple to get enough bromelain to help a sprain, though. For best results, get your bromelain in capsule form from a health food store. Take 200 to 300 milligrams three times a day on an empty stomach, says Andrew T. Weil, M.D., director of the program in integrative medicine at the University of Arizona College of Medicine in Tucson and author of *Spontaneous Healing* and *8 Weeks to Optimum Health*.

Rub some arnica on it. Arnica is a plant from western North America that is crushed and soaked in alcohol and made

RESISTANCE TRAIN YOUR FOOT

The following exercise can help you strengthen the muscles around your ankle to rebuild your joint after an injury and to prevent future sprains, says Rochel Rittgers, head athletic trainer and director of the sports-medicine curriculum at Augustana College in Rock Island, Illinois. Once you can do 15 to 20 repetitions of this exercise in all four directions, you can safely advance to less ankle-friendly sports like walking, bowling, and tennis.

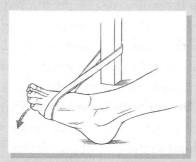

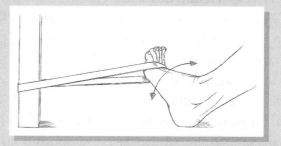

Readjust your foot in the tubing so you can press your foot from side to side.

Sit down close to something stable, such as a heavy table. Take rubber tubing (many sporting goods stores carry it) and wrap it around the ball of your injured foot. Hook the other end of the tubing around the leg of the heavy table. Push the ball of your foot forward, relax, and repeat.

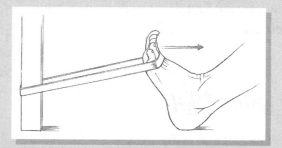

Finally, readjust the tubing to pull backward, toward your body.

into a cream. Sold at health food stores and in some drugstores, this herbal cream may relieve pain, especially while you are sleeping and unable to ice your sprained joint, Dr. Weil says.

Move it. If you've sprained a joint before, a doctor may have put you in a cast or had you use crutches for a few weeks. No more. Treatment recommendations have changed over the years. As long as you haven't fractured a bone, you want to start using the injured joint as soon as possible. Just be sure to check with your doctor first. "The earlier you start rehabilitating it, the better," says Dr. Fredericson.

Start with moving your joint in the widest circles you can, says Rochel Rittgers, head athletic trainer and director of the sports-medicine curriculum at Augustana College in Rock Island, Illinois. If it's your ankle that's sprained, you can make things interesting by using your big toe to trace the letters of the alphabet.

PAIN PREVENTERS

Curl a towel. Once the swelling has gone down, you want to strengthen the muscles near the joint to prevent future sprains and to encourage your bones to stay aligned. If you've sprained an ankle, one of the easiest exercises you can do early on is a towel curl, says Rittgers. Sit in a chair and place a towel flat on the floor, just in front of your bare feet. Then use your toes to drag the towel bit by bit under your feet. Repeat until your feet and lower leg muscles get tired.

Pick up marbles. In addition to the towel curl, you can also strengthen your foot and ankle muscles with this little exercise. Pour a bunch of marbles or other small objects on to the floor. Sit in a chair and use your toes to pick up the marbles and place them in a bucket one by one, says Rittgers.

Sunburn

It seems like it ought to be a divine right of older men and women. After decades of hard work, you deserve a literal place in the sun. There's a reason southern and Pacific states are filled with retirees. The warm weather and hot sun feel wonderful, loosening stiff joints, taking the ache out of your bones.

But as wonderful as the sun feels, you know it's possible to get too much of a good thing. Sun that felt so good during the day may come back to haunt you by nightfall, as your skin starts to redden and all the signs of sunburn start to make themselves known.

Sunburn is caused by overexposure of the skin to the ultraviolet rays of the sun or a sunlamp. The symptoms do not begin until 2 to 4 hours after the damage has been done. The peak reaction of redness, pain, and swelling is not seen for 24 hours, and prolonged sun exposure can cause blistering.

Some may think it a small price to pay for a day in the sun, but over time sunburn can lead to some serious problems. A history of sunburns is associated with an increased risk of skin cancer. So first, here is some advice from the experts on what to do to ease your current pain, followed by some tips to ensure that next time you won't get caught with your sunscreen down.

For Fast Relief

Try some tea bags. If your arms, legs, or face is sunburned, you can ease the pain with a couple of tea bags and an old wash-cloth or towel, says Sheila Roit, R.N., a spokesperson for the American Nurses Association in Washington, D.C. Heat 2 to 3 cups of water until it reaches a tepid (not boiling) temperature of about 90°F. Add two regular tea bags to the water once it has been heated; let it steep for 10 minutes. Herb tea does not work since it does not contain the necessary tannic acid found in regular tea. Moisten the towel or washcloth with the tepid tea water and apply the damp towel directly to the burned area for about 10 minutes. You may remoisten the towel and reapply two or three times.

"The tannic acid in the tea will combine with the enzymes that your skin produces when it is burned, and you'll get some instant relief," Roit says.

For Lasting Relief

Apply a compress. Following a burn, your skin is inflamed. Try cooling it down with a cold-water compress. Fill a sink with cold water from the faucet and add a few ice cubes if the water isn't cool enough to provide relief to your burning skin, says Roit. Dip a cloth into the cold water and lay it over the burn. Repeat every few minutes as the cloth warms. Apply the compresses several times a day for 15 minutes at a time.

Take a bath. As an alternative to compresses, especially for larger burned areas, Roit suggests throwing ¼ cup of baking soda into a tepid bath. Then, instead of drying off with a towel, let the baking soda dry on your skin. The baking soda will help your skin retain some of its moisture, which will help in the healing process.

Treat yourself to some aloe vera. Apply pure aloe vera to the sunburned area to ease the pain and to promote healing, says Andrew T. Weil, M.D., director of the program in integrative medicine at the University of Arizona College of Medicine in Tucson and author of *Spontaneous Healing* and *8 Weeks to Optimum Health*. Aloe plants can be purchased at most nurseries and are easy to grow.

To use the fresh plant to ease the pain of your sunburn, cut off a lower leaf, slicing close to the central stalk. Remove any spines along the edges, then split the leaf lengthwise. Score the gel with your knife and use your fingers to apply it to the burn. Do this as often as needed for the pain.

You can also use aloe products found in drugstores and health food stores. Read the label to determine the percentage of aloe gel before making your purchase.

Drink up. Older men and women are especially prone to losing fluids in warmer climates, and doubly so after getting sunburnt. So drink at least eight 8-ounce glasses of water per day after a sunburn to replace the fluids lost from the swelling of sunburned skin. Avoid caffeinated beverages like coffee, iced tea, or cola. "The caffeine in these drinks will actually further dehydrate you," says Roit. "And that may cause your skin to blister or may further aggravate the existing pain."

Make yourself a milk bath. Sitting in a bathtub containing 3 to 4 inches of cool water combined with a gallon of milk in a bathtub is still a widely recommended method of easing the soreness of sunburn, says Warren R. Heymann, M.D., professor of medicine and head of the division of dermatology for the Cooper Health System in Camden, New Jersey. Do this for 15 to 20 minutes several times per day. The protein in the milk acts as a soothing agent on the burnt skin.

PAIN PREVENTERS

Follow the rules. While the memory of the burn is still painfully fresh, brush up on your sun sense with these tips from Mona Saraiya, M.D., from the division of cancer prevention and control at the Centers for Disease Control and Prevention in Atlanta.

▶ About 30 minutes before going outdoors, generously apply a sunscreen with a sun protection factor (SPF) of at least 15. Reapply it frequently throughout the day, especially after swimming or exercise. Don't forget to protect your lips, hands, ears, and the back of your neck.

▶ Take extra care between the midday hours of 10:00 A.M. and 3:00 P.M. (11:00 A.M. to 4:00 P.M. during daylight savings time), when the sun is at its hottest and ultraviolet (UV) rays are at their strongest and most dangerous. Dr. Saraiya suggests that when you're outdoors during these peak hours, it is wise to seek shade under trees and beach umbrellas or in tents. Use these options to prevent a burn, not after you need relief. If you can't avoid the midday sun or find shade, at least try to take a break from the sun during the day.

▶ Use your head because not all sun protection comes in a bottle, says Dr. Saraiya. Wear a wide-brimmed hat to protect your face, ears, scalp, and neck from the sun's rays. A hat with a 4-inch brim provides the most protection. She warns that up to 80 percent of the most common skin cancers (known as non-melanoma skin cancers) occur on the head and neck. So if you choose a baseball cap, she also suggests that you use a sunscreen with an SPF of at least 15 to protect your exposed ears and neck.

To help shield your skin, wear protective clothing when you're enjoying your favorite outdoor activities. Melanomas, the deadliest skin cancers, occur most frequently on the trunk in males and the lower limbs in females. A shirt, a beach cover-up, or pants with a tight weave are all good choices for cover. Keep in mind, however, that a typical T-shirt has an SPF that is much lower than the recommended SPF 15. So add some shade or sunscreen—especially if your clothes don't completely cover your skin.

Grabbing a pair of sunglasses is more than cool, it's also the best way to protect your eyes from harmful UV rays. Sunglasses protect the tender skin around your eyes and reduce your risk of developing cataracts. For maximum protection, look for sunglasses that block both UVA and UVB rays.

Be aware of photosensitivity. Many prescription drugs don't mix well with prolonged exposure to sunshine, cautions Dr. Heymann. "Before taking a vacation to a warm-weather resort, check with your doctor to make sure that your medications won't make you more sensitive to sunlight."

Some everyday drugs that often cause such reactions, which are called photoreactions, include:

Tetracycline, quinolone, and sulfonamide (sulfa) antibiotics

Thiazide diuretics

Tricyclic antidepressants

Cancer-treatment drugs

Diabetes drugs taken orally

Certain high blood pressure drugs

Nonsteroidal anti-inflammatory drugs, generally in dosages used in the treatment of arthritis

Antiwrinkle creams and acne medications containing tretinoin (Retin-A)

Swimmer's Ear

You don't have to swim to get swimmer's ear.

In fact, you don't have to go anywhere near an ocean or pool. That's because swimmer's ear—also called otitis externa (a fancy medical term for an infection of your ear canal)—can arise from any type of moisture trapped inside your ear, whether it be drips from shower water or from a pool. It's called swimmer's ear because swimmers are more prone to the infection, for obvious reasons.

Germs love warmth, darkness, and moisture. At times—like right after a shower or a dip in a swimming pool—the small passageways in your ears provide all three ingredients. When water gets into your ears and doesn't drain out right away, these tiny germs multiply like crazy. This germ infestation first makes itself known with that telltale itch you can't quite scratch. But as the tissue in your ears swell, your ears will hurt like the dickens, and your hearing may become muffled.

Swimmer's ear is a common cause of ear pain. "It's very painful, especially if the infection has had time to set in. The ear canal can actually swell shut and totally cut off hearing," says James Reibel, M.D., assistant professor of otolaryngology at the University of Virginia Health Sciences Center in Charlottesville.

People over 60 are no more or no less prone to swimmer's ear than those younger. The only way to cure swimmer's ear is to see your doctor for prescription antibiotic ear drops. Without them, the infection may spread through your eardrum and inner ear. In rare cases, it can spread to the brain, causing partial paralysis of your face, especially in elderly people with diabetes, says Jack A. Shohet, M.D., assistant clinical professor of neurotology and skull-base surgery at the University of California, Irvine.

Meanwhile, you can try the following pain-relieving remedies.

For Fast Relief

Get cheeky with papaya. Papaya enzyme is a natural anti-inflammatory that can reduce swelling of your outer and inner ear, swiftly reducing pain. "The enzyme helps antibiotics penetrate an ear more effectively," says Murray Grossan, M.D., an otolaryngologist at Cedars-Sinai Medical Center in Los Angeles. You can buy chewable papaya-enzyme tablets at health food stores. Place a tablet between your cheek and gums while it dissolves. Do this one to four times a day until your symptoms clear.

For Lasting Relief

Use garlic and oil for more than pasta. Garlic is a natural germ fighter, says Andrew T. Weil, M.D., director of the program in integrative medicine at the University of Arizona College of Medicine in Tucson and author of *Spontaneous Healing* and *8 Weeks to Optimum Health*.

You can easily make your own garlic oil by crushing a few cloves into some olive oil and setting it aside in the refrigerator for a couple of days. To use it, strain the oil and warm it slightly in your hand. Then, using a medicine dropper, put a few drops in your hurting ear and loosely plug it with cotton. You can also buy garlic oil at your local health food store.

Try the mullein cure. This common weed, which can be purchased at health food stores, can help kill off a mild infection. Make an oil from it by steeping mullein flowers in olive oil for a few days. Strain any residue and then warm the oil in your hand. Use a medicine dropper to put a few drops in your ear, then loosely plug your ear with cotton, suggests Dr. Weil. You can also buy mullein oil or a combination garlic-mullein oil at health food stores.

Cool it down. Wrap a wet washcloth around a small bag of ice and place it on your ear for 20 minutes at a time. This will reduce swelling and pain, says Don R. Powell, Ph.D., founder and president of the American Institute for Preventive Medicine in Farmington Hills, Michigan.

Sit up while you sleep. Get some comfortable pillows and build yourself a nest in bed that will help you comfortably sleep upright. This will help the fluid that has built up around the infection in your ears to drain, reducing pain, says Dr. Powell.

Suck on hard candy. You've heard that sucking on hard candy or chewing gum can help with ear pain when you're on an airplane. The same can also help when you wake up in the middle of the night with pain from an ear infection. The facial muscles used to suck on the piece of candy or chew gum force air into your Eustachian tube, the canal that connects the middle ear to the throat. This action encourages the drainage of germs and fluid from your ear, says Dr. Powell.

PAIN PREVENTERS

Leave wax alone. If you can look beyond it's greasy, yellow, ugly appearance, you can learn to appreciate earwax for all its goodness. This natural anti-infective debris produced by your body provides a barrier to the germs that do make their way into your ears. It's good stuff. Leave it there and let it do its job.

Besides removing one of your body's natural defenses to germs, rooting through your ear with a cotton swab or other small-tipped device can cause small abrasions to the delicate skin inside your ear. These tiny nicks set up the perfect nesting ground for germs, explains Dr. Reibel. Trying to clean your ear can also push earwax far back into your ear, trapping water and letting an infection run rampant.

If you use cotton swabs to scratch an itchy inner ear, you probably don't have enough earwax. This leaves your skin dry and flaky—and more prone to swimmer's ear. Dr. Reibel suggests a better solution for itchy ears: Put a few drops of mineral or baby oil in your ears once a day. "More oil is not necessarily better," he cautions.

Cock your head to one side. Instead of using a cotton swab to dry out water stuck in your ear, simply turn your head to one side and lean it against a towel. Pull on your earlobe while your clench your jaw and the water should come right out, says Dr. Reibel.

Buy an over-the-counter solution. Products such as Swim Ear contain substances that will keep your ear dry. Use a few drops after swimming or showering, says Dr. Shohet.

Use your vinegar for more than salad dressing. Plain, cheap vinegar mixed in a one-to-one solution with distilled water will do the same thing as those store-bought ear drops, but it costs less money.

"This is the poor man's antibiotic," says Dr. Shohet. Vinegar creates an acidic environment that repels infec-tions. This solution will keep for a week. You should throw away any solution that remains.

Wear earplugs when wet. If you swim, Dr. Shohet recommends that you consider having the plugs custom-made by a hearing specialist, which will cost around $20. If you're a land lover who just needs to keep the water out of your ears while you shower, you can buy a few pairs of foam earplugs from the drugstore for less than $10.

Tongue Pain

You wouldn't think of the tongue as an area of your body that generates much in the way of pain. That is, until you're chewing along one day and accidentally bite it.

Bites, burns, and abrasions are all common tongue injuries that can be uncommonly painful at the moment they happen and for days afterward. Relief for most tongue pain is as close as your kitchen, however, says Louis Abbey, D.M.D., professor of oral pathology at Virginia Commonwealth University School of Dentistry in Richmond.

But there is another type of tongue pain—an incessant burning sensation—that's not so easy to resolve. Glossodynia, or burning tongue, afflicts mostly postmenopausal women over the age of 50 with an intense burning on different areas of the tongue. For some, it's the top, says Dr. Abbey; for others, the bottom or sides. Some patients report mild discomfort, but others experience an unquenchable fire that leaves them anxious, irritable, and in chronic pain.

If you have persistent burning-tongue pain that lasts for a number of weeks, see your family doctor, advises Roy S. Rogers III, M.D., professor of dermatology at the Mayo Clinic in Rochester, Minnesota. "Burning tongue can be a flag for several disorders," he says, such as anemia, a vitamin B_{12} deficiency, or Sjögren's syndrome, an autoimmune disease characterized by dryness in normally moist areas of the body.

Whatever pain has got your tongue, here are some ways to ease it.

FIGHT FIRE WITH FIRE

A fiery spice seems a strange remedy for extinguishing tongue pain, but using Tabasco sauce to reduce your pain may be the answer to your problems, says David Edelberg, M.D., founder of the American Whole Health Center in Chicago.

A drop or two of Tabasco sauce on your tongue can relieve burning-tongue syndrome by triggering a counterirritant effect, says Dr. Edelberg. Counterirritants enrage tissue on contact, distracting attention from the original irritation, he explains. Adding a little Tabasco to your food may inflame your tongue, but when the sensation abates, your burning-tongue syndrome will be less as well.

For Fast Relief

Go for the cold. Whether your tongue pain is caused by ill-fitting dentures, too-hot food, or an unknown ailment, sucking on ice chips may bring you immediate relief, says Dr. Abbey.

Ice numbs the pain and keeps your mouth moist, he says. Be sure to use ice chips rather than cubes, says Dr. Abbey, since you can easily move them around in your mouth, which will help avoid damaging the skin due to the ice sitting too long in one place. Hold them against the painful area as much as possible.

As an alternative to ice, you can hold cold low-fat yogurt or ice cream in your mouth for several minutes, says Dr. Abbey.

For Lasting Relief

Keep your mouth moist. People with burning tongue often have dry mouth as well, says Dr. Rogers, and the two conditions tend to make one another worse.

He suggests that you carry around a water bottle or make frequent trips to the water fountain. "Take a drink of water, swish it around to wet your whole mouth, then spit it out so you're not going to the bathroom all the time," advises Dr. Rogers.

There are also several over-the-counter preparations that moisten the mouth, like Optimoist and Oralbalance toothpaste.

Employ positive thinking. Many times, nothing physical can help patients with burning tongue, but there are some mental techniques that can help.

Dr. Abbey suggests meditation or positive thinking. Distraction therapy also helps. "Try to focus your attention on something else," he says. "By taking your mind off the pain, you thereby reduce it." Treat yourself to something you enjoy, something that you know will fully engage your attention—take yourself out to a funny movie or show, call your best friend or your grandchildren. The more engaging and distracting it is for you, the greater the chance it will minimize the pain.

Try flower power. To relieve tongue pain from injury like an abrasion or a bite, try tincture of calendula, suggests Dana Ullman, director of Homeopathic Educational Services in Berkeley, California, and coauthor, with Stephen Cummings, M.D., of *Everybody's Guide to Homeopathic Medicine.*

Calendula, also known as common marigold or pot marigold, has long been considered a valuable topical remedy for burns, bruises, cuts, and rashes.

Rinse your mouth with this tincture two or three times a day to stimulate natural healing, says Ullman.

PART FIVE

Pain Makers—
Chronic Illnesses

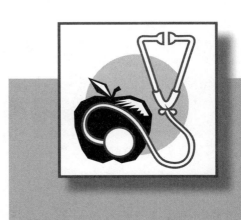

Easing the Pain of Illness

Let's face it. The longer you live, the greater your odds of developing chronic pain. It's the cost of doing time on this Earth.

Maybe you worked with your hands all your life, and now you have arthritis in your fingers. Perhaps that knee injury you got back in the war is acting up again on cold, damp days. Or perhaps you've developed a chronic disease such as diabetes, osteoarthritis, heart disease, or osteoporosis. Joints creak and nerves sometimes crackle with pain. You have your good days and your bad days.

That doesn't mean that you have to give in to the pain or give up all the activities you once enjoyed, says Frederick Goldstein, Ph.D., professor of clinical pharmacology at the Philadelphia College of Osteopathic Medicine.

"There is a tendency for people to get accustomed to pain. When they do that, they may develop a lifestyle around it, even though it means changing the way they want to live," says Dr. Goldstein. "It doesn't have to be that way. Pain can usually be dealt with in some way—first, with nondrug therapies and, only if necessary, with medications."

Of course, you're not always going to be able to rid yourself of all pain. Sometimes, you do just have to learn to live with some of it. And therein lies the sinister nature of chronic pain. Not only does it hurt often, it seems to sneak up on you. It endures.

The hurt may stem from an old injury. It made be due to an overwrought nervous system that keeps firing weeks, months, and even years later. Chronic pain can become a vicious circle. It adds to mental stress and keeps you away from the activities you love. Sometimes, it even recycles itself into more pain.

Pain can get you down, but it doesn't have to. You need to take control.

While discussing options with your doctor is a starting point, the management of chronic pain is ultimately in your hands. All the advice and therapies come to naught unless you're willing to take control.

What you will find in the following chapters is advice meant to help you take control of the most serious type of pain—the kind that comes from chronic health problems and illness. You'll learn about down-to-earth strategies and take-charge advice that allows you to work in complementary fashion with your doctor's recommendations.

"What you want to do is maximize the body's strength and healing power. And then if you still need medications, by all means use them," says Dr. Goldstein. "There's a lot that can be done to relieve pain. You don't have to give in to it and accept a lesser quality of life."

Blepharitis

Blepharitis describes an inflammation of the eyelids that's caused by a number of underlying conditions, among them, blocked glands, bacterial infections, dandruff, and an overproduction of oily substances in the skin. It's also called granulated eyelids because of the crusting and scaling that occurs along the margins of the lids.

But if you have it, you may know it by just one word: annoying.

Although it can become a chronic condition, blepharitis usually can be controlled by simple hygiene techniques in conjunction with some topical medication. It depends on which type of blepharitis you have, says David Kozart, M.D., an ophthalmologist at the University of Pennsylvania Health System in Philadelphia.

Staphylococcal blepharitis tends to occur more frequently in younger patients. It's caused by an infection of staph bacteria, a common bug on your skin.

When you're older, you're more likely to get seborrheic blepharitis. It occurs because the sebaceous glands around your eyes secrete too much sebum, an oily substance that moisturizes your skin. The sebum builds up and doesn't melt away. Instead, it crusts up and plugs small glands along your eyelids.

Chronic irritation from dandruff of the eyebrows and eyelashes are causes of seborrheic blepharitis. If you get blepharitis from this type of dandruff, you nearly always have dandruff of the scalp as well, says Edward Yu, M.D., an ophthalmologist at the Wilmer Eye Institute at John Hopkins University in Baltimore.

When you have meibomitis, another type of blepharitis, your eyelids tend to have an oily appearance and greasy deposits along the lashes and lid margins. The chronic irritation of the excess sebum leads to the inflammation, says Dr. Yu.

"In reality, there are different combinations of blepharitis types. One can sort of blend into the other," says Dr. Yu. "If you have blocked pores and crustiness, you may also tend to get a bacterial infection in the area."

Dry eyes, a very common condition with elderly patients, can make blepharitis worse. Dry eyes are characterized by lack of the tears that ordinarily lubricate the eyes. Sometimes, this dry up can happen on its own, or it may be caused by a number of diseases, including rheumatoid arthritis, says Dr. Kozart. "If you have dry eyes, you tend to rub your eyes. That mechanical irritation just makes matters worst. Your eyelids can get really inflamed from the irritation."

Although blepharitis is a condition that you can take care of yourself, you should see a doctor if your eyelids are red and have never been inflamed before, says Dr. Kozart. You could have an infection that may require a prescription antibiotic ointment or even an oral antibiotic.

Otherwise, the following tips may be all you need to control the inflammation and relieve most or all of the symptoms.

For Fast Relief

Loosen up the gunk. The key to easing the pain and irritation is to get the crusty buildup off your eyelids. The simplest, fastest way to do that is to soak a clean washcloth in warm water, wring it out, and place it across your closed eyes for about 5 minutes. Do it in the morning and again at night, instructs Dr. Yu. You should rinse the washcloth with clean water after use and replace it with a clean washcloth every 2 days. The warmth and moisture loosen up the oily materials, open up pores, and help wash the crust from the eyelashes and lid margins.

"You should do this every day on a long-term basis, not just as needed. That way, you'll be able to prevent a problem before it actually gets started," he says.

Be forewarned, though, that you may actually have more symptoms the first week or two of using compresses. That's because you're drawing or squeezing out more sebum, but eventually the condition should improve, says Dr. Yu.

For Lasting Relief

Shampoo your lids. Warm compresses can be used alone, but they are usually the first step of a self-treatment known as lid hygiene. Lid hygiene unplugs blocked ducts and cleans away any dandruff and oily debris, says Dr. Yu.

After you've taken off the compresses, mix up a dilute solution of water and baby shampoo—2 or 3 drops of shampoo to 3 ounces of water. Then, dip a cotton swab or cotton ball into the solution and gently scrub your eyebrows and lids for about 2 minutes. As you scrub, don't squeeze your lids tightly, but close them gently as if you were asleep, he says.

Next, look into a mirror and carefully scrub along your eyelashes and lid margins. It makes no difference if you brush horizontally or vertically, the idea is simply to loosen and remove the granular debris trapped in your eyelashes.

Afterward, rinse off with cool tap water and wipe your eyes clean with a fresh towel. You should do this twice a day, or more often if you have lots of crusting and dandruff accumulation.

"The shampoo acts like a mild detergent. It cleans up the oily materials that may be blocking the pores," says Dr. Yu.

"Make sure you pick a mild shampoo because some can cause more irritation and worsen the inflammation."

Make do without the makeup. Sometimes, blepharitis is the result of an allergic reaction to a substance: a cosmetic, hair spray, perfume, soap, or shampoo.

"We often see problems with women wearing mascara or eyeliner," says Dr. Kozart. "If you get any kind of rash or reaction, stop using the product." Or look for a hypoallergenic alternative.

Tear up. When your eyes can't make their own tears, you can get the artificial kind over the counter at the drugstore. These drops, generically known as artificial tears, act as lubricants.

If you have sensitive eyes or severe dryness and need to use tear supplements more than four times a day, you may want to examine the label of an artificial-tear product and choose a type that does not contain a preservative. Preservative-free tears are clearly labeled and come in small vials instead of bottles; however, their cost is higher. Some brands to look for include Tears Naturale and Refresh Drops. These can be used throughout the day as needed, says Dr. Yu.

Surprisingly, you can have dry eyes and still have a lot of tearing. That's because there are two tear-production systems in the eye. One, the basic tear, lubricates the eyes; the other is a reflex tear that is produced with irritation or emotion.

If you're deficient in basic tears and have dry eyes, you may still have a lot of reflex tears. In fact, the sensation of dryness often stimulates reflex tears. By using artificial tears, the irritation from dry eyes is eliminated and reflex tears are not produced. The common symptom of dry eyes is the sensation of a foreign object in the eye.

Wet the air. Dry eyes are more common during the winter months, when humidity is low, particularly within enclosed spaces like your home or automobile. Low humidity tends to dry out all mucous membranes, including the eyes, says Dr. Kozart.

During dry months, set out a pan of water or run a humidifier or vaporizer in your home and bedroom to get more moisture into the air. Also, when you're driving, don't direct the dry air coming out of your car vents directly at your face. "Better to leave the window open a crack or blow the air at your feet," he says.

Carpal Tunnel Syndrome

Knit one, purl two. Knit one, purl two.

Repeat 15,000 times a day—as you might if you were hand-knitting a sweater for a new grandbaby—and you may end up with clumsy fingers, pain that shoots up your arms, and a strange numbness or tingling in your hands that wakes you from sleep.

Knitters are notoriously at high risk for developing carpal tunnel syndrome, as are needlepointers, dairy farmers who milk by hand, musicians, and other folks who are involved in tasks that require repetitive motion.

Carpal tunnel syndrome is an injury that develops over time. It occurs when the median nerve in your wrist becomes compressed within the carpal tunnel, a narrow passageway formed by bones and a liga-

ment in the wrist. This tunnel also happens to be the passageway for the tendons of your fingers and thumb.

When you overuse these tendons, they can become swollen and inflamed. Surrounding tissue may swell with fluid, a process known as edema. All of this puts the big squeeze on the median nerve, which carries temperature, pain, and touch information between your hand and your brain.

"The swelling affects the nerve's conductivity. It slows down the velocity of signals and delays transmission," says Hubert Rosomoff, M.D., professor and chairman emeritus of the department of neurological surgery at the Comprehensive Pain and Rehabilitation Center at the University of Miami. "If you find yourself with a numbness and tingling in the thumb and first

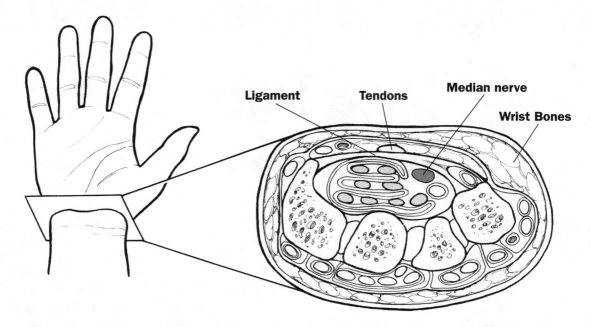

Ligament **Tendons** **Median nerve** **Wrist Bones**

When the tendons swell up in the already-crowded carpal tunnel of your wrist, squeezing your median nerve, pain and tingling is the result.

two fingers, you may be headed toward a serious problem."

Folks with carpal tunnel syndrome may be unable to unscrew bottle caps, turn keys, fasten buttons, or finger the change in their pockets and tell quarters from dimes.

Carpal tunnel often disappears with simple self-help treatments such as rest, exercise, and proper body mechanics. If the problem persists for more than a week, however, you should see a doctor. As a last resort, there are surgical methods to relieve pressure on the nerve, Dr. Rosomoff says.

For Fast Relief

Chill out. When your wrist is painful, swollen, and inflamed, ice is the great equalizer, says Dr. Rosomoff.

Cold shrinks the swollen tendons and tissues surrounding the median nerve, thus relieving some of the pressure. Because cold also slows down and deadens the pain messages being pumped out by the irritated nerves, you get some fast pain relief, he says.

What you want to avoid, however, is putting pressure on the median nerve while icing your wrist. You don't want to rest a heavy bag of ice on your wrist or strap on an ice pack with an elastic bandage.

Instead, rest the back of your hand on a table, place a thin cotton towel over your skin, and set a small plastic bag of crushed or slushy ice on the inside of your covered wrist. To make the ice even colder and thus more able to penetrate to the nerve, add a couple of spoonfuls of rubbing alcohol to the mix, he says.

Most people don't leave ice on long enough so that the cold penetrates to the nerve, says Dr. Rosomoff. He recommends a minimum of 30 minutes, and longer is better.

For Lasting Relief

Stop what you're doing. If possible, temporarily avoid the trauma that is causing pain by refraining from activities that aggravate your wrist, says Lisa Wolford, a physical therapist assistant at the Pain and Rehabilitation Clinic of Chicago.

That may mean taking a few days off from painting, woodworking, or knitting. Or, you may be able to simply take frequent breaks that include stretching activities and avoid overusing the tendons, she says.

Splint it. Bending your wrist puts pressure on the median nerve. If it's already inflamed and painful, that's the last thing you need to do.

To keep your wrist straight, use plastic or aluminum splints. The splints hold your hands in a neutral position—essentially straight—so there's no pressure on the nerve. Although splints may limit your wrist movements, you can still use your fingers, says Dr. Rosomoff.

You can buy splints off the shelf at a drugstore or medical supply store. It may be better, however, to get them fitted by a physical or occupational therapist to make sure that you're immobilizing the joint and getting a proper fit, says Wolford.

"It's a good idea to wear them at night so you don't bend your wrists while you're sleeping," she says. "Depending on the severity of the problem, you can wear them during the day, too."

Squeeze for strength. As the pain lessens, slowly resume activities and begin stretching activities. For example, squeeze a tennis ball, a sponge, or a hunk of clay to

TENDON TAMERS

Here are some stretches that experts recommend you do to warm up and loosen your tendons before you start doing repetitive work with your hands. You can also do these stretches intermittently while you're working. It's important to do these stretches after completing the activity as well.

Wrist flexion. Hold your right arm out in front of you at shoulder height, with your palm down. Keep your elbow straight, but not locked. Place the fingers of your left hand across the front of the fingers of your right hand and slowly bend your right wrist by pulling up and back on your fingers. Hold for 20 to 30 seconds. You'll feel the stretch in the front of your wrist. Do two or three repetitions. Then, repeat with your left hand.

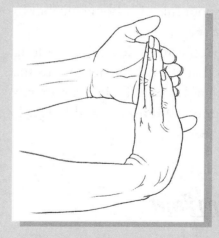

build up the grip and flexor muscles in your affected arm, suggests Wolford.

If you have been inactive on account of the pain of carpal tunnel, your arm muscles probably have weakened from disuse. By building stronger upper-arm and forearm muscles, you may make your carpal tunnel less likely to recur, she says.

Start off by squeezing the ball 20 times twice a day. "You can do it while you're watching television or reading," she says. Let pain be your guide. If your wrist is still hurting, stop squeezing.

Wrist extension. Hold your right arm out in front of you at shoulder height, with your palm down. Relax your wrist so that your fingers point down. Keep your elbow straight, but not locked. Place your left hand across the back of the fingers of your right hand and pull toward your body, slowing bending your wrist down. Hold for 20 to 30 seconds. Do two or three repetitions. Then, repeat with your left hand. If this stretch causes pain, avoid it.

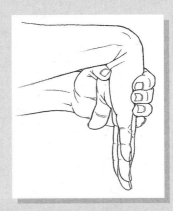

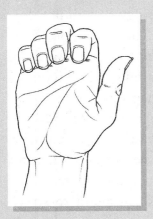

Tendon glides. Hold your right hand upright in a neutral position, with your hand open and in line with your arm and your palm facing toward you. Slowly fold in your fingers and make a fist, keeping your thumb immobile. Hold for 10 to 20 seconds. Return to the open palm position and repeat 10 times. You'll feel the stretch in the front of your wrist. Then, repeat with your left hand.

Straighten up. Use proper body mechanics, and you will decrease the likelihood that you will get carpal tunnel syndrome. In the case of this condition, proper body mechanics means keeping your wrist straight while doing an activity, says Wolford.

It may seem strange at first, but eventually, you can train yourself to hold a tool like a knife or a knitting needle in a way that does not bend your wrist and compress the nerve. "It's a matter of maintaining that neutral position," she says. "If you do it often enough, it becomes second nature."

Fibromyalgia

In people who have fibromyalgia, what hurts are the fibrous tissues of their bodies—muscles, ligaments, tendons, and fasciae (the sheets of connective tissue). People with fibromyalgia often have difficulty sleeping and may barely have sufficient energy to make it through the day.

Typically, lab tests show nothing wrong, but some poking around reveals tenderness at specific points of the body. These points may include the inside edges of the shoulder blades, the base of the head, the outer forearms just below the elbows, and the insides of the knees—places that don't usually hurt from simple wear and tear.

Some researchers think that the problem is related to pain neurochemicals, says I. Jon Russell, M.D., Ph.D., of the section of rheumatology and clinical immunology at the University of Texas Health Science Center at San Antonio. Researchers have found elevated levels of spinal fluid substance P, a kind of pain amplifier; lower-than-normal levels of serum serotonin, a biochemical that helps to regulate pain and sleep/wake cycles; and low production of cortisol, a hormone that helps our bodies respond to stress. Other findings include changes in energy metabolism in red blood cells and muscle cells, he says.

Conventional medicine is not all that helpful for this condition, says Terry Grossman, M.D., a doctor practicing in Lakewood, Colorado. But there are some nonconventional ways to manage the pain of fibromyalgia.

For Fast Relief

Sip ginger tea. Ginger is a good alternative to aspirin to relieve minor aches and pains, says Andrew T. Weil, M.D., director of the program in integrative medicine at the University of Arizona College of Medicine in Tucson and author of *Spontaneous Healing* and *8 Weeks to Optimum Health*. Steep 1 teaspoon of the grated root in 8 ounces of hot water for 10 minutes. Strain and add honey, if you like. You also can try taking, with food, 1,000 to 2,000 milligrams of powdered ginger a day in capsule form, he says.

For Lasting Relief

Take a few deep breaths. There is a direct connection between how you breathe and the amount of tension you hold in your body, says Caron Goode, Ed.D., codirector of the International Breath Institute in Boulder, Colorado. When you're feeling stress, your muscles tighten, and your breath becomes shallow and faster. That actually changes the ratio of gases in your bloodstream, which can contribute to more muscle tension and, consequently, more fibromyalgia-related pain. Taking full, deep, slower breaths reverses the stress response and helps muscles to relax.

Sit up straight, loosen your clothes if necessary, and exhale fully, emptying your lungs. On this full exhale, your breathing muscles pull in tight under your rib cage and sternum. Then, inhale fully, filling your abdomen with air, like a balloon. Expand your breath into your rib cage. Focus on your breathing and let your thoughts drift away. Do this for a few minutes whenever you feel muscle tension beginning to build, Dr. Goode suggests.

Find pain relief at your fingertips. If specific tender points are particularly painful, you can use acupressure to help calm them down, says Joseph Carter, a licensed acupuncturist and acupressurist, and an instructor at the Acupressure Institute in Berkeley, California. Simply find the spot with your fingertips and press, gradually increasing the pressure. The spot may initially feel sore, but within a few seconds, the pain should start to ease off, and you will actually feel the muscle relax, he says. For hard-to-reach places on your back, you can lie down and roll your back on a tennis ball.

Mind your magnesium and malic acid. Some people with fibromyalgia have found that taking daily doses of 500 milligrams of magnesium and 2,000 milligrams of malic acid reduces their fatigue and exhaustion at the end of an active day, says Dr. Russell. With the extra malic acid and magnesium, they can handle exercise and still get out and about the next day. "That suggests that the combination is helping their bodies handle physiologic stress better," he says. "I know of no one with fibromyalgia who has tried it with effective doses who isn't continuing it."

People with heart or kidney problems should check with their doctors before taking supplemental magnesium.

Get aerobic. In several studies, aerobic exercise—the kind that makes you sweat and breathe hard—has provided relief for people with fibromyalgia. Exercise was found to raise serotonin levels, which probably contributes to its benefits, Dr. Russell says.

Many people with fibromyalgia are seriously out of shape and may need to start working out at a snail's pace. Dr. Russell has people start with as little as 5 to 15 minutes every other day, working up to 20 minutes every other day. The every-other-day routine was designed to allow time for muscle repair. "People with fibromyalgia have low levels of growth hormone that helps to repair the muscles we all injure

during exercise," he explains. "They need a longer time to recover."

Dr. Russell recommends low-impact water walking. "I tell them to get into a swimming pool with the water level to their upper chest and then walk, moving their arms and legs against the resistance of the water." If you don't have access to a pool, riding an exercise bike and walking are reasonable substitutes.

Be kneaded. A study of people with fibromyalgia done by the Touch Research Institute at the University of Miami School of Medicine found that those who got 30 minutes of massage two times a week for 5 weeks had less anxiety and depression and lower levels of stress hormones, and over time they reported less pain and stiffness, less fatigue, and less trouble sleeping.

Take a good multivitamin/mineral supplement. In addition to magnesium, many vitamins and minerals play crucial roles in energy metabolism, Dr. Grossman says. They also are important for the body's production of hormones. Look for a multi that offers the full Daily Value of the B vitamins, 200 to 400 IU of vitamin E, 500 milligrams or more of vitamin C, and important trace minerals like selenium, manganese, and zinc.

Add in some oils. The fats that we consume determine whether our bodies make inflammatory or anti-inflammatory prostaglandins, which are hormonelike substances. Eating fatty fish like salmon or mackerel or taking fish-oil capsules shifts our bodies' production toward anti-inflammatory prostaglandins, which may be helpful for people with fibromyalgia, Dr. Grossman says. You can eat fish a few times a week, or you can take two to four 120-milligram fish-oil capsules a day. Do not take this supplement if you have a bleeding disorder or uncontrolled high blood pressure, if you take anticoagulants (blood thinners) or use aspirin regularly, or if you are allergic to any kind of fish.

Zero in on enzymes. Certain enzymes that break down protein, called proteolytic enzymes, can also help to reduce inflammation because they also direct the body to produce anti-inflammatory prostaglandins, Dr. Grossman says. You can find these enzymes in pill form at drugstores and nutrition stores. They include papain and rutin, amylase, lipase, trypsin, and chymotrypsin, often in combinations of "multi-enzyme" capsules. These capsules should be taken on an empty stomach for optimum anti-inflammatory effect. "You can take from three to five capsules three times a day," he suggests.

Gallbladder Pain

There are two ways people become aware of their gallstones. Sometimes, a doctor performs an ultrasound or x-ray diagnostic test for another condition and discovers stones in the gallbladder. Not to worry, though. Most of these are probably asymptomatic gallstones that rarely cause any significant problem.

In fact, 16 million to 22 million people have gallstones, with people over 60 at a higher risk of developing them than younger people. "Most gallstones are silent. Most people never know they have one," says Roger Gebhard, M.D., a gastroenterologist and professor of medicine at the University of Minnesota in Minneapolis.

The other way you learn about gallstones is when they make you sick—and they can make you very sick when a stone obstructs the ducts that carry bile to and from the gallbladder.

The mildest form of gallbladder disease is biliary colic, a cramping pain in the upper abdomen that usually occurs in the evening, several hours after eating. Sometimes accompanied by vomiting, it typically lasts just a few hours or overnight.

The cause is probably a stone lodged in the duct exiting the gallbladder. Bile flow is interrupted, so tension builds up in the gallbladder. Usually, when the stone falls back into the gallbladder or passes further along the system, the tension lessens and the pain eases. Because the stone is still in your system, however, you may get other attacks.

If the biliary attacks are prolonged and frequent, the gallbladder may become inflamed. "In that case, your pain is not as vague. It's much sharper and more localized," says Dr. Gebhard. "You push near the rib cage, and it's tender."

Along with the inflammation and pain, you may have an infection, fever, and chills. "This is potentially a much more serious condition. You ought to be seeing a physician," he says.

Finally, if a stone blocks the main bile duct, your entire liver may become involved. Then, bile can't flow at all. Not only will you have fairly severe pain, the whites of your eyes may yellow with jaundice.

"If you get jaundice, you need to get to an emergency room. This could lead to a life-threatening condition," says Dr. Gebhard. "You may need to have the bile duct drained or the gallbladder removed."

Nearly all gallstones consist of cholesterol, the same fat that can clog arteries. Not surprisingly, you're more likely to get gallstones if you're overweight and eat a high-fat diet. You also have a greater chance if you're female, particularly if you've ever been pregnant—even decades ago.

Once you have gallstones, there isn't much you can do about them—except to hope they stay put and never cause you pain. Severe pain or repeated attacks of pain are signs that you should see your doctor. But there may be ways to ease the discomfort of biliary colic and perhaps prevent stones from forming in the first place.

For Fast Relief

Eat beet greens. Beet greens contain betaine, a substance that stimulates the production of bile. It also thins the bile and makes it flow more easily, says William Warnock, N.D., a naturopathic physician in Shelburne, Vermont.

"Betaine gets the gallbladder to contract and gets bile flowing. It really moves things along." He recommends steaming the greens to retain the vitamin A, minerals, and betaine. Eat ½ cup of beet greens a day during a flare-up.

"I've had patients get really effective relief from gallbladder pain with beet greens," he says. "It works."

For Lasting Relief

Don't pig out. Want to avoid that queasy, achy pain of a gallbladder attack? Then avoid high-fat meals. Although it has not been proven scientifically, the traditional advice that doctors give to gallstone

GALLBLADDER SURGERY: A KINDER CUT

Having your gallbladder out used to be a big deal.

When Lyndon Johnson had his removed in 1965, his recovery was so painful that he cut back his schedule at the White House for several weeks. One day, he shocked his aides but delighted news photographers by hiking up his shirt to display a long, ugly scar running across his belly.

If Johnson were showing off gallbladder scars today, he probably wouldn't have much to show, and he would be back at his desk within days, not weeks, says Roger Gebhard, M.D., a gastroenterologist and professor of medicine at the University of Minnesota in Minneapolis.

It's not that gallbladder surgery has become routine, but laparoscopic techniques—inserting instruments into small holes punched into the abdomen—have made it much less

patients is to lower the amount of fat in their diets, says Dr. Gebhard.

"It makes good sense. Don't pig out on a fatty meal," he says. "It seems that biliary colic often comes on after a rich, high-fat meal."

Fiber up. Many alternative medical practitioners believe that the best defense against gallstones probably lies with diet. Cut back on the fat and add more fiber, advises Kristin Stiles, N.D., a naturopathic physician at the Complementary Medicine and Healing Arts Center in Vestal, New York.

Fiber absorbs lots of water and helps to bulk up the stool. A well-hydrated stool absorbs many of the by-products of digestion, including a small amount of fat, says Dr. Gebhard.

You can increase dietary fiber by eating

painful and invasive. On most patients, there's no need for doctors to do the major surgery that people used to undergo. The new techniques are much less painful to recover from simply because the doctor makes several small punctures rather than a big incision, says Dr. Gebhard. "Usually, you're out of the hospital in just a day or two."

During the procedure, which is known as a laparoscopic cholecystectomy, the surgeon pumps in a gas to expand the abdominal cavity, inserts a scope to watch the operation on a video screen, and manipulates the surgical instruments—clamps and lasers—through a couple of other holes. The surgeon snips off the gallbladder, seals off bleeding, and pulls out the diseased organ. The doctor may also look for stones in nearby ducts and remove them if necessary, says Dr. Gebhard. It may not be the most natural or drug-free way to ease pain, but if you do ever need gallbladder surgery, this is the most painless way to have it.

more fruits and vegetables, bran, and whole grains like wheat, brown rice, millet, barley, quinoa, and oats.

Lose weight gradually. If you're obese, you're more likely to get gallstones. Watch your weight and slim down if necessary, says Dr. Gebhard.

If you're going to diet, make sure you use a sensible program designed to decrease weight very gradually. Rapid weight loss and extremely low fat diets have been linked to the formation of gallstones.

Here's why: When you lose weight, you draw cholesterol out of tissues where it has been stored during the weight gain. That extra cholesterol concentrates in bile, where it can crystallize and precipitate out as a stone.

"Cholesterol is not very soluble, and it doesn't take much to upset the balance in the bile," says Dr. Gebhard. "You put more cholesterol into the bile, and you quickly overwhelm its carrying capacity."

Let's say you're losing that weight by denying yourself fat. Unless you're eating some fat, there isn't much reason for your gallbladder to contract and release bile. Bile is what breaks down fat and removes the excess from the body.

With an extremely low fat diet, bile just sits there—in stasis—so there's a greater chance of it crystallizing and forming a stone, says Dr. Gebhard.

"If you're not contracting the gallbladder, you're not washing out those little crystals," he says. "The moral is don't try to keep all the fat out of your diet. You need some for the gallbladder to work." He suggests eating 8 to 10 grams of fat per meal, about the same as in a tablespoon of butter.

Don't smoke. Some studies show that smoking may be associated with gallstone formation, says Dr. Gebhard. "This is an easy piece of advice. Don't smoke."

Supplement with lecithin. Dr. Stiles sometimes recommends taking a nutritional substance called lecithin, or phosphatidylcholine. Lecithin occurs naturally in the body and in bile, where it helps make cholesterol mix more easily with water.

Some naturopaths believe that people with low levels of lecithin are more prone to forming stones, because their bodies are not breaking down and removing the fat, she says. If you supplement with lecithin, you may improve the solubility of cholesterol.

"Lecithin won't dissolve the stones you may already have, but it may help prevent any new ones from forming," says Dr. Stiles. She recommends taking between 500 and 1,000 milligrams in capsules or 1 to 2 teaspoons of granulated lecithin daily over a period of several months. You can also get lecithin from soybeans, wheat germ, and peanuts.

Contract the gallbladder. Milk thistle is an herb with a long folk history of improving digestion, particularly of fats. It's alleged to have chloretic properties—meaning, it stimulates gallbladder contraction and bile flow.

Boost the flow of the bile, and you may flush out small crystals and "gravel" before they become a problem. Milk thistle can help dissolve certain types of stones, says Dr. Warnock. Be aware, though, that you may have to take the herb for 3 to 6 months before it has a beneficial effect.

Look for a standardized extract that contains 80 percent silymarin, the primary active ingredient in milk thistle, says Dr. Warnock. Depending on the concentration of the product you buy, the dosage may range from 70 to 210 milligrams per day.

Inflammatory Bowel Disease (IBD)

Inflammatory bowel disease (IBD) describes two similar but distinct conditions: Crohn's disease and ulcerative colitis. Though different, these diseases share many of the same symptoms, including abdominal pain, cramping, fatigue, and diarrhea.

Crohn's disease is an inflammation that can occur anywhere in your gastrointestinal tract. Often, the inflammation, which can penetrate all layers of bowel tissue, occurs in patches in between sections of healthy tissue. Ulcerative colitis affects only your colon and the inner lining of the colon tissue. Both diseases can be controlled by medication. In severe cases, diseased tissue may need to be removed through surgery.

Other types of bowel inflammation may also occur because of allergies, bacteria, parasites, and even stress, says Ron Parks, M.D., a specialist in complementary and nutritional medicine at St. Vincent Hospital in Indianapolis. "Or your immune system may be weakened to the point that you can't fight off parasites and bacteria."

If you suspect that you have IBD, or if you have any change in bowel habits, you obviously want to be seen and correctly diagnosed by a doctor. You may be prescribed anti-inflammatory drugs and, perhaps, antibiotics to clear any infections. During flare-ups of IBD, you can control some of the pain and discomfort you'll feel.

For Fast Relief

Combine heat and massage for abdominal aching. Some people with abdominal discomfort feel better when they apply warmth and light massage to their aching midsections, says Alison Lee, M.D., a pain-management specialist in Ann Arbor, Michigan.

Dr. Lee recommends a *qigong* (Chinese) massage technique in which you lightly press your fingers on the skin of your abdomen. "You make clockwise rotations out from the navel," she instructs. "Sometimes, you barely touch the skin."

Other people prefer the same motion but find more relief with greater pressure, she says. For warmth, you can use a hot-water bottle wrapped in a thin towel or a warm compress. Neither should be hot, just warm.

For Lasting Relief

Keep your flora in check. Sometimes, your bowel becomes inflamed when over-populated by the wrong bacteria or yeast. "It's a common side effect of taking antibiotic medication. You kill off the bad bacteria with the medications, but then you upset the balance of flora (bacteria) in the bowel," says Dr. Parks.

Dr. Lee concurs. After a course of antibiotics, which are sometimes needed for an IBD problem, she tells her patients to repopulate the good bacteria in the gut by taking an acidophilus supplement, available in health food stores and drugstores. Usually, a dose of 1-billion- to 10-billion-active-organism count per day is enough to colonize the gut, she says. But because the concentration of each product is different, the best thing to do is to simply follow the directions on the bottle. She suggests taking the supplement for 2 to 4 weeks after the antibiotic treatment.

Dr. Lee says that some acidophilus preparations may be bothersome to people with lactose intolerance or milk allergy. If you have one of these conditions, check product labels carefully and purchase supplements that are specially formulated to be less irritating to milk-sensitive people.

Calm with ginger. If nausea accompanies your pain and abdominal distress, you can treat it with ginger. Shred about a teaspoon of fresh gingerroot and steep it in hot water for 3 to 5 minutes to make ginger tea, says Dr. Lee. Drink the tea as needed.

"Fresh ginger is better than dried because it contains compounds that may be removed during the drying process," she says.

Fight inflammation with flax. Your body knows how to fight inflammation, but it needs all the help it can get. Dr. Parks suggests taking a daily dose of 1 tablespoon of flaxseed oil or three to six 500-

milligram capsules of fish oil, rich in omega-3 fatty acids. Both of these supplements improve your body's ability to reduce swelling and inflammation. He says that you can take these supplements for as long as they are helpful.

Some individuals may also need to supplement their diets with other beneficial fats such as omega-6, found in evening primrose oil or borage oil. Talk to your doctor before starting this program, especially if you are on blood thinners. People with diabetes should not take fish oil because of high fat content.

Ease gut problems with glutamine. Glutamine, an amino acid supplement, has some beneficial effects on the intestines, says Dr. Lee, who recommends it to patients with irritable bowel syndrome. It seems to accelerate the healing of lesions and ulcers.

"You can take 500 milligrams per day for as long as you want," she says. "Or you might consider just eating more plants from the cabbage family. These are also rich in glutamine." You can also find glutamine supplements in most health food stores.

Press the point. Acupressure not only helps with pain and discomfort associated with IBD, it may normalize gastric acid levels in your stomach and other gastrointestinal functions, says Dr. Lee. The point known as Stomach 36 (ST36) is especially helpful.

To locate it, travel four finger-widths below your kneecap and one finger-width to the outside of your shinbone. ST36 lies where you feel a large depression. If you are at the correct spot, you should feel tension in the muscle as you move your foot up and down.

"It's a large point, but deep. You can try pressing in with your finger, but to get the full effect, you probably need to percuss the point—meaning, lightly tap it," says Dr. Lee. Tap the point lightly with the side of your fist 10 to 30 times, or until you feel a radiating sensation down your leg. Do this three to five times a day.

PAIN PREVENTERS

Avoid fat. Some studies have suggested that if you eliminate meat, refined carbohydrates, and saturated fats from your diet, you may be able to reduce your IBD pain. Saturated fats may actually add support to the inflammatory pathways in your body, Dr. Parks says.

Kidney Stones

Unless you've had a kidney stone before the age of 60, it's unlikely you'll ever get one.

Most people get their first stones by their forties and have a 50 percent chance of developing more stones within 10 years. The propensity for forming kidney stones tends to run in families but also can be the result of chronic dehydration or an intestinal illness. Men are three to four times more likely than women to form stones.

If you've had a kidney stone already, you know that there is nothing quite like it in terms of pain, so we won't belabor the point. Suffice it to say, the pain is extreme and usually comes on very suddenly as the stone leaves your kidney and begins its descent down your urinary tract. In addition to the pain, you also may have blood in your urine and severe nausea, says Greg Downer, M.D., a nephrologist at West Michigan Nephrology in Muskegon.

"The pain is mostly in the flank, but it can extend further down into the genital area," he says. For this kind of pain, you'll likely be prescribed heavy pain medications.

Other than drinking a lot of fluids, there really isn't much you can do except wait for a kidney stone to pass. That usually occurs within about 48 hours. Depending on its size and shape, the stone may pass on its own, or the doctor may need to intervene, using surgical tools to snare it or shock waves (lithotripsy) to break it into smaller, easier-to-pass chunks.

There are four types of stones: calcium, uric acid, struvite, and cystine. The vast majority—about 80 percent—are the calcium kind.

These stones form because you have

too much calcium in your urine. No one really knows why except that some people have that tendency. If the urine is laden with calcium salts, they can crystallize and eventually form a stone.

Although you can't do much about a stone once you have one, there are some prevention strategies. Here are suggestions for avoiding the formation of calcium stones.

For Lasting Relief

Drink up. No matter what type of stone you're prone to form, you should drink 8 to 12 glasses (8 ounces each) of fluid every day. At least half of this volume should be plain old water, says Dr. Downer.

Fluids, especially water, reduce the concentration of minerals in your urine so they have less of an opportunity to form a stone, he says. Also, if you're in the throes of passing a stone, a high fluid intake can help.

Try to spread your fluid intake out over the entire day, he says. Drink a glass of water at each meal, between meals, before bed, and during the night if you wake up to urinate. That way, you keep your urine from concentrating minerals. To judge if you're drinking enough, watch the color of your urine. It should be pale, nearly watery. If it is dark and yellow, drink more.

"Maintaining a high fluid intake around the clock is the single most important thing that you can do to protect yourself from kidney stones," says Steven Scheinman, professor and chief of nephrology at the State University of New York Health Science Center in Syracuse.

Catch the stone. You'll need to know exactly what kind of stone you have to prevent them in the future. Urinate into a strainer or cup with a mesh bottom fine enough to catch sand, and save any bits of stone you may excrete. Have the doctor send them off for analysis, says Dr. Downer. Any stone that is small enough to pass on its own is going to measure less than 5 millimeters, or about one-half the width of your little finger.

Drink milk. Forget that old wives' tale about not drinking milk if you're prone to kidney stones, says Dr. Scheinman. Once, that seemed like a good idea because most stones are made up of calcium, but it was later found that less milk or calcium in your diet actually increases your risk for forming stones.

Here's why. Calcium in your diet binds with oxalate and keeps you from absorbing oxalate from your food. Oxalate is a substance present in many fruits and vegetables that binds with calcium and becomes insoluble. The more oxalate that binds with calcium, the less you'll have in your urine. "So drinking milk can actually protect you from kidney stones," he says. It doesn't have to be milk. You can also eat cheese, yogurt, and other dairy products.

Go on a diet. You may want to consider cutting back or eliminating oxalate-rich foods from your diet. These include spinach, chocolate, nuts, rhubarb (late in the season), tea, all berries, darker lettuce such as Romaine, and many fruits, such as bananas, grapefruits, and oranges.

Supplement with magnesium. Magnesium binds with calcium salts and makes it more likely that they will stay in your system rather than forming stones, says Dr. Downer. He recommends taking 250 milligrams of magnesium per day.

Try B$_6$ to reduce oxalates. If dietary restrictions don't bring down the amount of oxalate in the urine, Dr. Scheinman tells people to take 100 to 200 milligrams per day of vitamin B$_6$. There are no conclusive studies that this is effective, but it does appear that B$_6$ can reduce oxalate, he says. Doses above 100 milligrams, however, must be taken under medical supervision.

Restrict your salt intake. When your kidneys excrete salt, that raises the amount of calcium in your urine and makes it more likely that you'll form a stone. So if your doctor tells you that you have too much calcium in your urine, avoid salt.

"If you eat less salt, you'll retain more calcium, and more will be available for your bones," says Dr. Scheinman. He recommends no more than 2,000 milligrams per day.

Mental Pain

Most of us know physical pain when we feel it. But there are other types of pain that are hard to recognize as such. Emotional distress, anxiety, worry, depression. These are types of pain, too.

It was once thought that mental anguish—being down in the dumps, feeling sad or lonely—was a normal part of growing old. It certainly is not, but the perception lingers. Many people, even doctors, dismiss mental and emotional pain and anguish in the elderly as mere grumpiness or crankiness.

But all too often, it's a form of anxiety or depression and, therefore, a form of pain.

Anxiety can be difficult to define. It may be excessive worry, uneasiness, apprehension, or an overwhelming feeling of dread. It can be rational or entirely irrational, and intense enough to cause breath-lessness, trembling, heart palpitations, and even a choking sensation—some of the physical symptoms of a panic attack.

"There are many different kinds of anxiety and many different ways of dealing with it. Sometimes, it will resolve itself; sometimes, you have to take steps to deal with it," says Shirley N. Gruen, Ph.D., a clinical psychologist practicing in Sugarland, Texas.

True depression—beyond the normal blues we all sometimes feel—is more serious. You might experience sleep and appetite problems, difficulty focusing, lack of energy, and weight loss. Or, you might feel sad or irritable, lose interest in activities you once enjoyed, or experience aches and pains without medical cause. If these symptoms last for more than 2 weeks, or if your thoughts turn to suicide, you should see your doctor immediately, she cautions.

However minor or severe it might be, we consider mental anguish to be a type of pain all its own. And it's one you can ease.

people out there who have the same symptoms and problems, it's not so scary or embarrassing to let others know how they feel."

For Fast Relief

Don't be the Lone Ranger. The first, best step to easing mental pain and anguish is to share it with someone else: a family member, a friend, a pastor, a spiritual advisor, or perhaps a therapist. Just that act of opening up can go a long way toward easing the pain you're feeling.

"The first step is to recognize that there is a problem and then talk to someone about it," says Dr. Gruen. "They probably won't be able to fix your problem, but sometimes just getting your thoughts out into the air tends to dissipate the seriousness of your situation. It may not be as bad as you thought."

Obviously, another person can offer advice, give solace, and let you know you aren't alone in all this. It's not unusual for people under mental anguish to believe that they are the only ones who ever had this problem, that they are truly alone and unique, she says.

"You think, 'It's just me. I'm the weird one,'" she explains. "Then, when they find out that there are lots of

For Lasting Relief

Take the high road. Clouded thinking can shift into pessimistic thinking. Some people get carried away with worry and construct a line of negative thinking that ends with the worst-case scenario, says Michael Keane, Ph.D., a clinical psychologist and yoga teacher at New Directions for Yoga Health and Psychotherapy in Brookline, Massachusetts.

"It's like a fork in the road. You can go down one path toward negative thinking, or you can find another, less destructive route that is more realistic and helpful," he says. "Sometimes, that's all up to you."

With professional guidance, you can learn to find these forks in the road of your thinking. On your own, he suggests that you write down all your personal feelings on a piece of paper: How you feel about yourself, your situation, your future.

If you start seeing phrases such as "I'm no good," "Nothing can help," "Why should I bother?" or "Nobody cares," then you are definitely going down the negative fork in the road. If you can't see any alternatives, you may be clinically depressed and in need of professional help. Take yourself seriously. If you are stuck, get help, says Dr. Keane. It is very hard to change alone. Therapy plus some active movement such as yoga or tai chi can help to shift your perspective of being stuck and helpless.

When you're able to rationally examine many of these negatives, you may find that they aren't very true. Rather, they are products of worry, things entirely out of your control or still in the future. They aren't real, and what you're left with instead are the facts, he says.

"This type of thinking shouldn't run your life. Better to deal with the facts and look at reality. You may not like the facts—of being alone or facing some crisis—but at least you can do something about them or decide how to react to them. It isn't always easy to do, but it's important that you reframe your thinking and take a different road," adds Dr. Keane. "If you do this work, you will be proactive in life instead of reactive. You will find freedom of choice in your emotional, mental, and physical experience."

Avoid downers. When you're feeling low, the last thing you need is someone who's going to bring you down further.

"Avoid negative people. It's as simple as that," says Dr. Gruen. Sometimes, of course, you can't avoid these folks because they're coworkers, friends, neighbors, even your spouse. If you can't beat them, don't join them. Let them know that you're not buying into their negative way of thinking. The most diplomatic method is via an "I" message, because no one can argue with your feelings.

For example, instead of telling your spouse, "Your pessimism really makes me feel bad. I hate when you make me feel that way," it would be better to say, "I feel bad when I hear negative things. It really brings me down." Even though you're not being direct, the other person will certainly get the message, says Dr. Gruen. "They may not like what they hear, but at least you're not accusing them of causing your problem."

Shake a leg. Although it won't take away the root causes of anxiety and depression, exercise will relieve some of the physical symptoms: stress, fatigue, sleeplessness, and inertia, says Dr. Gruen. Also, it will increase blood circulation and flood your system with endorphins, hormones that reduce pain in your body and act as a natural mood lifter.

"It's like a short-term fix," she says. "But it could be just the 'magic' to help you focus your energy in a more productive direction."

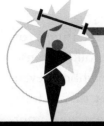

SEEKING A PROFESSIONAL EAR

Although some mental and emotional problems can be treated on your own and by nondrug means, there certainly is a role for professional help, and you shouldn't be the least bit embarrassed about seeking it, says Shirley N. Gruen, Ph.D., a clinical psychologist practicing in Sugarland, Texas.

Depression and anxiety are legitimate medical concerns, and the pain and anguish they cause are all too real. Seeking help from a trained mental-health professional can help you determine the root of the problem. Dr. Gruen suggests that you look for a therapist who is licensed by the state regulatory board for that profession.

You should first see a licensed psychologist or psychiatrist, who will have a Ph.D. or M.D. degree and the professional qualifications to provide proper diagnosis of whether you have

Aerobic exercise—cycling, walking, or swimming—is probably better than anaerobic activity, such as strength training. But the type of exercise is less important than just getting out and doing something. "Walking is fine, 20 to 30 minutes a day," Dr. Gruen says. "If you can schedule a walk with a friend, better yet.

That way, you can get your exercise and do a little talking, too."

Eschew the brew or java. Sitting around stewing in your thoughts and drinking coffee, cola, or cocktails will just make matters worse, says Dr. Gruen.

Alcohol is a depressant. After an initial high of 20 to 30 minutes, the drug works

clinical depression, suggests Marta Peck, executive director of the Berks County Mental Health Association in West Reading, Pennsylvania. She urges that you then check with your insurance provider to see which type of psychotherapist it covers: Some will cover psychologists, others will include social workers and other licensed counselors. Either way, your insurance will have a list of people among whom you can choose for treatment.

Sometimes, mental anguish can be caused by a chemical imbalance in your brain, interactions between different medications, or other physical conditions that can be remedied surprisingly quickly. The point is, says Dr. Gruen, you won't know that unless you ask for help from a professional.

You can obtain information on where to get a free confidential depression screening in your area by writing to the National Mental Health Association, Attn.: Campaign on Clinical Depression, 1021 Prince Street, Alexandria, VA 22314-2971.

the opposite way. "You're going to end up lower than you started," she says.

Caffeine, on the other hand, fuels anxiety. You're already keyed up and on edge; you don't want to add to it.

"A lot of people just don't realize how much caffeine they're taking in," notes Dr. Gruen. "They come in to see me, wondering why they are so anxious, and I find out they are drinking 8 to 10 cups of coffee every day." For the sake of your moods, try to cut back a little each day, getting down to a maximum of 2 cups per day. Also, she advises, remember the caffeine in chocolate.

Get back on your horse. If you've had a panic attack from anxiety, you may find yourself changing your daily behavior, says Dr. Gruen.

For example, if you had the attack in a grocery store, you may refuse to shop. Or if you panicked in a crowd, you may start avoiding crowds. This is how phobias get started, and you'll want to nip any of these tendencies in the bud. "It really becomes a fear of the fear, and you can't let it control your life,"she says.

Go back to the grocery store. Force yourself to be with people. And if an attack comes, ride it out, knowing that you will get to the other side. The actual panic attack lasts only about 7 minutes. You can convince yourself to hang in there for that length of time. If need be, take along a friend to help you through it.

"Where an anxiety attack happens has nothing to do with it. It's not the cause. It's whatever is going on in your life," she says.

Join up. Sitting around moping by yourself is never going to make you feel better, says Roy Grzesiak, Ph.D., a psychologist at the New Jersey Pain Institute and Robert Wood Johnson Medical School in New Brunswick.

Volunteer at your church or a local charity. Enroll in a group exercise class. Learn to dance. Take up a hobby. Get out there and do something with other people. "There's no techniques or secret to this.

You just have to be doing something and get with people," he says.

Unfortunately, a lot of older people give up their hobbies and things they used to like doing. That's really a mistake. "It can isolate you from other people and leave you with too much time on your hands," he says.

Think about the beach. Imagine it's a summer day; you're lying on the beach with your eyes closed. Warm sand is beneath your towel; the sun is orange and bright against your eyelids; and the surf's rhythm is mesmerizing your brain. You're relaxed, almost about to fall asleep.

It's not real, but for a moment your mind is focused not on your troubles but on this soothing image. Guided imagery is a way to take a vacation from your anxiety.

"Imagery can really help you relax. Your body releases endorphins, blood circulation increases, and you become more alert, more into the moment," says Dr. Grzesiak. "It has a lot of long-term benefits, too, in terms of stress relief."

Pick a favorite place, imagine yourself relaxing there, and then repeat a cue word, such as *beach* or *relax*. Eventually, you will associate the word with the image and will be able to relax more quickly by invoking the cue word. "Then, say it to yourself anytime you're feeling anxious," he says.

Raynaud's Disease

If you have Raynaud's disease, a hypersensitivity to cold and sudden drops in temperature, you understand the phrase "turn blue with cold."

During a Raynaud's attack, the blood vessels near the surface contract, shutting off the blood supply to your skin and extremities and shunting it deeper into your body. In a severe attack, your fingers, feet, kneecaps, ears, and nose may turn blue. An eerie, bluish lacework may mottle your arms and legs. The pain you'll feel as a result can last from minutes to hours.

If your condition is primary Raynaud's, you've likely had it for years and have learned to deal with it. Primary Raynaud's nearly always occurs in women between the ages of 15 to 40, and it doesn't seem to be part of any underlying disease.

Secondary Raynaud's occurs in older people and can be a symptom of a serious underlying disease such as lupus, scleroderma (hardening and thickening of the skin), vasculitis (inflammation of blood vessels), and atherosclerosis (hardening of the arteries). It also may be brought on by drugs that constrict the blood vessels, such as those for high blood pressure. If necessary, contact your doctor to discuss the possibility of changing your medication.

Although you can take precautions to try to minimize the manifestation of secondary Raynaud's, the main treatment is to address the underlying disease, says Fredrick M. Wigley, M.D., a Raynaud's researcher and medical director of the division of rheumatology at Johns Hopkins University School of Medicine in Baltimore.

Because another disease is involved and older people are often already using other medications, you should first try nondrug therapies to control the Raynaud's, says Dr. Wigley. But for severe cases of Raynaud's, a doctor may prescribe vasodilating drugs, such as calcium channel blockers, to open up bloodflow to the skin and extremities. In addition to drugs, there are steps you can take to control the pain.

For Fast Relief

Get toasty. You may be able to ward off a Raynaud's attack or shorten it by quickly warming your hands. At the first sign of an attack, you can place them in warm water, put them beneath your armpits or in your crotch, or simply sit on them. In an emergency, some folks carry hand-warmers used by hunters and outdoorsmen. You can find them in sporting goods stores.

For Lasting Relief

Put your hands through the spin cycle. Get blood flowing to your hands (the most common site of Raynaud's pain) by swinging your arms in a circle, says Dr. Wigley. That gets the blood moving and

opens up your blood vessels. Gravity and centrifugal force pushes blood back toward the extremities and will help warm them up.

"Any kind of exercise will dilate blood vessels. Walking or running in place usually helps," he says.

Watch those temperature drops. It isn't just cold that brings on Raynaud's; it's also rapid changes in temperature, such as when you walk from a parking lot on a hot summer day into an air-conditioned store. The drop in temperature may be just 20 degrees, but it's enough to set off the Raynaud's trigger, says Dr. Wigley.

Avoid the frozen-food section at the grocery store. Wear gloves when you reach into the refrigerator. Don't sit in front of or walk near an air conditioner. If you live in the North, warm up your car on a winter day.

Use space heaters to maintain a higher temperature in the cold spaces of your home or workplace. Don't abruptly change the cooling or heat regulation in your home.

Take a niacin supplement. You could try taking niacin, a powerful vasodilator (something that will expand your blood vessels). Niacin will cause a wave of heat from your head to your toes, says Andrew T. Weil, M.D., director of the program in integrative medicine at the University of Arizona College of Medicine in Tucson and author of *Spontaneous Healing* and *8 Weeks to Optimum Health*.

He recommends starting with 100 milligrams of niacin daily and eventually working up to 200 to 300 milligrams per day over a 2-week period. Do not take time-released niacin, however, cautions Dr. Weil. Consult with your doctor before taking this much niacin.

Try ginkgo. Ginkgo biloba is touted by herbalists as a vasodilator and a particularly potent herb in opening up the small capillaries in the extremities and near the skin. Some Raynaud's patients feel that ginkgo is helpful. There have been no scientific studies, however, showing it to be so, says Dr. Wigley. Still, it may be worth trying. The usual dose is 120 milligrams per day, not to exceed 240 milligrams.

Condition yourself. You may be able to condition yourself to be less cold-sensitive. Dr. Weil suggests dressing lightly for the indoors and immersing your hands for 2 to 5 minutes in very warm water, around 120°F. Then, go outside or to an air-conditioned room (somewhere under 70°F) and again immerse your hands in 120°F water. Go back inside and do the immersion again. Repeat this procedure up to six times a day for 10 days.

PAIN PREVENTERS

Wear your mittens. Most of the blood vessels involved with Raynaud's are on your fingers, ears, nose, and toes, so it's especially important to wear a hat and gloves and keep your feet dry and warm to ward off a Raynaud's attack. But keeping the rest of your body warm is important too.

Always wear layered, loose-fitting clothing when you go outside. You'll create dead air space in between the layers and avoid a body chill.

"Humidity is a concern, too. Cold, damp days are the worst for getting a body chill," Dr. Wigley says. "And that chilled perception from the body may trigger a Raynaud's attack."

Keep the blood flowing. You want to avoid anything that constricts blood vessels. That means no smoking. Nicotine in cigarettes is a powerful vasoconstrictor, says Dr. Weil. Also, ask your doctor about the vasoconstricting qualities of prescription and over-the-counter cold remedies. Many drugs can constrict blood vessels, including beta-blockers given to heart patients, says Dr. Weil. There may be alternative medications.

Although not studied in depth, there may be a link between some estrogen-replacement therapies and Raynaud's. Dr. Wigley has examined several women who started to get Raynaud's-like symptoms after starting the therapy. "It's an unproved association, but an interesting one," he says. "If you're taking estrogen and getting these symptoms, it may be something to discuss with your doctor."

Reflex Sympathetic Dystrophy (RSD)

Reflex sympathetic dystrophy (RSD) is an illness that causes chronic pain as a result of some kind of previous physical injury or trauma. Another name for this condition is complex regional pain syndrome, or CRPS (pronounced "crips").

Whatever the name, this illness often begins after a minor injury or operation. Sometimes, the cause is unknown, but the symptoms are unmistakable. A severe, burning pain is the most constant symptom of the illness, and it's usually much more painful than the initial injury. Another distinguishing symptom is what's called allodynia—the limb becomes supersensitive to stimulation. Just the touch of clothing may cause pain.

Early in the disease, chemicals in the nervous system that used to send all sorts of messages about touch, joint position, and temperature are now sending only messages of pain, explains David Flemming, M.D., a pain-management specialist at American Whole Health in Chicago and director of medical services at the Center for Integrated Therapy in Chicago, a clinic that focuses on RSD.

Over time, people with RSD tend to use their affected limb less and less, which only makes the condition worse, as muscles waste away. The condition also gets harder and harder to treat successfully, says Bradley Galer, M.D., codirector of the program for pain due to nerve injury and director of clinical studies in the department of pain medicine and palliative care at Beth Israel Medical Center in New York City. That's why if you think you have this condition, it's important to seek

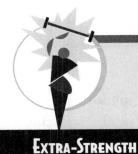

MINDING YOUR PAIN

Believe it or not, if you have reflex sympathetic dystrophy, you can learn to control the pain in your affected limb by using a combination of biofeedback and visualization, says Nanny Christie, a certified biofeedback therapist at the Forest Park Institute in Fort Worth, Texas. Biofeedback is a technique that uses sensitive monitoring devices to help you learn skills that allow you to override automatic body responses.

More specifically, a form of biofeedback that uses a visualization technique called hand warming can be used to dilate the blood vessels in hands or feet, which actually raises the temperature of the limb, Christie says. And once you've learned this technique, you can use it to moderate your pain.

Close your eyes and visualize what it feels like to hold your hands in front of a fire or to hold a warm drink in your hands. People who have the opposite problem—whose hands or legs feel hot—can imagine a cooling breeze or experience the burning pain as pleasurable warmth.

"People see that they do have some control over what's happening to them and that there are things they can do to reduce the pain," she says. And just as they consciously controlled the temperature of a limb, people who are having painful muscle spasms can use biofeedback to consciously relax specific muscles and to begin again to use the muscles in their affected limbs.

out appropriate medical treatment as soon as possible. This may mean that you need to contact a nearby university hospital for a pain specialist who's up-to-date on treating RSD.

You also want to be sure that your symptoms are due to RSD and are not the result of nerve entrapment; a spinal cord injury; an unhealed, undiagnosed fracture; or some other treatable problem, Dr. Galer says.

These days, RSD is best treated with a multidisciplinary approach. Physical therapy is a must. "The doctor's role is to provide symptom relief that makes doing the physical therapy easier," Dr. Galer says. Drugs are the front line of treatment. One currently popular drug, gabapentin (Neurontin), is an antiseizure drug that provides about one-third of people with significant relief. Doctors may also use a temporary nerve block to provide pain relief during initial physical therapy sessions. Permanent nerve blocks should be avoided. "They just don't work very well," he says.

If these treatments don't help enough, there are many others available. For the most part, these treatments haven't been studied enough to know how helpful they may be in dealing with RSD pain. But some doctors believe that they are worth trying.

For Fast Relief

Get the lowdown on rubdowns. Massage can be very helpful for inducing muscle relaxation, easing muscle spasm, improving bloodflow, reducing sensitivity to touch and pain, and helping your body heal itself, says Joy Flemming, a certified massage therapist in Chicago. For best results, see a therapist who has a national certification issued by the American Massage Therapy Association. "You need to find someone you can trust to follow your agenda. Work that is too strong can increase your pain," she says. "If massage hurts so much that you guard against it, the massage will make your condition worse."

For Lasting Relief

Use it or lose it. Unfortunately, utilization really is the bottom line for limbs affected by RSD. "You absolutely *must* gradually increase your use of the affected limb," Dr. Galer says. The key word here is *gradual.* "If you go too fast, you exacerbate the problem. You are always toeing the line between increasing activity and avoiding a flare-up," he says.

The payoff for all this hard work is a

working arm or leg and less pain. "Over time, the physical therapy actually reduces your pain and helps to resolve your symptoms," Dr. Galer says.

A good physical therapist is vital to the process. To find one, you may want to contact a pain specialist at a nearby university hospital.

Feed your muscles. No specific nutrients or nutritional deficiencies have been associated with RSD. Still, your body can't work right, or heal itself, unless it is properly nourished, Dr. Flemming says. For instance, muscles need magnesium to be able to relax, and they need certain trace minerals, such as manganese.

He suggests that his patients with RSD take a nutritional supplement called Fibroplex (by Metagenics). Per tablet, it contains 75 milligrams of magnesium, 2.5 milligrams of manganese, 300 milligrams of malic acid, and 25 milligrams each of thiamin and vitamin B_6. Patients might take 2 to 5 of these tablets a day. Check with your doctor to see which dosage is best for you. Other manufacturers make similar products.

Get help for sleep problems. "Poor sleep has a profound effect on mood and ability to cope with illness," Dr. Flemming says. If your pain is making sleep scarce, talk with your doctor about it. "We may try valerian, a calming herb; or melatonin, a nutritional supplement that aids sleep. But if that doesn't work, certain antidepressants are very good at helping people get the healing sleep they need," he adds.

Bag the butts. Not all doctors say that they see a connection between smoking and RSD pain, but Dr. Flemming does. "Nicotine stimulates the sympathetic nervous system, and it stimulates muscle spasms, which are a major part of this disease," he says. "My patients never get well if they continue smoking."

Temporomandibular Disorder (TMD)

Temporomandibular—whew, it almost hurts your jaw to say it.

Perhaps that's only fitting. That multi-syllabic monster of a word refers to a multifunctional joint that hinges your lower jaw, allowing it to move whenever you chew, talk, or swallow. Muscles and ligaments are connected to that joint, too, and they stretch across your face, up the side of your head, and down into your neck.

If you have a problem with that joint, you may feel pain in a lot of places around your head and neck. The problem, known as temporomandibular disorder (TMD), comes in two varieties. One involves a malfunctioning or inflammation of the joint—often due to osteoarthritis; the other stems from tight muscles and ligaments surrounding the joint. Cramping of the masseter muscle, which runs from your cheekbone to your lower jaw, is another major cause of TMD.

TMD pain tends to be a dull, chronic ache made worse by cold, wet weather. Or, because it affects the joint, the pain can also be quite sharp, says Larry Z. Lockerman, D.D.S., a dentist at the University of Massachusetts Memorial Hospital in Worcester.

"If you press your thumb on the joint and get shooting pain, that's usually a problem with the joint," says Dr. Lockerman. Although TMD is most prevalent among younger women between the ages of 25 and 45, it also happens to older folks, usually showing up as head and neck pain.

TMD is usually a temporary condition and doesn't require invasive treatment like surgery, says Dr. Lockerman. A softer diet, alternating warm and cold compresses, and

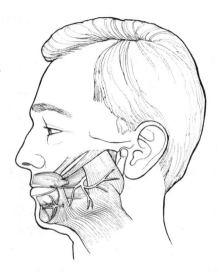

With so many muscles and nerves intersecting at this one spot on the jaw, it's easy to see how temporomandibular pain might be felt all over the head, face, and neck.

muscle-relaxation techniques will soothe the pain.

For Fast Relief

Ice it. When the pain is in the joint, the quickest way to douse it is with an ice massage. Simply rub ice directly on the skin right over the site of the pain. Rub gently, keep the ice moving for 5 seconds, and then remove it so that the skin won't freeze. Repeat, continuing for 5 to 10 minutes in total, says Noshir R. Mehta, D.M.D., chairperson of the department of general dentistry and director of the Gelb Craniomandibular Orofacial Pain Center at Tufts University School of Dental Medicine in Boston.

The ice knocks back the pain and begins to reduce the inflammation and soreness that's usually present whenever the pain involves the joint, says Dr. Mehta.

"Doing an ice massage two or three times a day is enough to reduce inflammation," he says. "But you need to be careful that there is no whitening of the skin. When you're older, it's easier to get frostbite." If you think you may have frostbite—your skin is white or waxy and numb, and when it warms, it looks red, swollen, and blotchy, and it hurts—seek medical attention right away.

For Lasting Relief

Hold the steaks and bagels. Since chewing hurts, you'll want to turn to softer foods for a time. Perhaps for a week or as much as a month, avoid chewing gum and foods that require a lot of jaw work, says Dr. Lockerman. "Sometimes, all your jaw needs is a little rest, and the pain and inflammation will ease."

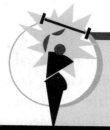

EXTRA-STRENGTH PAIN RELIEF

GUARDING AGAINST GRINDING

If you clench or grind your teeth at night, you're increasing your risk of temporomandibular disorder (TMD) pain. But a dental appliance known as a night guard may be just what's needed to guard against TMD pain. This plastic device keeps you from biting down hard and prevents grinding when you bite down. Some people simply buy the type of mouth guard used by football players, but it's better to go to a dentist so that you can be properly fitted, says Noshir R. Mehta, D.M.D., chairperson of the department of general dentistry and director of the Gelb Craniomandibular Orofacial Pain Center at Tufts University School of Dental Medicine in Boston.

You know you're a grinder if you wake up with a sore jaw—sorer than when you went to bed, if your dentist detects wear on your teeth, or, of course, if your bed partner has lodged a complaint about it.

Get fitted. Ill-fitting dentures or gaps in the rows of your natural teeth can create an unnatural bite. Over time, that bite may lead to TMD. See your dentist if your dentures are loose, says Dr. Lockerman.

"As you age, you lose the ridge of bone that the dentures ride on," he says. "If your false teeth shift around, they aren't holding your jaw in the correct position."

Wear your dentures. Without teeth, your bite tends to overclose in an unnatural way. That puts an extra strain on your joint and the surrounding muscles. It may be enough to set off TMD pain.

"At first, I tell people to wear their dentures 24 hours a day—even at night, so their jaws won't slip out of position," says

Dr. Lockerman. A night guard can replace the dentures to take pressure off.

Exercise your jaw. If you have tight, cramped muscles in your jaw and face, do some stretches, says Dr. Mehta. He suggests doing one set of each of these exercises two or three times a day or as needed.

First, put your thumb underneath

Mastering "Point M"

One of the biggest sources of temporomandibular disorder (TMD) pain is jaw muscles that are too tight. A helpful acupressure technique utilizes a spot known as Point M and can ease that tension—and the pain that goes with it, says Albert G. Forgione, D.D.S., Ph.D., director of research at the Gelb Craniomandibular Orofacial Pain Center at Tufts University School of Dental Medicine in Boston. This technique is adapted from Dr. Forgione's booklet *Acupressure for the Control of Muscle Tension Pain*.

Lay your left hand, palm side down, on a table. Place two fingers below the fold of your left elbow. Point M lies below your middle finger. Wiggle the middle finger of your left arm. You should feel a ligament moving.

Press down firmly with your forefinger or knuckle until you find a particularly tender area, then press down as hard as you can and apply a rotating pressure for 15 seconds. You may have to stimulate the point for three 15-second periods before you feel a warm tingling in your cheek. That's the signal that the muscle is starting to relax. Repeat the maneuver on your right arm.

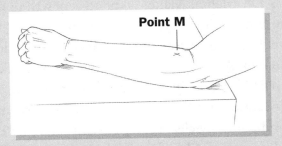
Point M

your chin and slowly open your jaw while you lightly resist the movement.

"In all of these exercises, you don't push with your fingers but maintain gentle pressure and resist the jaw motion," he says.

Next, put your finger on the right side of your chin and move your jaw slowly to the right and then back to the left. Switch to the other side of your face and repeat the motion but in the opposite direction.

Finally, place two fingers on the front of your chin under your lip and gradually jut your jaw forward.

As you reach the end of the movement for each exercise, hold for 5 seconds and then relax.

"These passive stretches are only used when muscles are the root of the problem," he says. "If the problem is more with the joint, they can actually make the pain much worse." Be sure to stop the exercises right away if your pain worsens.

Warm it up. Heat will break muscle tension. Hold a warm, wet towel on both sides of your jaw for about 5 minutes at a time, suggests Dr. Mehta. Make sure the towel isn't too hot. "What's more important is that it's wet heat, which seems to penetrate better to the muscles."

If the pain is more related to arthritis of the joint, heat will increase circulation, bring in fresh blood, and naturally cleanse the area of waste products created by in-flammation, says Dr. Lockerman. He recommends a hot-water bottle.

Release the tension. Folks clench their teeth all day without knowing it. Jaw, neck, and shoulder pain can be caused by stress and unintentional grimacing, says Roy Grzesiak, Ph.D., a psychologist at the New Jersey Pain Institute and Robert Wood Johnson Medical School in New Brunswick.

He advises sitting in a chair, closing your eyes, and quietly concentrating on the aching, tense muscles. Focusing on one group at a time—such as those in the neck—tense the muscles for a count of 10 and then release. Do this two or three times, says Dr. Grzesiak. Each time you release the muscle, it should revert to a slacker, more loose state.

Part of the mechanism is physical, but it's also psychological, says Dr. Grzesiak. "I tell people to focus on what the muscle feels like when it is relaxed. You can also repeat to yourself words like *slack* and *loose*, *warm* and *heavy*. These are suggestive words that will help you focus on relaxing."

Give it a jolt. Facial muscles tend to respond very well to transcutaneous electrical nerve stimulation (TENS), a common pain treatment used by doctors and physical therapists, says Dr. Lockerman. Relief is temporary but immediate. Portable TENS units for home use are available only by prescription. "I recommend a very low pulse for about 40 minutes once or twice a day," he says.

Ulcer Pain

Although most ulcers are caused by bacterial infection or the use of common painkilling drugs, the real damage is done by your own stomach—specifically, by the acid your stomach produces.

"It's strong stuff. If you spilled stomach acid on your skin, it could cause a chemical burn," says Roger Gebhard, M.D., a gastroenterologist and professor of medicine at the University of Minnesota in Minneapolis. "The only place stomach acid belongs is in your stomach because the stomach has the ability to protect itself."

The stomach, in essence, has a liner—a mucosal layer of tissues—that resists the acid. But a bacterial infection, such as one caused by the *Helicobacter pylori* bacteria, can eat away the lining and is thought to cause a vast majority of ulcers. Using too many nonsteroidal anti-inflammatory drugs (NSAIDs), such as aspirin and ibuprofen, also can break down the mucosal tissues. If that occurs in your stomach, you get a gastric ulcer. If it occurs in the duodenum, which is the small intestine just below your stomach, you get a duodenal ulcer.

The corrosive stomach acid then creates lesions in the underlying muscle tissue. In the case of a perforated ulcer, the acid can actually burn a hole through the entire wall, so the stomach contents leak into the surrounding area.

The typical ulcer symptoms are a burning, achy sensation in the mid-abdomen. The pain often happens on an empty stomach before meals or at bedtime. It might not occur before breakfast because that's when stomach acid is lowest. And

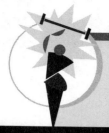

THE HOKU POINT IS NO HOKUM

If you're considering acupuncture for pain relief from ulcers, ask the practitioner to stimulate the Hoku, or Hegu, point, located between the thumb and forefinger, suggests George Ulett, M.D., Ph.D., clinical professor of medicine at St. Louis University School of Medicine.

Of all the Chinese acupuncture points on the body, this point, also known as Large Intestine 4 (LI4), is one of the strongest points to release endorphins, the body's own painkillers. "I use this point with almost any pain syndrome," he says.

Acupressure on the point might not be enough to stimulate the endorphin release. It could also be done with electro-acupuncture, says Dr. Ulett. Electro-acupuncture (which is different from acupuncture-like transcutaneous electrical nerve stimulation) is basically acupuncture without the needles, but it involves small amplitude electrical currents that come into contact with an adhesive conductive pad placed on the skin. The Hoku point, along with 80 other acupressure points on the body, has a direct physiological response on motorpoints—where the nerve enters the muscle—in this case, in the digestive area. "It has been shown that stimulating this point cuts down on the acid secretion in the stomach," he says.

with some ulcers, there may not be any symptoms at all.

If the cause of your ulcer is a bacterial infection, you'll likely be treated with antibiotics to kill the bacteria. If it is caused by NSAIDs, you'll need to look for other drug alternatives. You may also be given medications to suppress stomach acid. Tagamet or Zantac are two of the most popular over-the-counter acid suppressors. They aren't a cure and should only be used to relieve symptoms and to enable the ulcer to heal, says Dr. Gebhard.

Typically, these treatments help the mucosal lining heal itself within 4 to 8 weeks, says Dr. Gebhard.

Ulcers can get more complicated and severe. You should immediately see a physician if you vomit blood or see blood in your stools, or if pain is persistent or severe and associated with abdominal tenderness, fever, or chills, says Dr. Gebhard.

For Fast Relief

Eat a little. It's a quick fix, but ulcer pain can be relieved by eating. Food will quickly buffer the acid concentration in your stomach, but only for the short term, says Dr. Gebhard.

"The trouble with food is that it also stimulates acid secretion, so within an hour or so, you're back in the same situation," he says. "It can be a vicious cycle. Some people have told me that they gain weight when their ulcer is acting up. They say, 'I have to go feed my ulcer.'" But if you need an immediate reprieve from the pain, this can help.

For Lasting Relief

Quaff some cabbage juice. Cabbage juice is high in glutamine, an amino acid that helps stomach cells regenerate. It also stimulates your body to produce a substance that actually protects the stomach lining. A good way to get glutamine is through drinking about a liter of fresh raw cabbage juice every day, says Priscilla Skerry, N.D., a naturopathic and homeopathic physician in Portland, Maine. To make your own juice, she suggests slicing then juicing or blending a green cabbage. You can also find glutamine supplements in most health food stores. Take the dosage recommended on the label.

Mind the pain. No matter the site of the pain, you can always address the hurt, to a degree, with meditation and relaxation, says George Ulett, M.D., Ph.D., clinical professor of medicine at St. Louis University School of Medicine and professor at the Missouri Institute of Mental Health of the University of Missouri–Columbia School of Medicine.

Relaxation relieves pain by reducing the stimulation of the sympathetic nervous system, which goes into high gear whenever the body and mind are challenged.

"This is part of the whole fight-or-flight response," explains Dr. Ulett. "When your ulcer is hurting, you naturally have a fight response. Your muscles tense, blood pressure goes up, and your anxiety increases." It doesn't matter how you achieve that relaxation. It could be through yoga, guided imagery, hypnosis, transcendental meditation, or a simple deep-breathing exercise. The point is that you use your mind to relax your body.

Spare the spice. With nearly any kind of digestive problem, Dr. Ulett recommends avoiding spicy foods, acidic foods, and others that may cause you distress. It's also a good idea to eat more fiber—grains, vegetables, and fruits.

There is no standard diet, however, for someone with an ulcer. As Dr. Gebhard puts it, "If it bothers you, don't eat it. Listen to your stomach."

PAIN PREVENTERS

No suds, no smokes. Heavy alcohol use can literally burn a hole in the stomach mucosal tissues. Even moderate drinking can aggravate the painful symptoms once you have an ulcer.

Tobacco also affects the mucosal resistance of your stomach. Smokers have a higher rate of ulcers and recurrence of ulcers. There's no clear evidence whether it is the nicotine or tar in cigarettes that does the damage, but it's apparent that the chemicals are absorbed through the lungs. Dr. Gebhard says that these chemicals enter the circulation and then alter the mucosal barrier and acid secretion.

"Cut back on your drinking, or don't drink at all," says Dr. Gebhard. "That goes for cigarettes, too. Don't smoke."

Avoid the NSAIDs. This may not be easy to do if you're taking nonsteroidal anti-inflammatory drugs to control severe arthritis pain. Still, check with your doctor because there may be alternative medications, says Dr. Gebhard.

If you're self medicating, however, and taking over-the-counter NSAIDs, such as aspirin and ibuprofen for everyday aches, you should reevaluate why you're taking those drugs in the first place.

"Maybe you're taking one aspirin a day to protect against heart disease because you heard that's a good idea," suggests Dr. Gebhard. "That's usually okay. But sometimes, we see ulcer problems in people taking only a small of amount of NSAIDs—amounts that wouldn't seem to be a problem. When you're older, you can become much more sensitive to these medications."

In the case of aspirin, you may be able to avoid the problem by taking enteric-coated aspirin, which enables the medication to pass through your stomach before dissolving. Be aware, however, that not all damage done to the mucosal wall is by direct contact with NSAIDs; just absorbing the medications into your bloodstream can cause problems.

Urinary Tract Infections

It's thought of mostly as a women's problem, but the truth is, older men and women are both prone to urinary tract infections. In men, weak abdominal muscles and enlarged prostates make it harder to completely empty their bladders as they get older. So the bit of urine they just can't squeeze out acts as a breeding ground for bacteria.

In women, meanwhile, the protective mucous membranes lining their urethras and bladders depend on estrogen to stay healthy. When estrogen levels drop naturally over time, these tissues get dry, thin, and open to infection by bacteria or yeast. Hormone-replacement therapy or estrogen-containing creams help reduce the incidence of urinary tract infections in women past menopause.

Many older people have some bacteria setting up residence in their bladders but often have no symptoms of infection, says William Greenough, M.D., professor in the division of geriatric medicine at Johns Hopkins University School of Medicine in Baltimore. Antibiotics don't seem to knock out these bacteria completely, so these drugs are not used unless pain or fever indicates a flare-up. "For most people, the trick is to keep bacterial growth in check, and there are ways to do that," he says.

Here's what our experts recommend.

For Fast Relief

Ease pain with aloe vera or vitamin E. Use a cream that contains soothing aloe or break open a capsule of vitamin E and coat painful private areas, suggests Ellen Kamhi, R.N., Ph.D., of Oyster Bay, New York, a professional member of the American Herbalists Guild and host of the nationally syndicated radio show *Natural Alternatives.*

For Lasting Relief

Add uva-ursi. This antimicrobial herb is the classic herbal choice for urinary tract infections, says Eric Yarnell, N.D., a naturopathic physician in Sedona, Arizona, and chairperson of the department of botanical medicine at Southwest College of Naturopathic Medicine in Tempe. Make a tea using 2 to 3 teaspoons of dried uva-ursi leaves steeped for 10 minutes in a cup of hot water, then strained. You can drink three or four cups of the tea a day for up to a week to help knock out an infection.

Drink as much water as you can. You want to keep flushing out your bladder, so the more water you can get down, the better, Dr. Yarnell says. Aim for enough water so that you have to urinate every waking hour.

Welcome friendly flora and fauna. It's a war zone down there, and you can help the normal, healthy bugs hold their turf against bladder-infecting bacteria by taking acidophilus capsules with a 5-billion-live-organism count, Dr. Yarnell says. The amount people need to take varies, but two or three capsules a day is usually enough. He recommends taking it during antibiotic treatment and for about a month afterward. "This is a good way to get friendly flora firmly reestablished," he says.

Have a cup of marshmallow tea. Certain plants, such as marshmallow, couchgrass, and cornsilk, contain soluble fibers, ingredients that impart a slippery, soothing quality to liquids, Dr. Yarnell says. They seem to reduce irritation in the bladder by an indirect and as yet undetermined mechanism. Add a good tablespoon of any one of these herbs to a cup of just-boiled water, let it sit for 10 minutes, then strain and drink. You can drink as much of this as you want, but don't take it with other remedies because it may lower their absorption, he cautions.

PAIN PREVENTERS

Guzzle cranberry juice. Cranberry juice contains compounds that help to prevent bacteria from sticking to the bladder wall, where they can multiply. Instead, they get flushed out each time you urinate. "Cranberry juice is critical for prevention and can help in the treatment of urinary tract infections," Dr. Yarnell says. In fact, the only human studies done with cranberry juice were in older men and women; 10 ounces a day produced a 50 percent reduction of bacteria in the urine.

Dr. Yarnell recommends unsweetened cranberry juice because too much sugar suppresses your immune system. You can get unsweetened cranberry juice concentrate at health food stores. Drink 16 ounces each day.

Capsules of cranberry extract are also available. Each day, you should take two or three 400-milligram cranberry-extract capsules for prevention. "And you definitely need to go up to six or eight a day if you actually get an infection," he says.

Support your mucous membranes. The same kinds of dietary measures that help relieve hot flashes, vaginal dryness, and other symptoms of low estrogen levels can also make a woman's urinary tract healthier, Dr. Yarnell says. He recommends 10 ounces a day or so of soy foods such as tofu, soy milk, or roasted soy beans, whichever is your preference. If soy products aren't for you, try soy powder supplements that provide 100 milligrams of isoflavones per day. He also suggests 1 tablespoon of flaxseed oil and 400 to 800 IU of vitamin E.

Add immune power with echinacea.

Extracts of this plant, the pretty purple coneflower, can give your immune system enough of a boost to ward off bladder infections, Dr. Yarnell says. Some doctors prefer an occasional break from this herb, but he says, "I haven't sees any problems with long-term use." To prevent a recurrence, he recommends 1 teaspoon three times a day of echinacea tincture or fresh-pressed juice preserved in alcohol. To treat an active infection, up that amount to 6 to 7 teaspoons a day for up to a week.

Shift positions. If you feel that you aren't emptying your bladder fully every time you urinate, try this: Go as you ordinarily would, then stand up for a bit (if you're a man, sit down for a bit), then try to go some more, Dr. Greenough says. "Sometimes, the problem is positional, and changing position allows you to void more urine."

Put the pressure on. Some people also find that pressing just above their pubic bones assists their bladders in emptying, Dr. Greenough says.

Wash up. Surface bacteria can get up into moist areas, causing infection, so it's best to keep all of your private surfaces as clean as possible, says Dr. Greenough. He says that regular bathing down there with soap and water is helpful in keeping bacteria in check. Since you want to avoid spreading germs from your anus to your urethra, always wipe from front to back.

Resources

Your Guide to Safe Use of Essential Oils

Essential oils are inhaled or placed on the skin, but with few exceptions, never taken internally. One exception is peppermint oil in enteric-coated capsules. Evening primrose oil and borage oil are often taken internally, but they are not essential oils.

In general, never apply essential oils neat (undiluted). Before application, dilute them in a carrier base, which can be an oil (such as almond), cream, or gel. You can, however, apply lavender, tea tree, jasmine, and rose undiluted.

Many essential oils may cause skin irritation or allergic reactions in people with sensitive skin. Before applying any new oil to your skin, always do a patch test. Put a few drops of the essential oil mixed with the carrier oil on the back of your wrist. Wait for an hour or more. If irritation or redness occurs, wash the area with cold water. For future use, use half the number of drops or avoid the oil altogether.

Do not use essential oils at home for serious medical or psychological problems.

Store essential oils in dark bottles, away from light and heat and out of the reach of children and pets.

Before you try the essential oil remedies in this book, check the safety guidelines in the following list, which are based on the advice of experienced herbal healers. Then, you can enjoy the world of herbal healing with confidence.

557

Common Name	Botanical Name	Safety Guidelines and Possible Side Effects
Black pepper	*Piper nigrum*	Do not use more than 3 drops in the bath. Do not use at the same time as homeopathic remedies.
Clove	*Syzygium aromaticum*	Do not use for more than 2 weeks without the guidance of a qualified practitioner. Do not use more than 3 drops in the bath. Can be used undiluted for tooth pain.
Eucalyptus	*Eucalyptus globulus*	Do not use for more than 2 weeks without the guidance of a qualified practitioner. Do not use more than 3 drops in the bath. Do not use at the same time as homeopathic remedies. Do not apply externally to the faces of infants and young children.
Ginger	*Zingiber officinale*	Do not use more than 3 drops in the bath. Avoid direct sunlight because this oil can cause skin sensitivity.
Juniper	*Juniperus communis*	Do not use for more than 2 weeks without the guidance of a qualified practitioner. Do not use if you have kidney disease.
Lavender (true)	*Lavandula angustifolia*	Generally regarded as safe. Can be used undiluted, but keep it away from your eyes.
Lemongrass	*Cymbopogon citratus*	Topical use only—don't inhale.
Orange	*Citrus sinensis*	Avoid direct sunlight because this oil can cause skin sensitivity.
Peppermint	*Mentha piperita*	Do not use more than 3 drops in the bath. Do not use at the same time as homeopathic remedies. Do not apply externally to

Common Name	Botanical Name	Safety Guidelines and Possible Side Effects
		the faces of infants and small children. Peppermint oil can be used internally but may lead to stomach upset in sensitive individuals. If you have gallbladder or liver disease, do not use without medical supervision.
Rosemary	*Rosmarinus officinalis*	Do not use if you have hypertension. Do not use if you have epilepsy, due to the powerful action on the nervous system.
Tangerine	*Citrus reticulata* var. tangerine	Avoid direct sunlight because this oil can cause skin sensitivity.
Tea tree	*Melaleuca alternifolia*	May be applied undiluted to the skin.
Thyme (white, common)	*Thymus vulgaris*	This oil may irritate the skin if used in high concentration. If it irritates your skin, use more carrier base to further dilute it. Do not use more than 3 drops in the bath. Do not use if you have hypertension.

Your Guide to Safe Use of Herbs

While herbal home remedies are generally regarded as safe and cause few, if any, side effects, herbalists are quick to point out that botanical medicines should still be used cautiously—and knowledgeably.

First, if you are under a doctor's care for any health condition or are taking medication, do not take any herb or alter your medication regimen without your doctor's knowledge.

Keep in mind that some herbal remedies may cause adverse reactions if you are allergy-prone or have a major health condition. A reaction may also occur if you take prescription medication, take an herb for too long, take too much, or use the herb improperly.

Also, remember that the guidelines in this chart are intended for adults only and usually refer to internal use.

Since some herbs can cause a skin reaction when used topically, it's always wise to do a patch test before applying an herb for the first time. To perform a patch test, apply a small amount to your skin and observe it for 24 hours to be sure that you aren't sensitive. If redness or a rash occurs, discontinue use.

Before you try the herbal remedies mentioned in this book, check the safety guidelines and look for possible side effects noted in the following listings, which are based on the advice of experienced herbal healers. Then, you can add herbal healers to your arsenal of pain-relieving remedies.

Common Name(s)	Botanical Name(s)	Safety Guidelines and Possible Side Effects
Aloe	*Aloe barbadensis*	Do not use gel externally on any surgical incision; it may delay wound healing. Do not ingest the dried leaf, as it is a habit-forming laxative.
Arnica	*Arnica montana*	Do not use on broken skin.
Cayenne	*Capsicum annuum*; *C. frutescens*	May irritate the gastrointestinal tract if taken on an empty stomach. Don't use near eyes or on injured skin.
Chamomile	*Matricaria recutita*	Very rarely, can cause an allergic reaction when ingested. If allergic to closely related plants such as ragweed, asters, and chrysanthemums, drink the tea with caution.
Comfrey	*Symphytum officinale*	For external use only. Do not use topically on deep or infected wounds; may promote surface healing too quickly and not allow healing of underlying tissue.
Dandelion	*Taraxacum officinale*	If you have gallbladder disease, do not use dandelion root preparations without medical approval.
Devil's claw	*Harpagophytum procumbens*	Do not use if you have gastric or duodenal ulcers. Consult your physician if you have gallstones.
Echinacea	*Echinacea angustifolia*; *E. purpurea*; *E. pallida*	Do not use if allergic to closely related plants such ragweed, asters, and chrysanthemums. Do not use if you have tuberculosis or an autoimmune condition such as lupus or multiple sclerosis because echinacea stimulates the immune system.

Common Name(s)	Botanical Name(s)	Safety Guidelines and Possible Side Effects
Eucalyptus	*Eucalyptus globulus*	Do not use if you have inflammatory disease of the bile ducts or gastrointestinal tract or severe liver disease. May cause nausea, vomiting, and diarrhea in doses higher than 4 g a day.
Fennel	*Foeniculum vulgare*	Do not use medicinally for more than 6 weeks without supervision by a qualified herbalist.
Feverfew	*Tanacetum parthenium*	If chewed, fresh leaves can cause mouth sores in some people.
Flaxseed	*Linum usitatissimum*	Do not take if you have a bowel obstruction. Take with at least 8 oz of water.
Garlic	*Allium sativum*	Do not use supplements if you're on anticoagulants or before undergoing surgery, because garlic thins the blood and may increase bleeding. Do not use if you're taking hypoglycemic drugs.
Ginger	*Zingiber officinale*	Generally regarded as safe when used as a spice. May increase bile secretion. So if you have gallstones, do not use therapeutic amounts of the dried root or powder without guidance from a health-care practitioner.
Ginkgo	*Ginkgo biloba*	Do not use with antidepressant MAO-inhibitor drugs, such as phenelzine sulfate (Nardil) or tranylcypromine (Parnate); with aspirin or other nonsteroidal anti-inflammatory medications; or with blood-thinning

Common Name(s)	Botanical Name(s)	Safety Guidelines and Possible Side Effects
		medications, such as warfarin (Coumadin). Can cause dermatitis, diarrhea, and vomiting in doses higher than 240 mg of concentrated extract.
Goldenseal	*Hydrastis canadensis*	Do not use if you have high blood pressure.
Hawthorn	*Crataegus oxycantha*; *C. laevigata*; *C. monogyna*	If you have a cardiovascular condition, do not take hawthorn regularly for more than a few weeks without medical supervision. You may require lower doses of other medications, such as high blood pressure drugs. If you have low blood pressure caused by heart valve problems, do not use without medical supervision.
Licorice	*Glycyrrhiza glabra*	Do not use if you have diabetes, high blood pressure, liver or kidney disorders, or low potassium levels. Do not use daily for more than 4 to 6 weeks because overuse can lead to water retention, high blood pressure caused by potassium loss, or impaired heart and kidney function.
Marshmallow	*Althaea officinalis*	May slow the absorption of medications taken at the same time.
Parsley	*Petroselinum crispum*	If you have kidney disease, do not use large amounts because it increases urine flow in large doses of several cups a day. Safe as a garnish or ingredient in food.
Peppermint	*Mentha piperita*	If taken close to bedtime, it may cause heartburn by relaxing the esophagus.

Common Name(s)	Botanical Name(s)	Safety Guidelines and Possible Side Effects
St. John's wort	*Hypericum perforatum*	Do not use with antidepressants without medical approval. May cause photosensitivity; avoid overexposure to direct sunlight.
Sarsaparilla	*Smilax orata*	May speed elimination of prescription medications, thereby requiring an increase in the effective doses.
Turmeric; curcumin	*Curcuma domestica*	Generally regarded as safe when used as a spice. Do not use as a home remedy if you have high stomach acid or ulcers; gallstones; or bile duct obstruction.
Uva-ursi	*Arctostaphylos uva-ursi*	Do not use for more than 2 weeks without the supervision of a qualified herbalist. Do not use if you have kidney disease because it contains tannins that can cause further kidney damage. Tannins can also irritate the stomach.
Valerian	*Valeriana officinalis*	Do not use with sleep-enhancing or mood-regulating medications because it may intensify their effects. May cause heart palpitations and nervousness in sensitive individuals. If such stimulant action occurs, discontinue use.
Willow bark	*Salix alba*	Do not take if you need to avoid aspirin, especially if you are taking blood-thinning medication, such as warfarin (Coumadin), because its active ingredient is related to aspirin. May interact with barbiturates or sedatives such as aprobarbital (Amytal)

Common Name(s)	Botanical Name(s)	Safety Guidelines and Possible Side Effects
		or alprazolam (Xanax). Can cause stomach irritation when consumed with alcohol. Do not give to children under 16 who have fever or any viral infection; may contribute to Reye's syndrome, which affects the brain and liver.
Yellow dock	*Rumex crispus*	If you have a history of kidney stones, do not take without medical supervision as it contains oxalates and tannins that may adversely affect this condition.

Your Guide to Safe Use of Vitamins and Other Supplements

Vitamins are tiny, organic substances necessary for life. But like anything else, you can get too much of a good thing. Read and heed the safety guidelines below, from vitamin and supplement experts.

Vitamin/Supplement	Safety Guidelines and Possible Side Effects
Acidophilus (*Lactobacillus acidophilus*)	Take with food. If you have any serious gastrointestinal problems that require medical attention, check with your doctor before taking. Amounts exceeding 10 billion viable *L. acidophilus* organisms daily may cause mild gastrointestinal distress.

Vitamin/Supplement	Safety Guidelines and Possible Side Effects
Amino acids (carnitine, glutamine, lysine, methionine, phenylalanine)	Don't take amino acids without a doctor's guidance. The use of individual amino acids in large doses is considered experimental, and the long-term effects on health are unknown. Phenylalanine supplements can raise high blood pressure to dangerous levels, especially in people taking MAO inhibitors as antidepressants. Do not take phenylalanine if you have phenylketonuria.
Bee propolis	Do not take if you have asthma; it contains allergens that can worsen asthma. May also cause a rash when handled. Take with food.
Bromelain	May cause nausea, vomiting, diarrhea, skin rash, and heavy menstrual bleeding; may increase the risk of bleeding in people taking aspirin or anticoagulants (blood thinners). Do not take if you are allergic to pineapple. As a digestive aid, take with meals; for all other uses, take on an empty stomach.
Calcium	Doses above 2,500 mg must be taken under medical supervision.
Fiber	Do not take if you have trouble swallowing. Talk to your doctor before taking, especially if you have diverticulitis, ulcerative colitis, Crohn's disease, bowel obstruction, or any other serious gastrointestinal disorder or if you are taking any medications. May cause bloating or constipation. Do not take with food; always drink at least 8 oz of water for each tablespoon of fiber that you take.
Lecithin	Large doses of lecithin may cause upset stomach, sweating, salivation, and loss of appetite.

Vitamin/Supplement	Safety Guidelines and Possible Side Effects
Magnesium	People with heart or kidney problems should check with their doctors before taking supplemental magnesium. Supplemental magnesium may cause diarrhea in some people.
Manganese	Talk with your doctor before taking supplements above 10 mg per day.
Melatonin	Take no more than 1 mg daily. Causes drowsiness; take only at bedtime and never before driving. Do not use if you have an autoimmune disease such as rheumatoid arthritis or lupus, or a personal or family history of a hormone-dependent cancer such as breast, testicular, prostate, or endometrial cancer. Consult your doctor before using if you're on a prescription medication; rarely, interactions may occur. Do not take if you are pregnant or trying to conceive, and do not give it to children. May cause headaches, morning dizziness, daytime sleepiness, depression, and upset stomach. As a sleep aid, take ½ hour before bedtime.
Niacin	Doses above 35 mg must be taken under medical supervision. Excess niacin can cause flushing, itching, and other symptoms.
Omega-3 and -6 fatty acids	Increases bleeding time, possibly resulting in nosebleeds and easy bruising, and may cause upset stomach. Do not take if you have a bleeding disorder or uncontrolled high blood pressure, if you take anticoagulants (blood thinners) or use aspirin regularly, or if you are allergic to any kind of fish. Take fish oil, not fish-liver oil, which is high in vitamins A and D—toxic in high amounts. People with diabetes should not take fish oil since it has a high fat content.

Vitamin/Supplement	Safety Guidelines and Possible Side Effects
Phosphorus	Talk with your doctor before taking more than 3,000 mg per day.
Potassium	Talk with your doctor before supplementing.
Selenium	Doses above 200 mcg must be taken under medical supervision.
Thiamin	No known toxicity from oral doses; few, if any, undesirable side effects.
Vitamin A	Doses above 10,000 IU must be taken under medical supervision. Because of the risk of birth defects, pregnant women should avoid vitamin A in doses of 5,000 IU or more.
Vitamin B_6	Doses above 100 mg must be taken under medical supervision. Excess vitamin B_6 can cause sensory neuropathy with pain, numbness, and weakness in the limbs.
Vitamin C	Excess vitamin C may cause diarrhea in some people.
Vitamin D	Doses above 2,000 IU must be taken under medical supervision.
Vitamin E	If you are considering taking amounts above 400 IU, discuss this with your doctor first. One study using low-dose supplements showed increased risk of hemorrhagic stroke.
Vitamin K	Talk with your doctor before supplementing.
Zinc	Doses above 30 mg must be taken under medical supervision.

Index

Underscored page references indicate boxed text and tables. **Boldface** references indicate illustrations.

I

W